Haematology

Other books in the Biomedical Sciences Explained Series

0 7506 3256 9   Biochemistry *J. C. Blackstock*
0 7506 2879 0   Biological Foundations *N. Lawes*
0 7506 3254 2   Biology of Disease *W. Gilmore*
0 7506 3111 2   Cellular Pathology *D.J. Cook*
0 7506 2878 2   Clinical Biochemistry *R. Luxton*
0 7506 3255 0   Human Genetics *A. Gardner, R.T. Howell and T. Davies*
0 7506 3413 8   Immunology *B.M. Hannigan*
0 7506 3253 4   Molecular Genetics *J. Hancock*
0 7506 3415 4   Transfusion Science *J. Overfield, M. Dawson and D. Hamer*

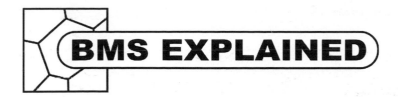

Haematology

Volume Author and Series Editor:

C. J. Pallister PhD MSc FIBMS CBiol MIBiol CHSM

Principal Lecturer in Haematology, Depatment of Biological and Biomedical Sciences, University of the West of England, Bristol, UK

A member of the Hodder Headline Group
LONDON

First published in Great Britain in 1999 by Butterworth Heinemann.

This impression published in 2001 by
Arnold, a member of the Hodder Headline Group,
338 Euston Road, London NW1 3BH

http://www.arnoldpublishers.com

Co-published in the USA by
Oxford University Press Inc.,
198 Madison Avenue, New York, NY10016
Oxford is a registered trademark of Oxford University Press

Whilst the advice and information in this book are believed to be true and
accurate at the date of going to press, neither the authors nor the publisher
can accept any legal responsibility or liability for any errors or omissions
that may be made. In particular (but without limiting the generality of the
preceding disclaimer) every effort has been made to check drug dosages;
however, it is still possible that errors have been missed. Furthermore,
dosage schedules are constantly being revised and new side-effects
recognized. For these reasons the reader is strongly urged to consult the
drug companies' printed instructions before administering any of the drugs
recommended in this book.

British Library Cataloguing in Publication Data
A catalogue record for this book is available from the British Library

Library of Congress Cataloging-in-Publication Data
A catalog record for this book is available from the Library of Congress

ISBN 0 7506 2457 4

1 2 3 4 5 6 7 8 9 10

Printed and bound in Malta by Gutenberg Press Ltd

What do you think about this book? Or any other Arnold title?
Please send your comments to feedback.arnold@hodder.co.uk

Contents

Preface

The study of the physiology and pathophysiology of blood has undergone a quiet revolution over the past decade or so. Our understanding of normal blood physiology and ability to explain, often in the minutest detail, pathological changes has expanded at a mind-boggling rate. This revolution has been fed by (and, in turn, has contributed to) the equally rapid expansion of knowledge of molecular genetics, biochemistry and cell biology.

Undergraduate students of the Biomedical Sciences often find difficulty in the early stages of learning about haematology, bedevilled as it is by the need for significant knowledge of underpinning disciplines to understand it properly. The problem is compounded by texts that concentrate exclusively on either the clinical or laboratory aspects of the subject. This book is intended to provide a review of the most important aspects of haematology, both clinical and laboratory based and to unite them by explaining the science which underpins these aspects. I have made no attempt to provide a 'how-to' book; laboratory and clinical practice are admirably described in other texts. Instead, I have aimed to provide a sound foundation for conceptual understanding of the physiology and pathophysiology of the blood. I believe that, once the fundamental concepts of haematology are firmly grasped, the student is able to 'think like a haematologist' and subsequent learning of the applied aspects of the discipline is easier.

The overall aim of the *Biomedical Sciences Explained* series is to provide a series of short, affordable, introductory texts, which assume little prior knowledge and which are written in an accessible style. They are designed to meet the needs of students on contemporary degrees in Biomedical Sciences, which demand knowledge of both applied and fundamental sciences. I sincerely hope you find this book, as well as others in the series, to be helpful to you in your studies.

Good luck with your studies and, remember, have fun!

C. J. Pallister

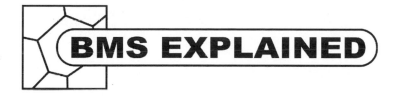

Series preface

The many disciplines that constitute the field of Biomedical Sciences have long provided excitement and challenge both for practitioners and for those who lead their education. This has never been truer than now as we ready ourselves to face the challenges of a new millennium. The exponential growth in biomedical enquiry and knowledge seen in recent years has been mirrored in the education and training of biomedical scientists. The burgeoning of modular BSc (Hons) Biomedical Sciences degrees and the adoption of graduate-only entry by the Institute of Biomedical Sciences and the Council for Professions Supplementary to Medicine have been important drivers of change.

The broad range of subject matter encompassed by the Biomedical Sciences has led to the design of modular BSc (Hons) Biomedical Sciences degrees that facilitate wider undergraduate choice and permit some degree of specialization. There is a much greater emphasis on self-directed learning and understanding of learning outcomes than hitherto.

Against this background, the large, expensive standard texts designed for single subject specialization over the duration of the degree and beyond, are much less useful for the modern student of biomedical sciences. Instead, there is a clear need for a series of short, affordable, introductory texts, which assume little prior knowledge and which are written in an accessible style. The *Biomedical Sciences Explained* series is specifically designed to meet this need.

Each book in the series is designed to meet the needs of a level 1 or 2 student and will have the following distinctive features:

- written by experienced academics in the biomedical sciences in a student-friendly and accessible style, with the trend towards student-centred and life-long learning firmly in mind;
- each chapter opens with a set of defined learning objectives and closes with self-assessment questions which check that the learning objectives have been met;
- aids to understanding such as potted histories of important scientists, descriptions of seminal experiments and background information appear as sideboxes;
- extensively illustrated with line diagrams, charts and tables wherever appropriate;
- use of unnecessary jargon is avoided. New terms are explained, either in the text or sideboxes;
- written in an explanatory rather than a didactic style, emphasizing conceptual understanding rather than rote learning.

I sincerely hope that you find these books as helpful in your studies as they have been designed to be. Good luck and have fun!

C. J. Pallister

Chapter 1
Content of the blood and haemopoiesis

Learning objectives

After studying this chapter you should confidently be able to:

Describe the cellular and fluid components of normal blood.

Describe the various sites of haemopoiesis throughout life.

Discuss the physiological significance of the haemopoietic stem cell compartment.

Outline the sequence of differentiation of the various blood cells.

Outline the mechanisms of regulation of haemopoiesis.

The blood is one of the largest organs of the body, with a volume of about 5 litres and a weight of 5.5 kg in an average 70 kg man. Blood circulates throughout the body, supporting the function of all other body tissues. Because blood and bone marrow are sampled easily, the haemopoietic system probably is the most intensively studied organ of the body. This has led to an explosion of knowledge about blood and blood-forming tissue in both health and disease.

Content of the blood

Normal peripheral blood is composed of three types of cell, **red cells**, **white cells** and **platelets**, suspended in a pale yellow fluid called **plasma**. The cells occupy about 40% of the total volume.

Red cells

Mature red cells, or **erythrocytes**, are the most numerous of the blood cells: about 5×10^{12} normally are present in each litre of blood. Red cells survive in the circulation for about 120 days before being sequestered in the spleen and consumed by the phagocytic cells of the reticuloendothelial system.

From the time of Hippocrates, curiosity about the blood and its functions combined with ignorance and mysticism to produce a plethora of mistaken beliefs, myths and legends. The aura of mystery which surrounds the blood has still not been completely dispelled. Examples of the vestiges of primitive belief abound in the work of poets, playwrights and authors.

Obvious examples include tales of vampires who must regularly imbibe the blood of virgins to sustain life and the constant reference to blood to symbolize murder and the pangs of conscience of the anguished Lord and Lady Macbeth following the murder of Duncan.

Our everyday language is enriched by expressions such as hot-blooded which denotes passion or 'cool as a cucumber'. Both are rooted in mediaeval beliefs about the power and properties of the blood.

Reference values for adults	
Men	
RBC	$4.4 - 5.9 \times 10^{12}/l$
Hb	$13.3 - 17.7\,g/dl$
Plt	$150 - 440 \times 10^9/l$
Women	
RBC	$3.8 - 5.2 \times 10^{12}/l$
Hb	$11.7 - 15.7\,g/dl$
Plt	$150 - 440 \times 10^9/l$

During its 120 days in the circulation, the average red cell travels about 300 miles around the body. The senescent red cells that are destroyed within the spleen are constantly replaced by juvenile cells synthesized and released by the bone marrow. An average 70 kg adult male produces about 2.3×10^6 red cells every second!

Reference values ($\times 10^9/l$)	
WBC	4.0 – 11.0
Neut	2.1 – 7.2 (55–65%)
Lymph	1.5 – 4.0 (20–40%)
Mono	0.2 – 0.8 (4–10%)
Eosin	0 – 0.45 (1–3%)
Baso	0 – 0.2 (0–1%)

The normal red cell is a biconcave discoid shape with a diameter of about 7.2 µm and a volume of about 85 fl. This characteristic shape imparts flexibility to the cell, allowing it to traverse the smallest blood vessels which have a diameter of about 3 µm and also facilitates gaseous exchange across the cell membrane by maximizing the surface area:volume ratio. The primary function of the red cell is to transport oxygen from the lungs to the tissues. The oxygen-carrying pigment **haemoglobin** is present in high concentration in mature red cells and is responsible for the characteristic red colour of the blood.

Platelets

The second most numerous type of cell in the blood is the platelet or **thrombocyte**: about 250×10^9 platelets are present in each litre of blood. Normal peripheral blood platelets are discoid, anucleate cells with a granular cytoplasm. They have a volume of about 7 fl, a diameter of about 3 µm and are about 1 µm thick. Platelets survive in the circulation for 10–12 days.

The primary role of the blood platelet is in the arrest of blood loss. Adequate numbers of functionally normal platelets are essential for optimal haemostasis. Platelets are also involved in the early stages of the development of atherosclerosis, which can lead to arterial disease and thrombosis.

White cells

The least numerous of the blood cells is the white cell or **leukocyte**: about 5×10^9 white cells are present in each litre of blood. There are five different types of white cell normally present in the peripheral blood: **neutrophils, eosinophils, basophils, monocytes** and **lymphocytes**. The neutrophils, eosinophils and basophils are characterized by the presence of cytoplasmic granules and so are known collectively as **granulocytes**. Conversely, lymphocytes and monocytes are known as **mononuclear leukocytes**.

Neutrophils

The neutrophil is the most numerous white cell in adults: about 60% of circulating white cells are neutrophils. The neutrophil nucleus is divided into a varying number of lobes, joined by a thin chromatin strand. Because of this, the neutrophil is sometimes called a **polymorphonuclear leukocyte**. Neutrophil cytoplasm contains numerous fine granules, which stain pale pink with Romanowsky dyes. The appearance of these cytoplasmic granules distinguishes the neutrophil from its granulocytic cousins.

Neutrophils spend about 8–10 h in the circulation before they exit to the tissues, where they are responsible for non-specific defence against bacterial and fungal infection.

Eosinophils

About 1% of the circulating white cells are eosinophils. This name is derived from the staining characteristics of the large cytoplasmic granules which stain strongly with the acidic dye eosin. Typically, the eosinophil nucleus is bilobed. Eosinophils circulate in the bloodstream for about 4–5 h before they exit to the tissues, where they are responsible for defence against parasitic infestation and also help to dampen the allergic response. Tissue eosinophils are also capable of responding, albeit inefficiently, to bacterial and fungal infection in a similar manner to neutrophils.

Basophils

Basophils are the least numerous circulating white cell: less than 1% of circulating white cells are basophils. The large cytoplasmic granules are characterized by their avidity for the basic dye methylene blue. Basophils are involved in anaphylactic, hypersensitivity and inflammatory reactions.

Monocytes

About 5% of circulating white cells are monocytes. The blood monocyte is a large cell (16–22 μm in diameter) with a kidney-shaped or distinctly cleft nucleus and a scattering of delicate azurophilic granules in the cytoplasm. Blood monocytes circulate for about 10 h before they exit to the tissues, where they mature into the actively phagocytic **tissue macrophages** which are responsible for the removal and processing of aged red cells and other debris. Tissue macrophages also play an important role in the processing and presentation of antigen to T lymphocytes.

Lymphocytes

Lymphocytes are the second most common white cell in the peripheral blood: about 33% of circulating white cells are lymphocytes. Typically, lymphocytes are much smaller than monocytes (10–12 μm in diameter) and have much less cytoplasm. In contrast to the monocyte, the lymphocyte nucleus is round and almost fills the cell. A few lymphocytes have more abundant cytoplasm. Lymphocytes have a variable lifespan of between a few days and many years.

There are different types of lymphocytes which play distinct roles in specific immunity. **T lymphocytes** account for 40–80% of the blood lymphocytes and are responsible for **cell-mediated immunity.** **B lymphocytes** normally account for 10–30% of the blood lymphocytes and are responsible for **humoral immunity.**

Romanowsky stains are produced by mixing alkaline methylene blue and eosin, producing complex dye mixtures. These stains have the useful property of being able to differentiate multiple structures by different colours in a single bath. For example, the phosphate groups in nucleic acids are highly basophilic and so stain purplish-blue, the cytoplasm of monocytes is mildly basophilic and so stains pale grey-blue and the haemoglobin in red cell cytoplasm is highly acidophilic or eosinophilic and stains bright pink. With careful technique and rigorous control of pH, Romanowsky stains can be used to reveal subtle details of cellular structure and function and are the mainstay of haematological morphologists.

Plasma

Plasma occupies about 60% of the total blood volume. It is a pale yellow aqueous solution of electrolytes, proteins and small organic molecules such as glucose. The major extracellular cation is Na^+, which has a plasma concentration of ~140 mmol/l. Other important plasma cations include K^+, Ca^{2+}, Fe^{2+} and Mg^{2+}, but these are all found at much lower concentrations. The relative concentrations of Na^+ and K^+ in the plasma contrast with their intracellular concentrations where K^+ is present at a higher concentration.

The major plasma anions are Cl^- and HCO_3^- although SO_4^{2-} and HPO_4^{2-} also are present at lower concentration. Plasma is always electrically neutral, i.e. the concentrations of anions and cations are always such that the total number of negative and positive charges exactly balance.

A large number of different plasma proteins exist but they fall into four distinct families:

- **Haemostatic proteins** such as the coagulation factors, fibrinolytic factors and their inhibitors.
- **Immunoglobulins** which are antibody molecules synthesized by plasma cells. There are five different classes of immunoglobulin (IgA, IgD, IgE, IgG and IgM) which are structurally related but perform distinct biological functions.
- **Complement** which consists of a family of plasma proteins important in the induction of inflammation and immunity against microbial infection.
- **Transport proteins** which ferry nutrients and waste products around the body.

Haemopoiesis

Under normal physiological conditions, the number of circulating blood cells is maintained within remarkably narrow limits. Since all blood cells have a limited lifespan, a dynamic equilibrium must exist between cell loss due to senescence or normal function and the synthesis and release of their replacements. Maintenance of this dynamic equilibrium requires a capacity for production of blood cells (haemopoiesis) of astonishing fertility, coupled with exquisite responsiveness to the changing needs of the body for blood cells.

Ontogeny of haemopoiesis

Haemopoiesis is conducted at a number of different anatomical sites during the process of development from embryo to adult (Figure 1.1). Changes in the primary site of haemopoiesis are accompanied by simultaneous changes in the morphology of the

An average 70 kg man has a total blood volume of about 5 litres which contains a total of 25×10^{12} red cells. Since normal red cells survive for an average of 120 days, maintenance of a constant cell number requires the replacement of more than 2×10^{11} red cells every day! If the destruction and replacement of the other blood cells is taken into account, the total daily requirement for new blood cells is about 5×10^{11}. This rate of production must be maintained without pause for an average of 70 years, during which time the bone marrow will have released more than 1×10^{16} mature blood cells!

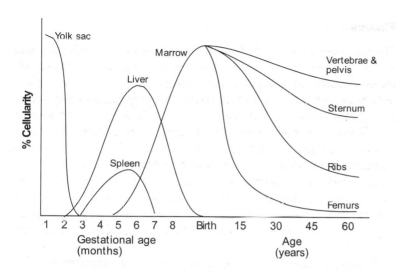

Figure 1.1 *Sites of haemopoiesis throughout life*

cells produced and in the types of haemoglobin molecule synthesized within the red cell precursors.

Embryonic haemopoiesis

The earliest recognizable red cell precursors are large, nucleated cells and are demonstrable in 2-week-old embryos. The major haemoglobin present in these cells is **haemoglobin Gower I** ($\zeta_2\varepsilon_2$). Leukopoiesis and thrombopoiesis do not commence until about 6 weeks into gestation when megakaryocytes and granulocytes can be seen in the yolk sac. In contrast to other blood cells, lymphocytes are not formed in the yolk sac, but in the lymph sacs, which begin to develop at about 7 weeks' gestation.

Foetal haemopoiesis

Haemopoietic activity is first demonstrable in the foetal liver at 6 weeks' gestation. This organ is the primary source of foetal blood cells until about 30 weeks' gestation. Hepatic haemopoietic activity ceases at about 40 weeks' gestation. The major haemoglobin synthesized during the hepatic phase of foetal haemopoiesis is haemoglobin F ($\alpha_2\gamma_2$).

The foetal spleen begins production of blood cells at about 10 weeks' gestation and continues throughout the second trimester of pregnancy. However, even at the height of its activity, the foetal spleen is of secondary importance as a haemopoietic organ.

Bone cavities begin to form at about 20 weeks' gestation and provide such an ideal environment for haemopoietic activity that the bone marrow rapidly becomes the sole source of blood cells in humans – a process complete by 40 weeks' gestation. This process is associated with a gradual replacement of haemoglobin F by haemoglobin A ($\alpha_2\beta_2$).

The earliest recognizable blood cell precursors are demonstrable in 2-week-old embryos. At this stage of development, the embryo consists of little more than two sacs – the **amniotic sac** and the **yolk sac** – separated by a wedge of tissue called the **embryonic plate**. As the embryo develops, the amniotic sac expands greatly to fill the entire uterus and the placenta is formed. The yolk sac becomes compressed by the expanding amniotic sac into a narrow stalk which forms the core of the umbilical cord. The embryo develops from the embryonic plate.

The first unequivocal demonstration of the existence of pluripotential stem cells came in 1961 when Till and McCulloch performed experiments to determine the sensitivity of mouse bone marrow to damage by irradiation. Briefly, mice were subjected to a dose of ionizing radiation sufficient to destroy their haemopoietic capacity and bone marrow cells from genetically identical mice were immediately transfused. After about 7 days the spleens of these mice had developed numerous macroscopic nodules which consisted of haemopoietic tissue. Subsequent experiments showed that these nodules were clonal in nature, i.e. each was derived from a single stem cell, which was given the name colony forming unit-spleen or CFU-S. Under different experimental conditions, CFU-S could be influenced to produce granulocyte-macrophage colony forming units (CFU-GM), erythroid colony forming units (CFU-E) or megakaryocyte colony forming units (CFU-Meg) or a mixture of more than one cell line.

Haempoiesis in the developing child and adult

At birth, haemopoietically active, or red, marrow completely fills the available marrow space. This means that infants have no reserve haemopoietic capacity that can be called upon in times of increased demand. The only response open to a neonate in such circumstances is to expand the marrow volume. This is the cause of the skeletal deformities that develop in severe dyserythropoietic states such as thalassaemia.

During early childhood, marrow volume increases in parallel with the increased marrow space made available by growth. The bone marrow volume in an average 3-year-old child has expanded to about 1500 ml. This is still entirely composed of active red marrow and is sufficient to meet the normal demands for blood cells of an adult. Thus, as the child grows into an adult, and the available bone marrow space expands, there is no requirement for a concurrent increase in volume of active red marrow. The expanding marrow space becomes progressively filled with inactive, or yellow, marrow. This process begins in the peripheral diaphyses of the long bones and continues until, in an adult, three-quarters of the red marrow is found in the pelvis, vertebrae and sternum.

Yellow marrow can readily be converted into its active counterpart during periods of increased demand for blood cells. This means that adults have a reserve haemopoietic capacity of about six times normal.

In conditions where the bone marrow is unable to meet the demands of the body for blood cells, e.g. when the bone marrow space is occupied by metastatic tumour, haemopoiesis may revert to foetal sites viz the spleen and liver. This phenomenon is known as **extramedullary haemopoiesis**.

Sequence of differentiation of blood cells

Blood cells are produced in vast numbers throughout life, with no apparent sign of exhaustion of their source. This requires the existence of a population of precursor cells that are capable of both self-renewal and differentiation – the **stem cell compartment**. The common ancestral cell of all mature blood cells in humans is the **totipotential stem cell** (Figure 1.2). This cell can differentiate to form either a **lymphoid stem cell** (CFU-L, colony forming unit-lymphoid) or a **non-lymphoid stem cell** (CFU-GEMM, colony forming unit-granulocyte, erythroid, macrophage, megakaryocyte). These cells are said to be **pluripotent**, i.e. they have the capacity to differentiate along several different cell line, but their choice is limited, as shown. These stem cells retain the dual capacity for self-renewal and differentiation. Pluripotential stem cells are capable of differentiating into a number of different **unipotential** stem cells. These are committed to differentiation along a single cell line, e.g. BFU-E (burst-forming unit-erythroid) can only differentiate into mature red cells.

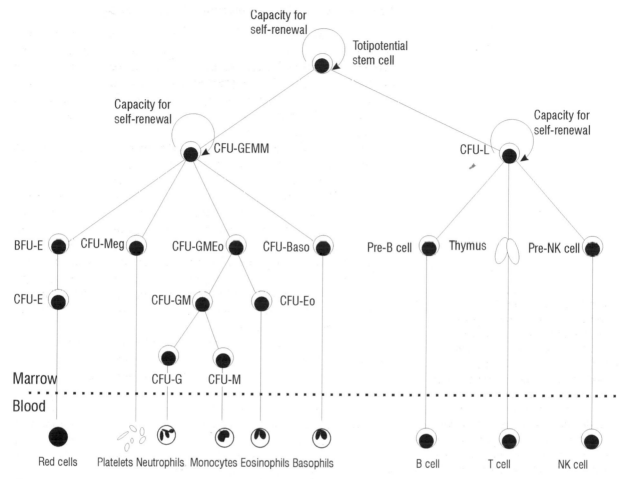

Figure 1.2 *Haemopoietic lineage tree showing the lines along which blood cells are produced*

Control of haemopoiesis

Haemopoiesis is closely regulated by a family of glycoproteins known as the haemopoietic growth factors. These substances fall into two main classes, the **colony-stimulating factors** and the **interleukins**. The main sites of action of these growth factors are depicted in Figure 1.3.

Erythropoiesis

Maintenance of the circulating red cell mass within the narrow limits seen in health is achieved by a feedback mechanism, which senses body oxygen demands and adjusts the rate of erythropoiesis accordingly. This feedback mechanism is mediated by the glyco-protein hormone **erythropoietin** as follows:

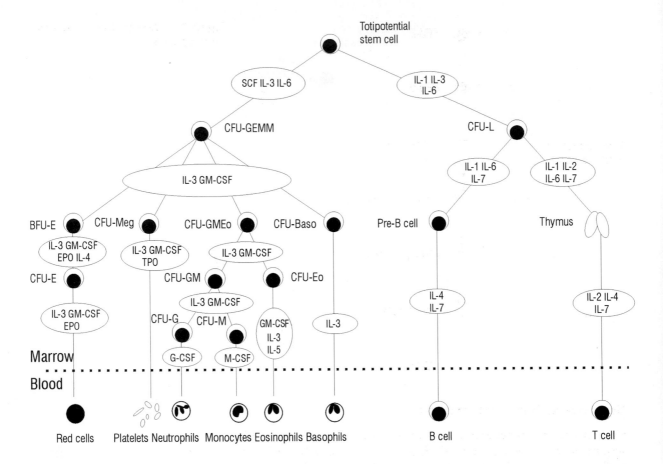

Figure 1.3 *Regulation of haemopoiesis by growth factors. IL, interleukin; SCF, stem cell factor; GM-CSF, granulocyte-macrophage colony stimulating factor; G-CSF, granulocyte colony stimulating factor; M-CSF, monocyte/macrophage colony stimulating factor; EPO, erythropoietin; TPO, thrombopoietin*

- A fall in the circulating red cell mass leads to decreased delivery of oxygen to the tissues and hypoxia develops.
- Tissue hypoxia is sensed by an enzyme-linked mechanism in the kidney and synthesis of erythropoietin (EPO) by the peritubular endothelial cells of the kidney is stimulated.
- EPO binds to specific receptors on BFU-E and CFU-E in the bone marrow, resulting in a shortening of cell-cycle time, an increased rate of maturation and an increased rate of release of red cells from the bone marrow.
- The increased red cell count improves oxygen delivery to the tissues, the hypoxia is corrected and EPO synthesis is switched off.

A lineage tree for normal erythropoiesis is shown in Figure 1.4.

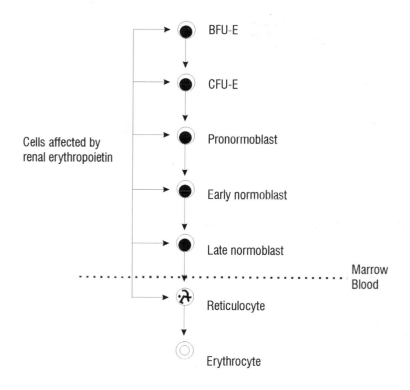

Figure 1.4 *Lineage tree for normal erythropoiesis*

Granulopoiesis and monopoiesis

Granulocyte and monocyte production is regulated by the combined actions of haemopoietic growth factors. IL-3 and GM-CSF act together on CFU-GEMM to stimulate production of CFU-GMEo and CFU-Baso. CFU-GMEo further differentiate to form CFU-GM and CFUEo. The action of G-CSF on CFU-GM stimulates neutrophil production, while M-CSF stimulates monocyte production and IL-5 stimulates eosinophil production. Basophil production is stimulated by the action of IL-3 on CFU-Baso. A lineage tree for normal granulopoiesis and monopoiesis is shown in Figure 1.5.

Thrombopoiesis

Megakaryoblasts are formed from CFU-Meg by a unique process called **endomitotic replication**. In this process, DNA replication and expansion of cytoplasmic volume occur but not cellular division. Thus, with each complete cycle of endomitosis, the cell becomes progressively larger and increasingly polyploid. Morphologically recognizable megakaryocytes may have up to 64n DNA content (i.e. 32 times the normal diploid (2n) content). Once endomitotic replication has ceased, the megakaryocyte nucleus becomes lobulated and the cytoplasm matures, with the formation of the structures that form the platelets and, finally, the platelets are shed into the venous sinus. This process is estimated to take from 2 to 3 days. Each

Figure 1.5 *Lineage tree for normal granulopoiesis and monopoiesis*

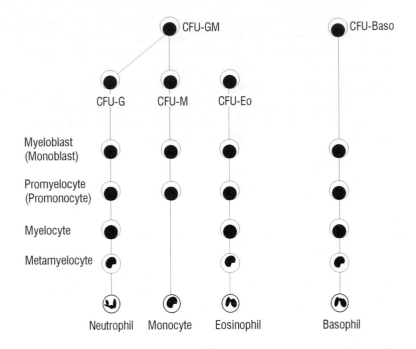

megakaryocyte is capable of producing between 2000 and 7000 platelets. A lineage tree for normal thrombopoiesis is shown in Figure 1.6.

Lymphopoiesis

In contrast to the other forms of haemopoiesis, lymphopoiesis is not a one-way process of differentiation and maturation into end-stage cells. Two distinct phases of lymphopoiesis are distinguishable:

- The lymphoid stem cell differentiates to form mature antigen-

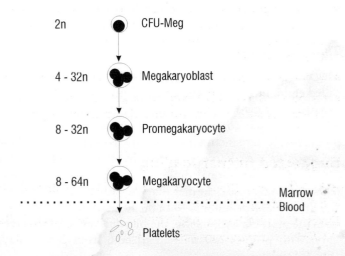

Figure 1.6 *Lineage tree for normal thrombopoiesis*

committed lymphocytes. This process occurs in the **primary lymphoid organs**. T lymphocyte differentiation occurs in the **thymus gland** while B lymphocyte differentiation takes place in the foetal liver and adult bone marrow.

- Antigen-dependent proliferation and development of mature T and B lymphocytes occurs in the **secondary lymphoid organs** such as the **spleen, lymph nodes** and **mucosa-associated lymphoid tissue.**

B lymphopoiesis

B lymphocytes are responsible for humoral immunity. Mature B lymphocytes carry surface receptors which recognize and bind to foreign (i.e. non-self) antigen, triggering cellular proliferation and differentiation into **plasma cells** which synthesize and secrete monoclonal antibody directed against the inducing antigen. A small number of lymphocytes revert to the quiescent state but are capable of mounting an extremely rapid response following further contact with the inducing antigen. These are known as **memory cells.**

T lymphopoiesis

Cellular immunity is mediated by T lymphocytes. The mechanism of activation of T lymphocytes also is antigen-specific but antigen must be processed and presented by macrophages for recognition and activation to occur. There are four main subsets of mature T lymphocytes which are defined in terms of their function and the presence of the adhesion molecules CD4 and CD8:

- Helper cells (T_H) help and induce activation of B lymphocytes. T_H are $CD4^+$ and synthesize the T lymphocyte growth factor IL-2; IL-3 which promotes the growth and maturation of various blood cell precursors, γ-interferon which activates macrophages and GM-CSF.
- T_{DTH} lymphocytes are involved in delayed type hypersensitivity reactions, secrete factors that attract and activate macrophages and inhibit their migration away from the site of inflammation. T_{DTH} are $CD4^+$.
- Suppressor T cells (T_S) act as a brake on T_H lymphocytes.
- Cytotoxic T cells (T_C) bind to target cells and release cytolytic substances such as perforin directly on to the target.

B lymphocytes are so called because, in chickens, they are 'educated' in a specialized organ known as the **bursa of Fabricius**. Glick and associates defined the importance of this organ in 1961, when bursectomized chickens were shown to fail to synthesize antibody and to succumb rapidly in response to Salmonella infection. In humans, B lymphocyte education occurs predominantly in the bone marrow.

The pivotal role of the thymus gland in cellular immunity was first demonstrated in 1961 when it was shown that thymectomized mice had a greatly impaired capacity to fight infection.

Suggested further reading

Bain, B.J. (1997). *Blood Cells. A Practical Guide*, 2nd edn. London: Gower Medical Publishing.

Eaves, C.J. and Eaves, A.C. (1997). Stem cell kinetics. *Bailliere's Clinical Haematology* **10**(2), 233–257.

Hannigan, B.M. (1999). *Immunology*. In BMS Explained (Series ed. C.J. Pallister). Oxford: Butterworth-Heinemann.

Hoffbrand, A.V., Lewis, S.M. and Tuddenham, E.G.D. (1999). *Postgraduate Haematology*, 4th edn. Oxford: Butterworth-Heinemann.

Self-assessment questions

1. What is the functional difference between red and yellow marrow? Where are these found?
2. Place the following in order of increasing maturity: promyelocyte; myelocyte; myeloblast; CFU-GEMM.
3. Which of the following cells are $CD4^+$: B lymphocyte; T_H lymphocyte; T_S lymphocyte; neutrophil?
4. Why is chronic renal failure associated with anaemia?
5. Place the following in order of increasing normal cell count in an adult: erythrocyte; neutrophil; platelet; monocyte; lymphocyte.

Key Concepts and Facts

Content and Function
- Normal blood consists of three cell types: erythrocytes, leukocytes and platelets, suspended in fluid plasma.

- Erythrocytes transport oxygen and carbon dioxide around the body.

- Platelets help to arrest bleeding after injury.

- Neutrophils defend against bacterial and fungal infection.

- Eosinophils defend against parasitic infestation and dampen allergic response.

- Basophils mediate inflammation.

- B lymphocytes mediate humoral immunity.

- T lymphocytes mediate cellular immunity.

Haemopoiesis
- Haemopoiesis is conducted at different sites throughout life.

- In adults haemopoiesis is sited in the bone marrow in health.

- All blood cell types are derived from the same totipotential stem cells.

- Blood cell counts are maintained within narrow limits in health.

- Haemopoiesis is governed by a complex network of growth factors such as erythropoietin, IL-3 and GM-CSF.

Chapter 2
Nutrition and the blood

Learning objectives

After studying this chapter you should confidently be able to:

Describe the importance of iron, vitamin B_{12} and folate for optimal blood cell production.

List the main dietary sources of iron, vitamin B_{12} and folate.

Describe the respective roles of iron, vitamin B_{12} and folate in the body.

Describe the site(s) and mechanism(s) of absorption of iron, vitamin B_{12} and folate from dietary sources.

Outline the luminal factors affecting inorganic iron absorption.

Discuss the daily requirements for iron, vitamin B_{12} and folate at various stages of life.

Discuss the plasma transport and storage of iron, vitamin B_{12} and folate.

Describe the roles of vitamin B_{12} and folate in DNA and RNA synthesis.

Adequate nutrition is an essential requirement for the maintenance of normal bodily function, growth and repair. The nutritional requirements for optimal blood cell production are similar to those of the other cells of the body. Because of this, nutritional deficiencies seldom cause problems that are restricted to the blood.

This chapter concentrates on iron, vitamin B_{12} and folic acid because an adequate supply of these nutrients is essential for maintenance of normal blood cell production and function. Deficiency of these nutrients is associated with the development of anaemia and other abnormalities of haemopoiesis, as described in Chapters 3 and 4.

The existence of essential nutrients in certain foods was suspected long before their identification. For example, the importance of citrus fruits in the prevention of scurvy and of the inclusion of unpolished rice in a diet dominated by rice in the prevention of beriberi were well known. It was not until 1911, however, that the essential factor in unpolished rice was identified by the Polish chemist Casimir Funk as thiamine. It was he who coined the term 'vital amine', from which the name vitamin is derived.

Iron

Iron plays a vital role in the normal function and metabolism of virtually every cell of the body. An adequate dietary intake of iron is essential for optimal health.

The role of iron within the body

Iron-containing compounds can be divided into two groups according to their role within the body: those that play a role in cellular metabolism and those that are required for iron transport and storage. Most of the iron-containing compounds that play a role in cellular metabolism contain iron in the form of a haem group. The haem-containing compounds include **haemoglobin** and **myoglobin**, the oxygen carrying pigments of red cells and muscle respectively and the **cytochromes**, which are a family of electron-transport enzymes that play a variety of roles in oxidative metabolism. Non-haem iron compounds such as the enzymes **nicotinamide adenine dinucleotide dehydrogenase (NADH)** and **succinic dehydrogenase** also are important in cellular metabolism.

Body iron distribution

A normal 70 kg male has a total body iron content of about 4 g. Almost three-quarters of this is found in the form of haemoglobin and myoglobin, while most of the remainder is held in reserve in the body stores (Figure 2.1). The tiny proportion of total body iron that is found in the cytochromes belies their pivotal role in oxidative metabolism within the body.

Daily iron requirements

Iron has been described as a 'one-way element' within the body. This means that iron is absorbed from the diet but that no substantial mechanism for iron excretion exists. On the contrary,

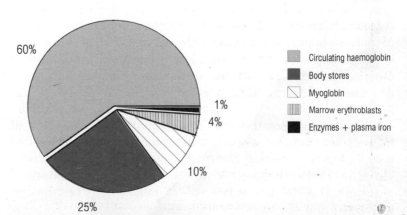

Figure 2.1 *Approximate distribution of iron within the body*

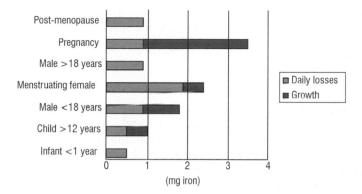

Figure 2.2 *Variations in the daily iron requirement throughout life*

the body possesses elaborate mechanisms to prevent loss of iron. In the normal steady state, daily iron requirements consist of the amount required to replace the small amount lost in sweat, tears, urine and faeces plus the amount required for growth (Figure 2.2).

The excess requirement in menstruating females is due to the monthly blood loss, which contains up to 30 mg of iron. The very high iron requirement in pregnancy consists of three components: the growth requirement of the foetus and placenta, the expansion in maternal blood volume and haemorrhage at delivery. The figure quoted is a representative average value: the actual daily requirements vary according to the stage of pregnancy.

Iron absorption

A normal, mixed daily diet in the UK contains about 18 mg of iron; far in excess of normal body requirements. The main dietary sources are liver, red meat, some green vegetables such as spinach, cereals (which are supplemented with iron during processing) and fish. Dietary iron falls into one of two categories: inorganic iron, which is mainly present in cereals and vegetables, and haem iron, which is found in the haemoglobin and myoglobin of meat products.

Inorganic iron in food is released by the combined action of proteolytic enzymes and hydrochloric acid in the stomach. The low pH environment of the stomach encourages the reduction of Fe^{3+} ions to Fe^{2+} ions, which are absorbed more readily. Iron is absorbed maximally from the duodenum and upper jejunum. Absorption of inorganic iron is enhanced by any factor that increases its solubility. For example, Fe^{2+} compounds generally are more soluble than their Fe^{3+} counterparts, so the presence of reducing agents such as ascorbic acid (vitamin C) improves absorption. Conversely, alkaline pancreatic secretions, phosphates and phytates decrease solubility and retard inorganic iron absorption.

The iron in animal products is absorbed by a different, and as yet improperly understood, mechanism. The luminal factors described

Copper is widely distributed in food and the daily requirement of 2 mg is readily met by the average Western diet. Deficiency of copper impairs iron metabolism and leads to a lack of usable iron in the blood.

Cobalt is required by micro-organisms for the synthesis of vitamin B_{12}. Cobalt deficiency does not appear to cause impairment of health in man but is associated with neurological problems in ruminant farm animals.

Small amounts of zinc are present in both red cells and plasma but its role remains obscure. Zinc deficiency is not associated with the development of anaemia but may predispose to microbial infection.

One of the most important sources of vitamins and minerals in the average, highly processed Western diet is breakfast cereals which are fortified with these nutrients during manufacture. An average (30 g) serving of cornflakes contains almost one-third of the recommended daily intake for an adult of iron and vitamins B_1, B_2, B_6, B_{12} and C.

above have much less influence on the absorption of haem iron. Haem groups are absorbed intact by the intestinal mucosal cell, and subsequently broken down for release into the portal bloodstream.

Control of iron absorption

Although iron is an essential nutrient, excess iron is highly toxic. Accumulation of iron is prevented by careful regulation of iron absorption from the gut. The precise mechanism of regulation remains controversial, but the most widely accepted model is the **mucosal block theory.**

When the intestinal mucosal cell is formed in the crypts of Lieberkühn, **ferritin** – a storage form of iron – is incorporated within the cell in direct proportion to the body stores of iron at the time. This intracellular ferritin is thought either to block absorption of iron from the gut or to interfere with the release of absorbed iron into the bloodstream. Thus, when body iron stores are low, the mucosal cells contain relatively little ferritin and absorption of iron from the gut is uninhibited. Conversely, in the presence of iron overload, high ferritin levels within the intestinal mucosae result in gross inhibition of absorption (Figure 2.3). Intestinal mucosal cells are relatively short-lived: they are constantly sloughed off into the faeces and replaced. This process provides a constantly updated indicator of body iron stores and acts as an effective and sensitive control mechanism for absorption of iron from the gut. This control mechanism is only effective in the presence of physiological

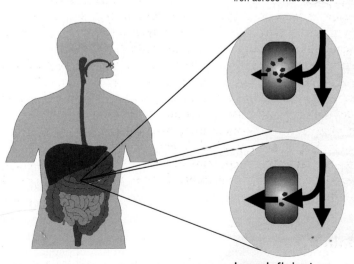

Iron replete
Stored ferritin blocks passage of iron across mucosal cell

Iron deficient
Lack of stored ferritin allows free passage of dietary iron

Figure 2.3   *The mucosal block theory of inorganic iron absorption*

amounts of iron. In the presence of much higher iron concentrations such as those encountered during iron replacement therapy, iron absorption occurs by passive diffusion across the gut wall and is not dependent upon body iron status.

Iron transport

Iron absorbed from the duodenum is released into the bloodstream where it is bound to a specific carrier protein called **transferrin**. Transferrin is a β globulin with a molecular weight of 74 000 which can carry up to two Fe^{3+} ions per molecule. Iron is transported to the bone marrow bound to transferrin where it is fed to developing erythroblasts for incorporation into haemoglobin. Normal plasma contains sufficient transferrin to bind about 300 µg of iron per decilitre. This figure is called the **total iron binding capacity (TIBC)** and is one of the useful measures in the assessment of iron status. Typically, plasma transferrin is about 33% saturated with iron.

Newly absorbed iron represents only about 5% of the iron utilized for haem synthesis. About 90% of the iron required each day for this purpose is derived by recycling iron from the haemoglobin of senescent red cells. Any shortfall in iron requirement is met by continuous slow release from the body iron stores.

Iron storage

About one quarter of the total body iron is in storage, mainly in the liver, tissue macrophages and bone marrow. Two forms of storage iron exist: **ferritin** and **haemosiderin**. Ferritin exists as a spherical structure with a diameter of ~ 5 nm and hydrated ferric (Fe^{3+}) phosphate at its core. Typically, ferritin contains about 25% of iron by weight. About two-thirds of body iron stores are present in this form. Different tissues are associated with slightly different forms of ferritin or **isoferritins**, which vary somewhat in their chemical and physical properties but share the same basic molecular shape. Plasma ferritin is derived from tissue macrophages and its estimation provides the single most useful indicator of iron status.

The other form of storage iron, haemosiderin, is not a single substance but a variety of different, amorphous iron–protein complexes. Typically, it contains about 37% of iron by weight. Haemosiderin probably represents ferritin in various stages of degradation.

Vitamin B$_{12}$

Vitamin B$_{12}$ can exist in a variety of different chemical forms, which together constitute the family of **cobalamins**. The cobalamins are organometallic complexes comprising three major structures: a

The most common method of assessing body iron stores involves the measurement of the serum concentration of ferritin. In most cases, this provides a fair reflection of the state of the body iron stores but serum ferritin is an **acute phase protein**, i.e. its concentration is (possibly markedly) increased during the acute phases of inflammatory conditions such as rheumatoid arthritis and cancer. In these circumstances, the serum ferritin concentration bears little relationship to the state of the body iron stores.

A definitive estimation of body iron stores is best obtained by taking a small liver biopsy. The iron content of the biopsy can be assessed by dehydration and acid digestion of the tissue, followed by colorimetric assay using bathophenanthriline sulphonate. Because of its invasive nature, this technique is reserved for suspected cases of iron overload, when it can be combined with microscopic examination to assess the level of tissue damage present.

Certain micro-organisms are incapable of synthesizing vitamin B_{12} or folate and so have an absolute requirement for exogenous supplies for growth. This fact has been exploited in the microbiological assay of vitamin B_{12} and folate. If suitable micro-organisms are maintained in a growth medium which contains all required nutrients except vitamin B_{12} or folate and a known volume of a test serum is added, then the rate of microbial growth is determined by the concentration of the missing nutrient in the test serum.

Examples of suitable test organisms include *Lactobacillus leichmanii* and *Euglena gracilis* for vitamin B_{12} and *Lactobacillus casei* for folate. Although universally used in the past, this method of assay is technically demanding and subject to severe practical limitations and has been almost completely superseded by radio-isotopic and immunological methods.

corrin nucleus and, bound at right angles to the nucleus, a nucleotide and a variable chemical group. The structure of the corrin nucleus is similar to that of haem in that it consists of four pyrrole rings with a Co^+ ion instead of an Fe^{2+} at the centre. The nucleotide comprises a base (5,6-dimethylbenzimidazole) bound to a phosphorylated sugar (ribose-3-phosphate).

The differences between the various cobalamins lie in the variable chemical group, which is bound to the central cobalt ion. In the physiologically active cobalamins, the variant chemical group is either a 5'-deoxyadenosyl group or a methyl group. **5'-deoxyadenosylcobalamin** is the predominant form of the vitamin encountered in the liver while **methylcobalamin** predominates in the plasma. Both 5'-deoxyadenosylcobalamin and methylcobalamin are unstable compounds which, on exposure to light, rapidly denature to form **hydroxocobalamin** which contains a Co^{3+} ion at its centre. Hydroxocobalamin is the main dietary form of the vitamin. **Cyanocobalamin** is a stable synthetic form.

The role of vitamin B_{12} within the body

In bacteria, vitamin B_{12} is involved in a relatively large number of metabolic reactions but, in humans, it is required as coenzyme for only two:

- **Conversion of L-methylmalonyl coenzyme A to succinyl coenzyme A.** 5'-deoxyadenosylcobalamin is required as a coenzyme in this isomerization reaction. A wide range of substances are catabolized via this reaction, e.g. cholesterol, odd chain fatty acids, the amino acids methionine and threonine and the pyrimidines uracil and thymine.
- **Methylation of homocysteine to methionine.** This reaction requires both methylcobalamin as a coenzyme and N-5-methyltetrahydrofolate as the methyl donor, and is important in the intracellular synthesis of folate coenzymes.

Daily vitamin B_{12} requirements and body stores

Vitamin B_{12} is synthesized exclusively by micro-organisms: the only source available to humans is from dietary sources such as liver, kidney, red meat, eggs, shellfish and dairy products. A typical mixed UK diet contains between 5 and 30 μg of vitamin B_{12} per day, depending on the quantity of meat included. Diets that exclude all animal products contain no intrinsic vitamin B_{12}. However, even strict vegans obtain small amounts of vitamin B_{12} from their diet as a result of bacterial contamination of their food. Vitamin B_{12} is relatively heat-stable; little loss occurs in cooking.

Typical daily losses of vitamin B_{12} are between 1 and 4 μg, primarily in the urine and faeces. Since there is no bodily consumption of vitamin B_{12}, the daily requirement matches daily losses.

Thus, a typical UK mixed diet provides more than enough vitamin B_{12} to meet requirements.

Normally, the body stores about 3–4 mg of vitamin B_{12}, primarily in the liver. This would be sufficient to meet the requirement for vitamin B_{12} for about 3 years if dietary intake ceased or if the ability to absorb the vitamin was lost.

Vitamin B_{12} absorption

Vitamin B_{12} absorption is an active process that occurs optimally in the terminal ileum. Vitamin B_{12} in food is liberated by gastric and duodenal proteolytic enzymes and rapidly complexes in a 1:1 ratio with a glycoprotein of molecular weight 45 000 called **intrinsic factor**. Intrinsic factor is synthesized and secreted by gastric parietal cells. The IF:B_{12} complex then progresses to the ileum where it binds, via the intrinsic factor part of the complex, to specific receptors on mucosal cells and is absorbed intact. Within the mucosal cell, vitamin B_{12} is released from its complex and, after a delay of about 6 hours, the newly absorbed vitamin is released into the portal circulation. Intrinsic factor is not recycled. Because of the finite number of ileal IF:B_{12} receptors, a maximum of about 2 µg of vitamin B_{12} can be absorbed from each meal, regardless of its content. After each meal, ileal receptors are unresponsive to further IF:B_{12} complex for up to 6 hours.

Excretion of vitamin B_{12} occurs mainly via the biliary system. A proportion is reabsorbed from the bile during its passage through the gut. This salvage mechanism is known as the **enterohepatic circulation** of vitamin B_{12}.

Vitamin B_{12} transport

There are three specific vitamin B_{12} transport proteins, known as **transcobalamins** (TCI–TCIII), normally present in plasma. The physiologically important transcobalamin is TCII which is a β globulin of molecular weight 38 000. It is synthesized primarily in the liver and ileum and binds to vitamin B_{12} in a 1:1 ratio. Developing blood cells carry specific surface receptors for TCII:B_{12} complexes which facilitate delivery of vitamin B_{12} to these cells. TCII binds newly absorbed vitamin B_{12} and delivers it rapidly to developing tissues such as the bone marrow: the plasma half-life of the TCII:vitamin B_{12} complex is about 12 hours. Congenital absence of TCII causes a severe megaloblastic anaemia within weeks of birth, despite normal vitamin B_{12} absorption and a normal serum vitamin B_{12} concentration.

Transcobalamins I and III are α globulins which are synthesized by granulocytes and have a molecular weight of about 58 000. They belong to a family of vitamin B_{12}-binding proteins known as **R-binders**, which are present in body secretions such as gastric juice, milk, bile and saliva. TCI and TCIII do not readily release

---

Key dates: vitamin B_{12}

1926
First demonstration by George Minot of Harvard University of the efficacy of eating raw beef liver in the treatment of pernicious anaemia.

1927
Identification by William Castle of Boston City Hospital that an 'extrinsic factor' in liver combines with an 'intrinsic factor' in gastric juice to produce this effect.

1930–47
Production of first clinically effective purified liver extract by Gänsslen in Germany.
Identification of **LLD factor**, **animal protein factor** and **ruminant factor**, all of which turned out to be cobalamins.

1947
Demonstration by Mary Shorb that clinically effective liver extracts contained an essential growth factor for *Lactobacillus lactis*.

1948
Crystallization of cyanocobalamin by Karl Folkers and co-workers at the Merck laboratories in the USA and E.L. Smith and co-workers, a few months later, at the Glaxo Laboratories in the UK.

vitamin B_{12} to developing cells. The plasma half-life of the TCI:vitamin B_{12} complex is about 9–12 days. Some 80–90% of the vitamin B_{12} present in plasma circulates bound to TCI, which is thought to act as a reservoir for serum vitamin B_{12}. Congenital absence of TCI causes no clinical disorder, despite a reduction in serum vitamin B_{12} concentration.

Folates

The parent of the folate family of compounds is folic acid (pteroylglutamic acid). Humans are incapable of synthesizing folate: all requirements must be met by dietary intake. The most common dietary forms of folate differ from the parent compound in three important respects:

- They exist in reduced form as dihydro- (DHF) or tetrahydrofolates (THF).
- They carry a single-carbon group (methyl, CH_3; formyl, CHO; formimino, CHNH; or methylene, CH_2) bonded to the N-5 or N-10 nitrogen atom.
- Most are conjugated with a series of glutamate residues, and are known as folate polyglutamates.

The role of folate within the body

The various forms of folate function as single-carbon group donor/acceptors in a variety of biosynthetic reactions:

- **Synthesis of methionine** from homocysteine involves donation of the methyl group from N-5-methylTHF and requires methylcobalamin as a coenzyme.
- **Pyrimidine synthesis.** The methylation of deoxyuridine-5′-monophosphate (dUMP) to thymidine-5′-monophosphate (dTMP) is the rate-limiting step in DNA synthesis and requires N-5,10-methyleneTHF as a coenzyme.
- **Purine synthesis** requires the presence of N-5,10-methyleneTHF or N-10-formylTHF as coenzymes.
- **Conversion of serine into glycine** involves THF acting as acceptor of a single-carbon group, becoming N-5,10-methyleneTHF in the process.
- **Histidine catabolism** involves its conversion into N-formiminoglutamic acid (FIGLU) and subsequent conversion into glutamate by donation of the formimino group to THF.

Daily folate requirements and body stores

Losses of folate amount to about 100 µg per day, mainly via faeces, urine, sweat and desquamated skin cells. Faeces contain a relatively large amount of both vitamin B_{12} and folate but these represent the biosynthetic activities of the gut flora rather than losses from body stores. Thus, the normal adult daily requirement for folate is about 100 μg.

Folates are present to some extent in most foods but liver, eggs, leafy vegetables, whole grains and yeast are particularly rich sources. Folate in food is extremely sensitive to heat: cooking can reduce the folate content of food by as much as 95%! A typical UK mixed diet may contain as much as 700 μg of folate per day.

Typical body stores of folate in a normal, healthy adult are about 10 mg and are located mainly in the liver. Thus, if dietary folate intake or intestinal absorption ceased, the body stores would become exhausted in less than 4 months.

Folate absorption and transport

Folates are absorbed maximally from the upper jejunum. Folate polyglutamates in food must be digested by the enzyme **γ-glutamyl conjugase** to form monoglutamates before they can be absorbed efficiently. Absorbed folates are converted within the jejunal mucosal cells into N-5-methyltetrahydrofolate monoglutamate and released into the portal bloodstream. Plasma folate circulates freely or loosely bound to a variety of plasma proteins. Once inside the developing blood cell, N-5-methyl-tetrahydrofolate is converted to tetrahydrofolate and reconjugated to the polyglutamate form. Conjugation facilitates the metabolic activities of folates and prevents leakage back into the plasma.

Role of vitamin B_{12} and folate in DNA and RNA synthesis

Synthesis of DNA and RNA requires a ready supply of the purines adenosine-5'-diphosphate (ADP) and guanosine-5'-diphosphate (GDP) and the pyrimidines cytidine-5'-diphosphate (CDP) and uridine-5'-diphosphate (UDP) as shown in Figure 2.4.

Folates are essential for optimal DNA and RNA synthesis: it is the cycling of folic acid between its various coenzyme forms which unifies the seemingly disparate biochemical reactions in which vitamin B_{12} and folic acid are involved within the body (Figure 2.5).

The folate taken up by dividing cells, N-5-methyltetrahydrofolate, cannot be conjugated with glutamate. First it must donate its methyl group to homocysteine, a reaction which requires methylcobalamin as coenzyme. In the absence of methylcobalamin, absorbed folate cannot be converted to a metabolically active form, a phenomenon known as the **methyltetrahydrofolate trap**. Thus, deficiency of vitamin B_{12} and/or folate results in failure of DNA synthesis and the development of megaloblastic anaemia.

Purines and pyrimidines such as adenine, guanine, cytosine, uracil, thymine and orotic acid are **bases**. The attachment of a sugar group (ribose or deoxyribose) to one of the nitrogen atoms of a base results in the formation of a **nucleoside**, e.g. adenine converts to adenosine and uracil converts to uridine. The addition of one or more phosphate groups to a nucleoside results in the formation of a **nucleotide**, e.g. adenosine diphosphate (ADP). The monophosphate form of a nucleotide can be designated as an '-*ylic*' acid, e.g. UMP is also known as uridylate. Nucleotides which contain a deoxyribose group are designated with a '*d*', e.g. dTMP.

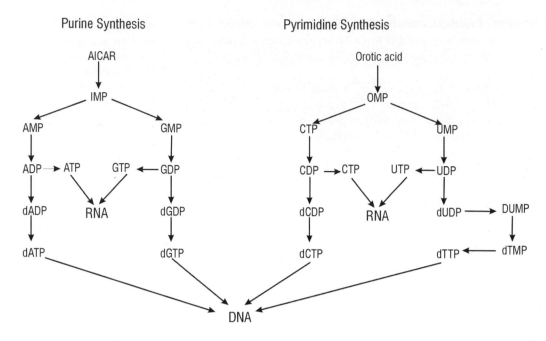

Figure 2.4   *DNA and RNA synthetic pathways. AICAR, amino imidazole carboxamide ribotide; IMP, inosine monophosphate; AMP, adenosine monophosphate (D, diphosphate; T, triphosphate); GMP, guanosinemonophosphate; UMP, uridinemonophosphate; CDP, cytidine-5′-monophosphate; dADP, deoxyadenosine-5′-monophosphate; dTMP, deoxythymidine-5′-monophosphate*

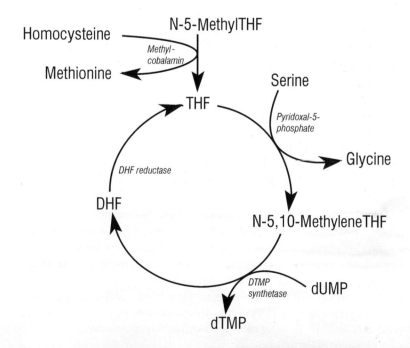

Figure 2.5   *The folate cycle*

Suggested further reading

Blackstock, J. (1998). *Biochemistry*. In BMS Explained (Series editor C.J. Pallister). Oxford: Butterworth-Heinemann.

Gilham, B., Papachristodoulou, D.K. and Thomas, J.H. (1997). Nutrition: iron and iron metabolism. In *Wills' Biochemical Basis of Medicine*, 3rd edn. (B. Gilham, D.K. Papachristodoulou and J. Hywel Thomas, eds) pp. 186–195. Oxford: Butterworth-Heinemann.

Gilham, B., Papachristodoulou, D.K. and Thomas, J.H. (1997). Nutrition: folate and vitamin B_{12}. In *Wills' Biochemical Basis of Medicine*, 3rd edn. (B. Gilham, D. K. Papachristodoulou and J. Hywel Thomas, eds) pp. 196–202. Oxford: Butterworth-Heinemann.

Goldenberg, H.A. (1997). Regulation of mammalian iron metabolism: Current state and need for further knowledge. *Critical Reviews in Clinical Laboratory Sciences* 34(6), 529–572.

Self-assessment questions

1. Where are iron, vitamin B_{12} and folate absorbed optimally?
2. Ascorbic acid is a reducing agent. Does it enhance or impair inorganic iron absorption? Why?
3. Where are the main body stores of iron, vitamin B_{12} and folate?
4. Why might severe iron deficiency be associated with breathlessness on exertion?
5. What effect do you think that surgical removal of the stomach would have on iron, vitamin B_{12} and folate absorption?
6. What effect does severe vitamin B_{12} deficiency have on folate utilization within the body?

Key Concepts and Facts

Function
- Iron (Fe^{2+}) is an essential part of the oxygen-carrying pigments of red cells (haemoglobin) and muscles (myoglobin).
- Vitamin B_{12} and folic acid are required for optimal DNA synthesis.

Absorption
- Inorganic iron is absorbed maximally as Fe^{2+} in the duodenum and upper jejunum.
- Only sufficient iron to meet current needs is absorbed.
- No substantial mechanism for iron excretion exists.
- Vitamin B_{12} is bound to intrinsic factor in the stomach and is then absorbed in the terminal ileum.
- Folic acid is absorbed maximally in the upper jejunum.

Transport
- Iron transport is mediated by the specific plasma protein transferrin.
- The physiological plasma transport of vitamin B_{12} is mediated by transcobalamin II.
- There is no known specific folate transport protein.

Storage
- Iron is stored in the liver and tissue macrophages as ferritin and, partially degraded, as haemosiderin.
- Estimation of serum ferritin provides a useful indicator of iron status.
- Vitamin B_{12} and folate are stored primarily in the liver.
- The body stores of vitamin B_{12} are sufficient to last for about 3 years if intake or absorption ceases.
- The body stores of folate are sufficient to last for about 3–4 months if intake or absorption ceases.

Chapter 3
Disorders of iron metabolism

Learning objectives

After studying this chapter you should confidently be able to:

Describe the process whereby a negative iron balance progresses to iron deficiency anaemia.

Describe the causes of iron deficiency anaemia.

Discuss the pathophysiology of iron deficiency.

Outline the differential diagnosis of iron deficiency, anaemia of chronic disorders and the sideroblastic anaemias.

Outline the classification of the sideroblastic anaemias.

Differentiate clearly the iron overload states.

Iron deficiency

Iron deficiency is by far the most common cause of anaemia worldwide. Most frequently, iron deficiency is observed as a secondary manifestation of another primary pathological state and may even be the presenting feature. Because iron is essential to the function of every cell of the body, iron deficiency causes a wide range of adverse physiological effects: anaemia is simply the best recognized of these.

The state of iron deficiency is defined as a reduction below normal limits of the total body iron content. Iron deficiency anaemia, the most severe manifestation of iron deficiency, develops slowly and insidiously through a series of successive stages, although progression from one stage to the next is not inevitable. When the rate of absorption of iron from the diet is insufficient to meet the daily requirement, iron is mobilized from the body stores to meet the shortfall. If this **negative iron balance** persists, the body iron stores become depleted, a state known as **latent iron deficiency**. In this state, the body is deficient in iron but erythropoiesis is still normal and no adverse physiological effects are present. Many people exist for prolonged periods in latent iron deficiency and never develop anaemia. If the negative iron balance persists once the body iron stores are exhausted, **iron deficient erythropoiesis** ensues

Spinach is commonly regarded as an extremely rich source of iron, calcium and vitamins A and C. In this regard, however, it is not particularly different from many leafy green vegetables. It is doubtful whether the iron content is assimilable because the leaves also contain a relatively high concentration of oxalic acid and iron oxalate is poorly absorbed.

and the characteristic changes that accompany severe iron deficiency gradually develop. The final stage in this sequence of events is the development of **iron deficiency anaemia**. Because iron deficiency anaemia develops gradually, the body is able to adapt to the falling haemoglobin level and clinical symptoms often do not appear until the anaemia is moderately severe.

Causes of iron deficiency

Iron deficiency arises where absorption of iron does not meet daily requirements. This can occur where the supply of iron is decreased or where the daily requirement for iron is increased.

Decreased supply of iron

A sustained decrease in the supply of iron to the body can be caused by two main conditions:

- Inadequate diet.
- Malabsorption of iron from the diet.

Inadequate diet

As described in Chapter 2, the average adult mixed diet in the UK provides about 18 mg of iron per day: more than enough to meet normal demands. For this reason, inadequacy of the diet is seldom the sole cause of iron deficiency in this age group, although it commonly is a contributing factor to the more rapid onset of iron deficiency due to another primary cause. Breast milk and its artificial substitutes are relatively deficient in iron. Newborn babies have significant body stores of iron which were accumulated *in utero*. Normally, these are sufficient to meet the relatively low demand for iron in the first weeks of life. However, introduction of a mixed diet that has a greater iron content is required to meet the increased demands imposed by growth. Prolonged breast or bottle feeding may lead to iron deficiency in toddlers. Inadequacy of the diet often is a significant contributory factor in the development of iron deficiency in the Third World, particularly when the iron demand is raised, for example in pregnancy.

The association between spinach and strength and vigour was brought to life for most people when Max Fleischer invented the cartoon character Popeye. The pugnacious sailor has been a popular character with children of all ages since the 1930s.

In 1971, Dr R. Hunter published in *The Lancet* his observations that laboratory animals fed on a high folate diet became tense and irritable. Perhaps it was the high folate content of spinach that caused Popeye to become so quarrelsome and to pick fights with Bluto!

Malabsorption of dietary iron

Iron deficiency secondary to malabsorption is a relatively common complication of diseases of the upper alimentary tract such as **coeliac disease**. Malabsorption of dietary folate commonly exacerbates the anaemia in this disorder. Partial gastrectomy predisposes strongly to the development of iron deficiency because the absence of stomach acid impairs absorption of dietary iron. The malabsorption is aggravated by the rapid gastrojejunal food transit times that result from removal of part of the stomach and by chronic antacid ingestion.

Increased requirement for iron

There are three main causes of an increase in daily iron requirement:

- Loss of blood.
- Growth and pregnancy.
- Loss of iron.

Blood loss

Chronic blood loss from the gastrointestinal and genitourinary tracts is the most common cause of iron deficiency. The effect of menstrual blood loss on iron requirements in adult females is described in Chapter 2. The most common cause of bleeding in tropical areas is infestation of the gut with the hookworms *Ancylostoma duodenale* or *Necator americanus*. It is estimated that about 500 million people carry hookworms in their guts. Each worm consumes a tiny quantity of blood from its host but infestations can be very heavy (a female *Ancylostoma* produces 30 000 eggs each day!).

Outside of the tropics, the most common causes of pathological blood loss are carcinoma, duodenal ulcer, hiatus hernia, haemorrhoids and menorrhagia. Frank blood loss commonly is absent in such cases: a loss of only 4–5 ml of blood per day, if sustained, will eventually lead to iron deficiency. Even smaller losses can result in iron deficiency if the diet is poor or if malabsorption is present.

Growth and pregnancy

The increased requirement for iron during periods of accelerated growth makes iron deficiency very common in adolescence and in pregnancy. For example, in a normal, uncomplicated pregnancy, maternal total red cell volume increases by between 20 and 40%. This imposes an extra requirement for iron of up to 500 mg. The developing foetus, which always has first call on available iron, requires about 300 mg of iron. These dual excess demands for iron are greatest during the second and third trimesters of pregnancy, when the daily demand for iron can rise to 6–7 mg! The delicate iron balance that this inevitably causes is compounded by maternal blood loss at delivery. Small amounts of iron are also lost in breast milk. The excess requirement for iron in pregnancy is offset partially by the temporary cessation of menstruation (amenorrhoea) which saves about 200 mg of iron.

In the seventeenth century, iron deficiency was known as 'the green sickness' or chlorosis and was believed to be associated with being in love. One common treatment for the condition was to drink wine (sherris) in which iron filings had been steeped. The effects of drinking this potion are described in Shakespeare's Henry IV Part 2:

Falstaff: '... for thin drink doth so over-cool their blood, and making many fish meals, that they fall into a kind of male green-sickness. ... A good sherris-sack hath a two-fold operation in it; it ascends me into the brain, dries me there all the foolish, and dull, and crudy vapours which environ it, makes it apprehensive, quick, forgetive, full of nimble, fiery, and delectable shapes, which delivered o'er to the voice, the tongue, which is the birth, become excellent wit. The second property of your excellent sherris is the warming of the blood, which, before cold and settled, left the liver white and pale, which is the badge of pusillanimity and cowardice. But the sherris warms it, and makes it course from the inwards to the parts extreme. It illumineth the face, which as a beacon gives warning to all the rest of this little kingdom, man, to arm, and then the vital commoners, and inland petty spirits, muster me all to their captain, the heart; who, great and puffed up with this retinue, doth any deed of courage. And this valour comes of sherris.'

Acute conditions (e.g. appendicitis) are of rapid onset and, usually, brief duration whereas chronic conditions (e.g. osteoarthritis) typically are of slower onset and longer duration.

Using the measured red cell parameters of haemoglobin (Hb), mean red cell volume (MCV) and red cell count (RBC), three red cell indices can be calculated:

Packed cell volume (haematocrit, Hct)

$PCV(l/l) = MCV(fl) \times RBC \, (\times 10^{12})$

Mean cell haemoglobin

$MCH(pg) = Hb \, (g \, dl^{-1})/RBC \, (\times 10^{12})$

Mean cell haemoglobin concentration

$MCHC \, (g \, dl^{-1}) = Hb \, (g \, dl^{-1})/PCV \, (l/l)$

Some analysers measure the PCV and calculate the MCV:

$MCV \, (fl) = PCV \, (l/l)/RBC \, (\times 10^{12})$

The suffix '-enia' implies a low number of the given cell type, e.g. thrombocytopenia means a low platelet count. The suffix '-osis' means an increased number of the given cell type, e.g. reticulocytosis means an increase in the reticulocyte count. The suffix '-plasia' means formation, e.g. erythroid hypoplasia means a reduction in the rate of erythropoiesis, erythroid hyperplasia implies an increased rate of red cell production and aplasia means a complete arrest of production.

Loss of iron

Chronic intravascular haemolysis can result in the loss of considerable amounts of iron as haemosiderin in the urine. In severe cases, this can contribute to the development of iron deficiency.

Pathophysiology

A wide range of clinical manifestations accompanies severe iron deficiency anaemia. These can be considered under three broad headings:

- Effects caused by the primary precipitating condition. These are beyond the scope of this book and will not be described.
- Effects which are manifest in the blood and blood-forming tissue.
- Effects which are manifest in other tissues.

Effects on the blood and blood-forming tissue

Depletion of the iron stores means that there is insufficient iron available for incorporation into the haemoglobin of developing erythroblasts and iron deficient erythropoiesis ensues. This is manifest as a reduced mean cell haemoglobin concentration (MCHC) and an increased concentration of free protoporphyrin within the cell. The major determinant of the volume of a mature red cell is the number of mitotic divisions it undergoes before the nucleus is poisoned by the increasing concentration of haemoglobin. In iron deficiency, haemoglobin synthesis is retarded and an extra mitotic division occurs before the erythroblast nucleus dies. This results in a mature red cell that is smaller than normal. Thus, the anaemia which accompanies iron deficiency typically is hypochromic and microcytic.

The condition most likely to be confused with iron deficiency anaemia on morphological grounds is β thalassaemia. The diagnosis of β thalassaemia is described in Chapter 6. The main laboratory features of iron deficiency anaemia are shown in Table 3.1.

One of the biochemical hallmarks of iron deficiency is the combination of a raised total iron binding capacity (TIBC) and a reduced percentage of transferrin saturation. The relationship between total iron binding capacity and per cent transferrin saturation in a range of conditions is shown in Figure 3.1.

General effects of iron deficiency anaemia

There are three main types of generalized effect of iron deficiency:

- Changes which are directly attributable to anaemia and not specific to iron deficiency.

Table 3.1 *Laboratory and physiological features of iron deficiency*

Blood cell features:
  Microcytosis and hypochromia
  Reticulocytopenia
  Poikilocytosis (pencil forms)
  Defective neutrophil function
  Reduced % T lymphocytes in children
Bone marrow features:
  Erythroid hypoplasia
  Normoblasts have ragged cytoplasm
  Decreased stainable iron deposits
Biochemical features:
  Raised TIBC
  Decreased % transferrin saturation
  Raised catecholamine levels
  Reduced serum ferritin levels
Physiological features:
  Impaired ability to maintain body temperature
  Depressed muscle function
  Abnormal thyroid hormone metabolism

- Changes in epithelial tissue.
- Changes in behaviour.

A reduction in circulating haemoglobin causes a reduction in oxygen-carrying capacity and leads to the most widely recognized changes seen in anaemia, i.e. pallor of skin and mucous membranes and reduced exercise tolerance. The body responds

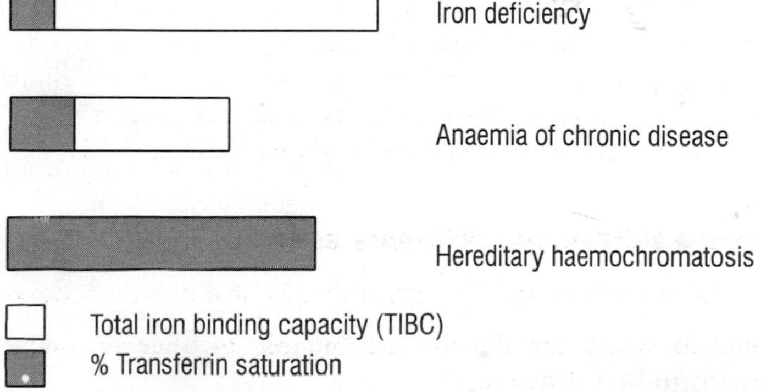

Normal

Normal pregnancy

Iron deficiency

Anaemia of chronic disease

Hereditary haemochromatosis

☐ Total iron binding capacity (TIBC)
▨ % Transferrin saturation

Figure 3.1 *The relationship between TIBC and % transferrin saturation in various conditions*

to anaemia by increasing cardiac output and increasing synthesis of red cell 2,3-DPG, thereby maintaining oxygen delivery to the tissues under basal conditions. However, there is an exaggerated response to exercise, which causes shortness of breath on exertion and palpitations, the most common presenting features of iron deficiency anaemia. Severe iron deficiency causes deficiency of iron-containing enzymes such as cytochromes in a wide range of tissues. The effect of this is manifest most severely in epithelial cells, which ordinarily are turning over relatively rapidly. Characteristic changes include:

- Koilonychia – flattening or 'spooning' of the finger nails.
- Angular stomatitis – atrophic lesions at the corners of the mouth.
- Glossitis – smooth, inflamed tongue.
- Atrophic gastritis – inflammation of the lining of the stomach.
- Achlorhydria – lack of hydrochloric acid secretion in the stomach.
- Dysphagia – difficulty in swallowing caused by the development of oesophageal webs. This rare condition is known as the **Plummer–Vinson syndrome** and may progress to oesophageal carcinoma.

Iron deficiency in early childhood is associated with impairment of intellectual ability and hyperactivity. Most studies have shown that these effects are at least partially reversed by suitable iron therapy.

Another characteristic but poorly understood behavioural abnormality in iron deficient subjects is manifest as a strong desire to eat unusual substances such as soil (geophagia), ice (pagophagia) or even carpet fluff. In some cases, this obsessive behaviour, known as **pica**, may exacerbate the iron deficiency. For example, ingestion of clay soil can impair intestinal absorption of dietary iron.

Iron deficiency is not a disease but, rather, it is a symptom of disease. Effective treatment of iron deficiency requires that the primary precipitating cause be removed. Excluding pregnancy and menorrhagia, the most common underlying cause of iron deficiency is occult blood loss from the gastrointestinal tract.

Replacement of body iron stores is best achieved by supplementation of the diet using ferrous sulphate or, less commonly, by intramuscular injection of iron-dextran. Appropriate oral supplementation should induce a reticulocyte response within 3 or 4 days and a sustained rise in circulating haemoglobin concentration. Failure of response to an adequate dose of oral iron suggests that the underlying cause has not been removed, that patient compliance is poor or that iron deficiency is not the cause of the anaemia. It should be remembered that iron deficiency is only one of many causes of microcytic, hypochromic anaemia.

It has been suggested that pica may be at least part of the explanation for the unusual dietary cravings experienced by some pregnant women. A number of studies have shown that the more exaggerated cases of this phenomenon correlate with depletion of the iron stores.

Anaemia of chronic disorders

Chronic inflammatory or malignant disorders frequently are accompanied by a normocytic, normochromic anaemia that is refractory to all treatment except that which causes regression of the primary condition. This form of anaemia is known as the anaemia of chronic disorders (ACD). Disordered iron metabolism is a common finding in ACD but its relative contribution to the development of the anaemia remains a matter of debate. Chronic inflammation causes activation of tissue macrophages with a consequent upregulation of surface apotransferrin receptors. Binding of significant quantities of apotransferrin to macrophages reduces the total iron binding capacity of the plasma as shown in Figure 3.1. Inflammation also stimulates neutrophils to synthesize and release large quantities of apolactoferrin, which acts as an iron-binding protein. The apolactoferrin is bound to specific surface receptors on activated tissue macrophages and acts like a magnet for circulating iron. Any iron that is bound to the apolactoferrin:receptor complex is internalized by the macrophage and stored as ferritin. Thus, tissue iron stores are increased. It is this apparent anomaly of reduced TIBC and % transferrin saturation accompanied by increased body iron stores which is the hallmark of ACD.

There is clear evidence of suppression of erythropoietic activity in ACD. There have been sporadic reports of the presence of specific inhibitors of erythropoiesis in individuals but in most cases the suppression is likely to be caused by the release of growth inhibitors such as interleukin 1, γ interferon and tumour necrosis factor in response to the primary condition. A slight reduction in red cell lifespan has also been reported in a minority of cases of ACD.

Sideroblastic anaemias

The sideroblastic anaemias are a heterogeneous group of disorders that are characterized by disordered incorporation of iron into haem within developing erythroblasts. The resulting toxic accumulation of iron within the mitochondria of late erythroblasts leads to some degree of ineffective erythropoiesis. Demonstration of iron-laden mitochondria encircling the nuclei of late erythroblasts, the so-called 'ringed sideroblast', is the hallmark of sideroblastic anaemia. However, ringed sideroblasts are not specific indicators of sideroblastic anaemia: they are frequently found in leukaemia, megaloblastic anaemia and alcoholism among other conditions. The sideroblastic anaemias are classified according to their aetiology as hereditary, secondary or idiopathic (unknown aetiology).

Hereditary sideroblastic anaemia

Most cases of hereditary sideroblastic anaemia have shown an X-linked recessive pattern of inheritance. Affected males have

Ineffective erythropoiesis means the production of red cells that die within the bone marrow, i.e. the production is ineffective because it does not increase the circulating red cell count.

hypochromic, dimorphic anaemia with mild ineffective erythropoiesis and erythroid hyperplasia. Many cases of hereditary sideroblastic anaemia have functional deficiencies of enzymes of the haem synthetic pathway, most commonly δ-aminolaevulinic acid (δALA) synthetase or ferrochelatase. The role of these enzymes in haem synthesis is described in Chapter 5. In some cases, however, the molecular defect remains to be determined. The anaemia responds to the administration of vitamin B_6 (pyridoxine) in about 50% of cases of hereditary sideroblastic anaemia. Such responses are, at best, partial and are usually temporary.

Secondary sideroblastic anaemia

Drug-induced sideroblastic anaemia

The most common cause of secondary sideroblastic anaemia is the administration of drugs such as isoniazid, chloramphenicol or alcohol. Isoniazid and alcohol inhibit biochemical reactions which involve pyridoxal 5'-phosphate, including synthesis of δALA, the first and rate-limiting step in the haem biosynthetic pathway. Chloramphenicol inhibits the synthesis of δALA synthetase and ferrochelatase. The blood picture in drug-induced or alcohol-induced sideroblastic anaemia closely resembles that of the hereditary form. All of the sideroblastic changes are reversible by withdrawal of the offending substance.

Lead poisoning

Chronic lead poisoning was a relatively common condition when most drinking water was supplied via lead pipes and lead pigments were commonly used in paints. Most cases nowadays are associated with occupational exposure. Lead is absorbed by ingestion or inhalation. Most absorbed lead accumulates in bone and bone marrow. In the bone marrow, lead is associated particularly with mitochondrial membranes of developing erythroblasts. The presence of lead in the mitochondria severely disrupts haem synthesis and leads directly to sideroblastic change. Lead also causes damage to red cell membranes and inhibits glycolytic activity. These two activities result in mild haemolysis which contributes significantly to the anaemia of chronic lead poisoning.

Typically, the blood picture in chronic lead poisoning is microcytic and hypochromic with prominent basophilic stippling and a reticulocytosis. The basophilic stippling is the result of the accumulation of pyrimidine nucleotides in the cell cytoplasm and is only present in the youngest red cells. The accumulation of pyrimidine nucleotides is caused by the inhibition of the enzyme pyrimidine 5'-nucleotidase by lead.

The ancient Romans made heavy use of lead. They used it in their water pipes (the name plumber is derived from the Latin for lead), their pottery drinking vessels were lead-glazed and their cooking utensils commonly were lined with lead. Archaeological evidence shows high concentrations of lead in bones found at Roman sites such as York and Cirencester. Some historians believe that the increasing sophistication of the Romans' use of lead contributed to the fall of the Roman Empire because of a presumed high incidence of lead-induced dementia.

Idiopathic sideroblastic anaemia

Idiopathic sideroblastic anaemia is primarily a disease of the elderly and is the most common of the sideroblastic anaemias. It is identical to the myelodysplastic syndrome refractory anaemia with ring sideroblasts (RARS). Characteristic dyserythropoietic changes include macrocytosis, poikilocytosis, basophilic stippling and the appearance of ringed sideroblasts affecting all stages of erythroblast development. In the early stages of the disease platelets and leukocytes appear normal. Cytogenetic abnormalities are demonstrable in about 50% of cases of idiopathic sideroblastic anaemia. About 10% of cases terminate as acute leukaemia, predominantly the M4 type.

Iron overload

There are three commonly seen forms of chronic iron overload:

- Hereditary haemochromatosis.
- Transfusion-associated haemosiderosis.
- Dietary causes.

Hereditary haemochromatosis

Hereditary haemochromatosis results from an irregularity of intestinal iron absorption in which feedback control over the rate of absorption of dietary iron is lost. The inexorable accumulation of iron within the body that results damages vital organs and, if untreated, is fatal. The condition is inherited in an autosomal recessive fashion: only homozygotes express significant disease. The gene for hereditary haemochromatosis is linked closely with the HLA portion of the MHC complex on chromosome 6 and is carried by about 1 in 16 individuals.

Absorption of dietary iron typically exceeds normal by about 2 mg per day in haemochromatosis homozygotes and is unrelated to iron requirements. Because of this, an affected adult male may have accumulated a total body iron content of over 20 g. However, in contrast to transfusion-associated haemosiderosis, bone marrow macrophages are not grossly overloaded with storage iron. Most of the excess iron is stored in the parenchymal cells of the liver and other organs.

Pathophysiology

One of the early signs of hereditary haemochromatosis is greatly increased saturation of circulating transferrin as shown in Figure 3.1. Thus, when iron is absorbed inappropriately and released into the portal circulation, some may be unable to bind to the iron-transport protein transferrin because it is already fully saturated.

A recent Swedish study demonstrated the potential dangers of iron fortification of food in developed countries. The iron status of 350 subjects was assessed. About 1 in 20 men carried iron stores above reference limits and almost half of these had iron stores approaching those of early haemochromatosis! Iron fortification remains a useful public health measure in underdeveloped countries where the average diet is deficient in iron.

Iron that cannot bind to transferrin circulates as hydrated complexes of ferrous and ferric ions until binding sites become available. About 30% of the circulating plasma iron exists as hydrated ionic complexes in haemochromatosis heterozygotes. These hydrated ionic complexes of iron can act as a catalyst for the formation of toxic oxygen radicals in the presence of NADPH. Oxygen radicals are short-lived and extremely reactive molecular species that are capable of causing extensive localized tissue damage. The principal villain in this regard is hydroxyl radical $(OH\cdot)$.

Accumulated organ damage results in the major clinical features of hereditary haemochromatosis: hepatic cirrhosis, skin pigmentation, diabetes and progressive congestive cardiomyopathy, which is the leading cause of death. In about 30% of cases, hepatic cirrhosis progresses to hepatoma. The laboratory features of hereditary haemochromatosis include a markedly raised serum ferritin concentration ($>500\,\mathrm{mg\,l^{-1}}$), accompanied by a raised serum iron and saturation of transferrin. If significant hepatic damage has occurred, macrocytosis and target cells may be present. Otherwise the blood picture is unremarkable.

Because the iron accumulates very slowly in hereditary haemochromatosis, tissue damage is seldom debilitating before the age of 30 years. If the diagnosis is made early, severe tissue damage can be avoided by a programme of weekly venesection involving the removal of at least 500 ml of blood on each occasion. The aim of this programme of venesection is to deplete the excess body iron stores over a 12–18 month period. Once depleted, a less energetic programme involving bimonthly venesection can prevent reaccumulation. Recent experience suggests that, provided that treatment is started early and controlled carefully, life expectancy is returned to normal.

Transfusion-associated haemosiderosis

As described in Chapter 6, β thalassaemia homozygotes are completely dependent on a programme of regular blood transfusion. Each transfusion of 400 ml of blood carries with it approximately 200 mg of iron which cannot be excreted. Steady accumulation of body iron results with similar consequences to those described above for hereditary haemochromatosis. The accumulation of iron in body stores is slowed appreciably by the administration of chelating agents such as desferrioxamine but, at present, these only delay the inevitable. The development of effective oral chelating agents would be a major advance in the treatment of the thalassaemia syndromes.

Dietary causes

Iron overload due to dietary causes was reported to be a serious problem in the Bantu people of Southern Africa. The cause of this was reputed to be the local habit of cooking exclusively in iron pots coupled with enthusiastic imbibing of strong, home-brewed beer, which had been brewed and illicitly stored in iron drums. For a number of reasons, **Bantu siderosis**, as this condition was called, appears to be on the wane.

Acute iron poisoning due to ingestion of a large number of iron tablets intended for therapeutic use is one of the most common causes of fatal poisoning in young children. If discovered early, gastric lavage and desferrioxamine therapy may prevent serious toxicity. Chronic use of iron supplements in the absence of iron deficiency can lead to iron overload because the large quantities of iron present are absorbed by passive diffusion across the gut wall, regardless of the state of the body iron stores.

Suggested further reading

Gilham, B., Papachristodoulou, D.K. and Thomas, J.H. (1997). Nutrition: iron and iron metabolism. In *Wills' Biochemical Basis of Medicine* 3rd edn. (B. Gilham, D.K. Papachristodoulou and J. Hywel Thomas, eds) pp. 186–195. Oxford: Butterworth-Heinemann.

Jazwinska, E.C. (1998). Hemochromatosis: a genetic defect in iron metabolism. *Bioessays* **20**(7), 562–568.

Worwood, M. (1997). The laboratory assessment of iron status – An update. *Clinica Chimica Acta* **259**, 3–23.

Worwood, M. (1998). Haemochromatosis. *Clinical and Laboratory Haematology* **20**(2), 65–75.

Self-assessment questions

1. Differentiate between the terms negative iron balance, latent iron deficiency, iron deficient erythropoiesis and iron deficiency anaemia.
2. List the three main causes of an increased iron requirement.
3. What are the main distinguishing features of an iron deficient red cell?
4. Why are iron deficient red cells microcytic?
5. Which of the sideroblastic anaemias is now considered to be a myelodysplastic state?
6. Differentiate between the pathogenesis of haemochromatosis and haemosiderosis.

Key Concepts and Facts

- Iron deficiency anaemia (IDA) is the most common anaemia worldwide.

- IDA is the result of a persistent negative iron balance secondary to a decreased supply of iron or an increased iron requirement.

- A decreased supply of iron results from inadequate diet or malabsorption.

- Increased demand for iron is present following chronic bleeding and in pregnancy.

- IDA is a microcytic, hypochromic anaemia and is associated with a range of physiological sequelae.

- Anaemia (ACD) is a common event in chronic inflammatory or malignant conditions.

- ACD is refractory to iron therapy.

- Hereditary sideroblastic anaemia results from deficiency of δALA synthetase or ferrochelatase and may respond to vitamin B_6 therapy.

- Secondary sideroblastic anaemia follows ingestion of certain drugs or lead poisoning.

- Idiopathic sideroblastic anaemia is synonymous with refractory anaemia with sideroblasts.

- Haemochromatosis and haemosiderosis are iron overload states.

- Haemochromatosis is a hereditary disorder of the feedback control of iron absorption.

- Haemosiderosis results from chronic transfusion regimes.

Chapter 4
Megaloblastic anaemias

Learning objectives

After studying this chapter you should confidently be able to:

Describe the mechanisms that predispose to deficiency of vitamin B_{12} and folate.

List some causes of megaloblastic change other then haematinic deficiency.

Describe the biochemical basis of the megaloblastic anaemias.

Outline the pathophysiology of the megaloblastic anaemias, including non-haematological manifestations.

The term megaloblastic anaemia relates to a group of disorders of haemopoicsis characterized by retardation of DNA synthesis but a normal rate of RNA synthesis. These disorders show distinctive morphological and biochemical features which reflect the resulting asynchrony between nuclear and cytoplasmic maturation in developing cells. All dividing cells of the body are affected: anaemia is but one of a wide range of manifestations of the megaloblastic anaemias. Most megaloblastic anaemias are caused by a deficiency of vitamin B_{12} or folic acid.

Vitamin B_{12} deficiency

Deficiency of vitamin B_{12}, in common with deficiency of all nutrients, can result from inadequate dietary intake, intestinal malabsorption, increased requirements which cannot be met from the diet or failure of utilization of absorbed vitamin.

Inadequate dietary intake

Deficiency of vitamin B_{12} attributable solely to inadequate dietary intake is uncommon for three main reasons:

- Vitamin B_{12} is present in a wide range of readily available foodstuffs.

The value of many haematological parameters fluctuates in an individual during the course of the day. This phenomenon is entirely normal and is known as **diurnal variation**.

The haemoglobin concentration and red cell count tend to be higher in the morning than in the evening. The platelet count and neutrophil count peak in the middle of the afternoon. The eosinophil count is at its lowest in the late morning and peaks just after midnight. Interestingly, these trends are reversed in night-shift workers.

In 1855, Thomas Addison first described a severe anaemia of unknown cause but uniformly fatal outcome and named it pernicious anaemia. The first real progress in the treatment of PA did not come for another 70 years when George Minot showed that the inclusion of 300 g of lightly cooked liver in the daily diet elicited a reticulocyte response and partial recovery of the haemoglobin concentration.

We now know that eating large amounts of liver provides massive doses of vitamin B_{12} which are absorbed from the gut by passive diffusion. Modern therapy consists of regular injections of hydroxocobalamin.

- Vitamin B_{12} is relatively heat-stable – cooking does not destroy it.
- Body stores of vitamin B_{12} are sufficient to meet the needs of the body for at least 3 years.

Dietary deficiency of vitamin B_{12} is restricted to vegans who eschew all animal and dairy products. Inadequate diet, however, frequently contributes to the development of vitamin B_{12} deficiency that is attributable mainly to other causes.

Malabsorption of vitamin B_{12}

Malabsorption of vitamin B_{12} is the most common cause of deficiency. A wide range of abnormalities exist which cause malabsorption of this vitamin:

- Lack of intrinsic factor.
- Gastrointestinal disease.
- Drug-induced malabsorption.

Lack of intrinsic factor

The most common cause of vitamin B_{12} deficiency in Northern Europeans is **pernicious anaemia (PA)** which is characterized by achlorhydria and a failure of gastric parietal cells to synthesize intrinsic factor. The disease is uncommon below the age of 45 years, is more common in women than in men and shows an association with blood group A.

Cytotoxic IgG antibodies directed against gastric parietal cells or intrinsic factor are present in the serum of about 90% of people with PA. In about 75% of these cases the antibody also is present in gastric juice. These anti-IF antibodies act in one of two ways:

- Preventing binding of vitamin B_{12} to IF (type I antibody).
- Inhibiting absorption of the IF:B_{12} complex (type II antibody). Type II antibodies are only found in association with type I antibodies.

About 30% of close relatives of people with PA also have anti-parietal cell antibodies in their serum but do not necessarily develop the disease. PA is associated with an increased incidence of other autoimmune diseases. A rare juvenile form of PA exists caused by congenital deficiency of IF or synthesis of a dysfunctional form of IF.

Gastrointestinal disease

Of this group of causes of vitamin B_{12} deficiency, the most obvious follows surgical removal of the source of intrinsic factor or the site of absorption of the vitamin.

- **Total gastrectomy** is associated with depletion of the vitamin B_{12} body stores. If vitamin B_{12} supplements are not given to these patients, megaloblastic anaemia develops within 5 years. The anaemia is frequently complicated by iron deficiency that also commonly follows gastrectomy.

- **Partial gastrectomy** involves removal of part of the stomach and refashioning the junction with the gut, creating an afferent blind loop of gut which becomes heavily colonized by bacteria. The vitamin B_{12} that these bacteria require for growth and metabolism is extracted from the gut, leading to reduced availability of the vitamin in the terminal ileum. This malabsorptive state is known as the **stagnant** or **blind loop syndrome**. Bacterial overgrowth also occurs in ileal diverticulae, with similar results.

Because of advances in the pharmacological treatment of gastric, peptic and duodenal ulcers, total and partial gastrectomy is performed much less often than in the past.

Ileal resection or **ileostomy** involving removal or bypass of the terminal ileum predisposes strongly to the development of vitamin B_{12} deficiency.

Generalized malabsorption of nutrients from the diet is a feature of intestinal disorders such as **Crohn's disease** (regional ileitis). Crohn's disease typically affects young adults in developed countries and leads to severe inflammation of the terminal ileum and ascending colon. Haematological complications of Crohn's disease include malabsorption of iron, folic acid and vitamin B_{12} leading to iron deficiency and megaloblastic anaemia. Chronic bleeding of the inflamed ileal mucosae frequently exacerbates the anaemia.

Infestation of the gut with the fish tapeworm *Diphyllobothrium latum* is acquired by eating infected raw fish. If the parasite lodges in the upper gastrointestinal tract, it is capable of extracting substantial quantities of vitamin B_{12} both complexed with intrinsic factor and as free vitamin from ingested food, thereby reducing the amount available for absorption.

Drug-induced malabsorption

A number of drugs have been reported to impair absorption of vitamin B_{12}, including the anticonvulsant phenytoin, the aminoglycoside antimicrobial agent neomycin, colchicine which is used in high doses in the treatment of gout and, most commonly, alcohol. Withdrawal of the drug usually reverses the malabsorption.

Increased requirements

The requirement for vitamin B_{12} is increased during pregnancy

---

The reference ranges for vitamin B_{12} and folate are as follows:
Serum vitamin B_{12}
    170–1000 pg/ml
Serum folate
    3–25 ng/ml
Red cell folate
    145–600 ng/ml packed RBC

because of the expansion of the blood volume and the foetal requirement. The increase is not sufficient to cause deficiency of vitamin B_{12} in a woman with normal stores prior to conception. It can, however, precipitate deficiency in a woman with previously borderline body stores of the vitamin. If a woman is severely vitamin B_{12} deficient throughout pregnancy, her baby is likely to have deficiency of the vitamin at birth, a situation seen most commonly in the Third World.

Failure of utilization

Failure of vitamin B_{12} transport

Congenital deficiency of transcobalamin II is characterized by the development of severe megaloblastic anaemia in the first weeks of life, despite the presence of a normal serum concentration of vitamin B_{12} and normal body stores of the vitamin. Early diagnosis is vital or severe neurological damage may result. Treatment requires very large doses of vitamin B_{12} by intramuscular injection.

Failure of vitamin B_{12} metabolism

A small number of examples of congenital failure to convert absorbed vitamin B_{12} to its active coenzyme forms have been described. Affected individuals fail to thrive and are mentally retarded. Only a minority of such cases develop megaloblastic anaemia, however.

Prolonged exposure to the anaesthetic nitrous oxide can induce megaloblastic change by inactivating vitamin B_{12} coenzymes due to oxidation of the central cobalt ion to the Co(II) state. Chronic exposure has been suggested as the cause of a mild neuropathy that has been described in dental surgeons.

Folic acid deficiency

Deficiency of folic acid can result from an inadequate diet, intestinal malabsorption, increased requirements or failure of utilization of absorbed vitamin.

Inadequate dietary intake

Nutritional deficiency of folic acid is relatively common for three main reasons:

- The ideal UK diet contains about 700 µg of folate of which about half is absorbed. The daily requirement for folate is about 100 µg.
- Folate is very heat-labile: cooking can destroy up to 90% of the folate present in food.
- Body stores of folate are only sufficient to last about 3 months.

Folate deficiency can develop rapidly where dietary intake is suboptimal, either because folate-rich foods are lacking from the diet or because of losses during cooking. An inadequate diet is often a contributory factor in the development of folate deficiency due to malabsorption or where the requirement for folate is increased.

Intestinal malabsorption

Intestinal malabsorption is a common cause of folate deficiency. The most common cause of malabsorption of folate in the UK is **coeliac disease**, which has an incidence of about 1 in 2000. This disease is characterized by intolerance of gluten in the diet, atrophy of intestinal villi and malabsorption of iron and folate from the duodenum and jejunum. The cause of coeliac disease is unknown but withdrawal of gluten from the diet reinstates jejunal absorption of iron and folate.

Tropical sprue is a similar condition to coeliac disease that is most common in the West Indies, the Indian subcontinent and in South-East Asia. The cause of the disease is unknown but malabsorption of folate commonly is present. **Crohn's disease** commonly causes folate deficiency, especially where the jejunum and upper ileum are involved. Surgical causes of folate malabsorption include ileal resection where the site of maximal absorption of folate is removed.

Increased requirement

Deficiency of folic acid is especially common in pregnancy because dietary intake often fails to meet the increased demand for folate imposed by the growth of maternal blood volume and the developing foetus. The daily requirement for folate can rise to 500 µg in the third trimester of pregnancy. In the absence of folate supplementation, about 60% of pregnant women have subnormal plasma concentrations of folate. Folate deficiency commonly is accompanied by iron deficiency in pregnancy. Because of the recently demonstrated association between folate deficiency in pregnancy and foetal neural tube defects, folic acid supplementation starting several months before conception is widely recommended. Prophylactic iron therapy may be given at the same time.

As described in Chapter 8, the compensatory increase in the rate of haemopoiesis in chronic haemolytic conditions imposes a sustained excess demand for folate. It is not uncommon for the rate of haemopoiesis to be increased by a factor of 10 in severe haemolytic conditions. When the increased demand for folate that this massively increased haemopoietic activity imposes exceeds the amount available from dietary sources, the development of folate deficiency is inevitable.

The first cytotoxic drug to be effective in the treatment of leukaemia was a folate antagonist called *aminopterin*. In 1948, Sidney Farber reported that 10 of 16 children with acute leukaemia responded to treatment with this drug. These remissions were only temporary but an important step towards successful treatment of a hitherto intractable disease had been taken. Antimetabolites like methotrexate are still in common use in the treatment of leukaemia today.

Drug-induced folate deficiency

A number of drugs have been reported to cause folate deficiency by interfering with folate absorption or metabolism. With some drugs, the antifolate effect is desired, while in others it is an unwanted side-effect. For example, long-term therapy with the anticonvulsant drug phenytoin is associated with the development of folate deficiency due to impaired intestinal absorption of folate. Alcohol is also thought to inhibit folate absorption and metabolism, although the most common cause of folate deficiency in alcoholics is inadequate dietary intake.

The cytotoxic drug **methotrexate** is an example of a drug that is used specifically for its antifolate properties. It is a close structural analogue of folic acid and acts as a powerful competitive inhibitor of the enzyme dihydrofolate reductase. Ingestion of methotrexate rapidly causes intracellular deficiency of folate coenzymes and depletion of thymidine and purine nucleotides. Methotrexate is used in the treatment of leukaemia.

Failure of utilization

Failure of folate metabolism

A number of rare enzyme deficiencies have been reported which cause impairment of folate metabolism. Most of these have been associated with megaloblastic anaemia and with some degree of mental retardation.

Causes of megaloblastic anaemia other than haematinic deficiency

There are three main circumstances associated with megaloblastic change that is not attributable to deficiency of vitamin B_{12} or folic acid:

- Treatment with cytotoxic drugs.
- Certain inborn errors of metabolism.
- In association with other haematological disorders.

Cytotoxic chemotherapy

Many of the cytotoxic drugs that are used in the treatment of malignant disease act by interfering with cellular metabolism. Three groups of cytotoxic drugs are associated with the induction of megaloblastic change of variable severity:

- Inhibitors of pyrimidine synthesis such as 5-fluorouracil and 6-azauridine.

- Inhibitors of purine synthesis such as 6-mercaptopurine and 6-thioguanine.
- Inhibitors of cellular enzymes such as hydroxyurea.

Megaloblastic change secondary to inborn errors of metabolism

A small number of inborn enzyme disorders show megaloblastic change of varying severity along with other, more serious, clinical problems. Two examples, **Lesch–Nyhan syndrome** and **hereditary orotic aciduria**, are described in the side-box on this page.

Megaloblastic change secondary to haematological disorders

Some degree of megaloblastic change is common in a wide range of malignant haematological disorders, e.g. in M6 acute leukaemia, the abnormal erythroblasts frequently show megaloblastic features in addition to the severe dysplasia which characterizes this disease. The cause of this megaloblastic change is unknown.

Megaloblastic features are common also in pyridoxine-responsive sideroblastic anaemia. The biochemical basis for the megaloblastic change is unknown. One possible explanation lies with the fact that both pyridoxal $5'$-phosphate and tetrahydrofolate are required as coenzymes for the conversion of serine to glycine, an important step in haem synthesis.

Biochemical basis of megaloblastic change

As explained in Chapter 2, an adequate supply of vitamin B_{12} and folate coenzymes is essential for optimal DNA and RNA synthesis. The most significant effect of a deficiency of either of these vitamins is to reduce the rate of conversion of deoxyuridine-$5'$-monophosphate (dUMP) to deoxythymidine-$5'$-monophosphate (dTMP), the rate-limiting step in DNA synthesis. The resulting asynchrony between DNA and RNA synthesis explains many of the morphological and biochemical features of megaloblastic anaemia.

Failure of dTTP synthesis results in an accumulation of dUTP relative to dTTP. DNA polymerases, the enzymes responsible for assembly of DNA from deoxynucleoside triphosphates, are unable to distinguish between dTTP and dUTP. The relative paucity of dTTP results in the misincorporation of uracil into DNA instead of thymine. An enzyme called **uracil-DNA-glycosylase** recognizes the aberrant uracils and excises them. Normally, a series of other enzymes mediate the repair of the mutilated DNA by incorporating thymine in place of the excised uracil. However, when thymine is in short supply, suboptimal repair of DNA leads to fragmentation of the helical structure, impaired mitosis and premature cell death.

Deficiency of the purine salvage pathway enzyme hypoxanthine-guanine phosphoribosyltransferase (HGPRTase) causes the **Lesch–Nyhan syndrome**, which is characterized by megaloblastic anaemia, hyperuricaemia, spasticity, mental retardation and self-mutilation. The disorder is very rare and shows an X-linked recessive pattern of inheritance.

Hereditary orotic aciduria results from a deficiency of either or both of the enzymes orotate phosphoribosyltransferase and orotidylate decarboxylase. This rare disorder of pyrimidine metabolism is associated with severe megaloblastic anaemia, growth retardation and excretion of large amounts of orotic acid in the urine. The anaemia is refractory to vitamin B_{12} or folic acid but responds well to the oral administration of uridine, which bypasses the enzyme block.

David W, an 18-month-old boy, was referred to the paediatric clinic at the Auchtermuchty Royal Infirmary for investigation of his failure to thrive after weaning onto solid food. Clinical examination revealed him to be pale, moderately underweight, weak and listless with poorly developed muscles and a distended abdomen. His mother reported that his faeces were abnormally bulky, pale and foul smelling. David was diagnosed as having coeliac disease, an intolerance of dietary gluten (a protein present in cereals such as wheat) which results in the loss of the villi in the duodenum and jejunum.
1. What do you think are the most likely causes of David's anaemia? Why?
2. Which laboratory tests would you recommend to investigate the cause(s) of the anaemia?

Pathophysiology

Individuals with megaloblastic anaemia typically display the physiological changes which are common to all types of anaemia i.e. pallor, weakness, shortness of breath on exertion, light-headedness, palpitations and congestive cardiac failure. In some cases, loss of appetite, weight loss and gastrointestinal disturbances also are present. In addition to these non-specific changes, a range of signs that are strongly suggestive of megaloblastic change may be noted. These typically affect the tissues that are most rapidly dividing and are attributable to impaired mitotic function. They can be grouped under three headings:

- General tissue manifestations.
- Neurological manifestations.
- Haematological manifestations.

General tissue manifestations

The effects of a deficiency of vitamin B_{12} or folate are manifest most clearly in rapidly dividing tissues such as bone marrow and epithelial cells. Disturbances of epithelial cell turnover are responsible for oral symptoms such as **angular stomatitis** (lesions at the corners of the mouth) and **glossitis** (inflammation and depapillation of the tongue). Disturbed epidermal growth promotes widespread melanin hyperpigmentation. Sterility is not uncommon. A variety of non-specific chromosomal changes such as random breaks are common in megaloblastic tissue, almost certainly due to uracil misincorporation as described above.

Neurological manifestations

Early neurological manifestations of vitamin B_{12} deficiency include a tingling sensation or loss of the sense of touch in the feet and fingers. This may progress to spasticity and degeneration of the spinal cord. Once established, neurological damage is irreversible. The mechanism of neurological damage is not fully understood but is probably due to secondary deficiency of S-adenosylmethionine. Some workers also believe that the accumulation of methylmalonyl-CoA that occurs in vitamin B_{12} deficiency promotes the incorporation of branched-chain fatty acids into myelin and leads to disturbed neurological function.

Folate deficiency in pregnancy is associated with an increased incidence of neural tube defects such as spina bifida and anencephaly in the foetus. It is also believed to lead to mild dementia and impairment of intellectual function.

Peripheral blood neutrophils normally have between one and five nuclear lobes, with an average of 2.8. A right shift is present when the average number of nuclear lobes is significantly increased. In practice, a rigorous lobe count (Cooke–Arneth count) is seldom performed. The presence of more than 3% of five-lobed neutrophils is used as a sensitive and readily discernible alternative indicator.

The presence of a right shift is not a reliable indicator of megaloblastic anaemia. This change is also seen in iron deficiency, uraemia, infection and even as an inherited abnormality (Undritz anomaly).

Haematological manifestations

Morphological changes

Typically, the megaloblastic bone marrow is hypercellular, with an increase in erythropoietic activity being especially prominent. There is an increased proportion of immature forms of all cell lines, reflecting the premature death of cells in the process of development. This combination of increased production of blood cells and increased intramedullary cell death is known as **ineffective haemopoiesis,** and is responsible for the pancytopenia that characterizes this condition.

The distinctive changes in blood and bone marrow cell morphology that accompany megaloblastic anaemia are the result of asynchrony between nuclear and cytoplasmic development. Megaloblastic red cell precursors typically display retarded maturation of the nucleus relative to the cytoplasm. This is exemplified by the appearance of the late megaloblast which features an open, lace-like chromatin network and a fully haemoglobinized cytoplasm. Circulating red cells typically are macrocytic but there is a marked variation in size and shape of individual cells. Macrocytosis results from a decrease in the number of cell divisions prior to loss of the nucleus and release into the circulation. In contrast to the macrocytes that accompany alcoholic liver disease, megaloblastic macrocytes typically are oval. Absolute reticulocytopenia is invariably present.

The twin abnormalities of megaloblastic leukopoiesis are the appearance of bizarre, giant metamyelocytes in the bone marrow and an increase in the average number of nuclear lobes in circulating granulocytes. Nuclear hypersegmentation probably results from structural abnormalities in the nuclear chromatin.

Morphological changes in megaloblastic megakaryocytes include an increase in cell size and failure to develop the characteristic cytoplasmic granulation. However, these changes often are difficult to detect.

Biochemical changes

The increased marrow cell turnover results in alterations in the biochemistry of the blood such as an increase in the concentrations of unconjugated bilirubin, lactate dehydrogenase and lysozyme. Bilirubin is one of the products of haemoglobin catabolism and so its accumulation in the blood reflects ineffective erythropoiesis. Similarly, the enzymes lactate dehydrogenase and lysozyme reflect ineffective erythropoiesis and ineffective leukopoiesis respectively. These changes in blood biochemistry are augmented by the shortened lifespan of circulating blood cells which is invariably present in megaloblastic anaemia.

Vitamin B_{12} deficiency is accompanied by specific biochemical changes in the blood, including a rise in the plasma concentration of homocysteine and methylmalonate and a fall in the plasma concentration of vitamin B_{12}. Alterations in the plasma concentration of homocysteine occur early in vitamin B_{12} deficiency and can be used as a sensitive marker of the condition. Folate deficiency is accompanied by a fall in red cell and plasma folate concentration.

Suggested further reading

Chanarin, I. (1990). *The Megaloblastic Anaemias,* 3rd edn. Oxford: Blackwell.

Gilham, B., Papachristodoulou, D.K. and Thomas, J.H. (1997). Nutrition: folate and vitamin B_{12}. In *Wills' Biochemical Basis of Medicine*, 3rd edn (B. Gilham, D.K. Papachristodoulou and J. Hywel Thomas, eds), pp. 196–202. Oxford: Butterworth-Heinemann.

Self-assessment questions

1. Why is vitamin B_{12} deficiency in pregnancy uncommon in the developed world even when the daily requirement exceeds supply?
2. Why is folate deficiency common in pregnancy?
3. Why does assay of red cell folate give a better guide to folate status than assay of serum folate?
4. Which of the following statements are true?
    (a) Dietary deficiency of vitamin B_{12} is common in the UK.
    (b) Folate deficiency inhibits RNA synthesis.
    (c) PA is an autoimmune condition.
    (d) Methotrexate is an inhibitor of folate absorption.
5. Why does the plasma concentration of homocysteine rise in vitamin B_{12} deficiency?
6. Why are chromosomal breaks common in megaloblastic tissue?

Key Concepts and Facts

- Megaloblastic anaemia is characterized by retardation of DNA synthesis but a normal rate of RNA synthesis.

- Dietary deficiency of vitamin B_{12} is restricted to vegans.

- The most common cause of vitamin B_{12} and/or folate deficiency is malabsorption due to gastrointestinal disease or drug treatment.

- Pernicious anaemia is an autoimmune disease characterized by failure to synthesize intrinsic factor.

- Dietary deficiency of folate is common.

- Deficiency of folic acid is especially common in pregnancy.

- Megaloblastic anaemia also is observed secondary to cytotoxic chemotherapy, certain inborn errors of metabolism or certain haematological disorders.

- Deficiency of vitamin B_{12} and/or folate slows the rate of conversion of dUMP to dTMP and so DNA synthesis is slowed.

- Deficiency of vitamin B_{12} is associated with irreversible neurological degeneration.

- Deficiency of folate in pregnancy is associated with neural tube defects.

- Megaloblastic anaemia is characterized by ineffective haemopoiesis, i.e. a hypercellular bone marrow with peripheral pancytopenia.

Chapter 5
Haemoglobin synthesis, structure and function

Learning objectives

After studying this chapter you should confidently be able to:

Outline the synthesis of haem and globins.

Describe the relationships between the structures of haem and globin and haemoglobin function.

Review the role of haemoglobin in gaseous transport within the body.

Describe the role of haem–haem interaction in oxygenation of haemoglobin.

Explain the effect of 2,3-DPG on haemoglobin oxygen affinity.

The haemoglobins are red globular proteins which have a molecular weight of about 64 500 and comprise almost one-third of the weight of a red cell. Their primary function is the carriage of oxygen from the lungs to the tissues. Over 400 different variants of haemoglobin have been described but all share the same basic structure of four **globin** polypeptide chains, each with a single prosthetic **haem** group.

Haemoglobin synthesis

Although haem and globin syntheses occur separately within developing red cell precursors, their rates of synthesis are carefully coordinated to ensure optimal efficiency of haemoglobin assembly.

Haem synthesis

Haem belongs to the class of pigments known as **porphyrins**. It is composed of four pyrroles linked by methene bridges each bound to a central ferrous ion (Fe^{2+}) as shown in Figure 5.1. Haem is synthesized to some extent in virtually all human tissues but the

Cyclic tetrapyrroles are extremely important structures in the maintenance of life in all its myriad forms. For example, **haem** is an essential component of the oxygen-transporting proteins of animals (haemoglobin and myoglobin), **chlorophyll** is central to photosynthesis which maintains plant life and acts as an important source of atmospheric oxygen and **vitamin B_{12}** is essential for DNA synthesis.

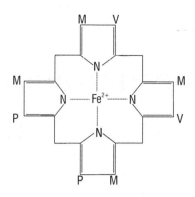

Figure 5.1 *The structure of haem. P, propionyl; M, methyl; V, vinyl*

most important sites are the liver (for incorporation into cytochromes) and red cell precursors.

The first step of haem synthesis is the rate-limiting reaction for the whole process and involves the combination of glycine and the succinic acid derivative succinyl-CoA to produce **δ-aminolaevulinic acid (δALA)**. The reaction is energy-dependent and occurs within the mitochondria. The catalyst for δALA synthesis is the enzyme δALA synthetase. The presence of free globin chains stimulates δALA synthesis while the presence of free haem groups is inhibitory, thus providing a control mechanism of the rate of haem synthesis and its coordination with globin synthesis. Several cofactors are required for δALA synthesis, including the vitamin B_6 derivative pyridoxal phosphate and the presence of free ferrous and copper ions. Synthesis of the enzyme δALA synthetase also is inhibited by the presence of free haem, providing a further feedback inhibition mechanism.

Two molecules of δALA condense asymmetrically to form a pyrrole called **porphobilinogen** (PBG) under the influence of the enzyme δALA dehydrogenase and glutathione. This and subsequent reactions occur in the cytoplasm of the cell.

The next step requires the synthesis of the porphyrin ring. The reactions involved in this process are extremely complex but can be summarized as the condensation of four PBG molecules to form the asymmetric cyclic tetrapyrrole **uroporphyrinogen III** (UPG III). Synthesis of UPG III requires the presence of two enzymes (uroporphyrinogen I synthetase and uroporphyrinogen III cosynthetase) and involves the formation of several short-lived intermediates.

UPG III is converted to **coproporphyrinogen III** (CPG III) by decarboxylation of the acetate side chains under the influence of the enzyme uroporphyrinogen decarboxylase. CPG III enters mitochondria where it is converted to **protoporphyrinogen IX** (PPG IX) by an unknown mechanism. This reaction is catalysed by the enzyme coproporphyrinogen oxidase. PPG IX is further converted within the mitochondria to **protoporphyrin IX**. It only remains for the central ferrous ion to be inserted to complete the synthesis of haem.

The porphyrias are a group of inherited abnormalities of haem metabolism and are characterized by accumulation of intermediates of haem synthesis. One of the rarest forms, congenital erythropoietic porphyria, is associated with severe photosensitivity (exposure to sunlight must be avoided), scarring, excessive hair growth, deformity of the fingers and fingernails, reddish discolouration of the teeth and chronic haemolysis. The teeth and urine fluoresce under UV light.

Many workers believe that the physical appearance and nocturnal habits of these unfortunate people could explain the popular legend of the werewolf.

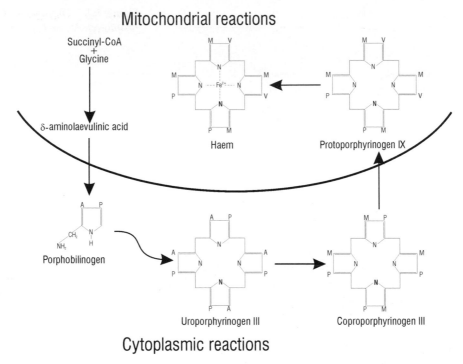

Mitochondrial reactions

Succinyl-CoA
+
Glycine

δ-aminolaevulinic acid

Haem

Protoporphyrinogen IX

Porphobilinogen

Uroporphyrinogen III

Coproporphyrinogen III

Cytoplasmic reactions

Figure 5.2   *The synthesis of haem. P, propionyl; A, acetate; M, methyl; V, vinyl*

This reaction is catalysed by the enzyme ferrochelatase and requires the presence of reducing agents. The synthesis of haem is depicted schematically in Figure 5.2.

Globin synthesis

The various globins that combine with haem to form haemoglobins are all single-chain polypeptides and, in common with all other proteins, their synthesis is under genetic control. Humans normally carry eight functional globin genes, arranged in two, duplicated gene clusters: the β-like cluster (β, γ, δ and ε globin genes) on the short arm of chromosome 11 and the α-like cluster (α and ζ globin genes) on the short arm of chromosome 16. These genes code for six different types of globin chains: α, β, γ, δ, ζ and ε globin. Functional haemoglobins all contain two α-like and two β-like globin chains.

Ontogeny of globin synthesis

Globin synthesis is first detectable in the primitive erythroid precursor of the yolk sac at about 3 weeks' gestation. At this stage of development, the embryonic globin genes ζ and ε are synthesized, resulting in the formation of **haemoglobin Gower I** $(\zeta\varepsilon)_2$. Activation of the α and γ genes occurs at about 5 weeks'

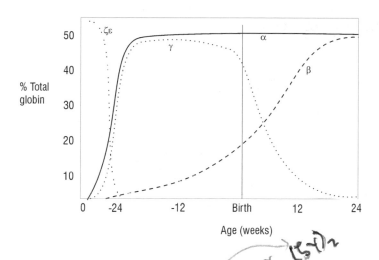

Figure 5.3   *Ontogeny of globin chain synthesis*

gestation when **haemoglobin Portland** $(\zeta\varepsilon)_2$ and **haemoglobin Gower II** $(\alpha\varepsilon)_2$ are synthesized. These three embryonic haemoglobins are undetectable by routine methods after about 10 weeks' gestation. This is coincident with the end of the yolk sac phase of erythropoiesis.

As the rate of synthesis of ζ and ε globins decreases, that of α and γ globins increases sharply. Thus, the predominant haemoglobin for the remainder of foetal life is **haemoglobin F** $(\alpha\gamma)_2$. At birth, approximately 50–80% of the haemoglobin content is of this type. Maximal synthesis of γ globin coincides with the hepatic phase of foetal erythropoiesis.

Synthesis of β globin begins at about the same time as α and γ globin but it remains a minor component until just before birth. The sharp increase in synthesis of β globin coincides with the establishment of the bone marrow as the main site of erythropoiesis. After birth, β globin synthesis continues to replace γ globin synthesis until 97% of the haemoglobin present is **haemoglobin A** $(\alpha\beta)_2$ and haemoglobin F accounts for less than 1%. This stage is usually reached by about 6 months of age. The remaining 2–3% of haemoglobin consists of **haemoglobin A$_2$** $(\alpha\delta)_2$. Synthesis of δ globin begins at about 30 weeks' gestation but remains a minor component throughout life. At present, the mechanism of switching from embryonic to foetal to adult globin chain synthesis is poorly understood. The relative rates of synthesis of the different globins throughout life are depicted in Figure 5.3.

Haemoglobin structure

Primary structure of globin

The primary structure of globin refers to the amino acid sequence of the various chain types. The position of individual amino acids is identified by numbering from the N-terminal end. Thus, the sixth

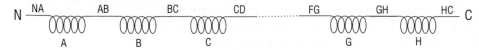

Figure 5.4 *The secondary structure of globin*

amino acid from the N-terminal end of the β globin chain is designated β^6. However, certain amino acids perform the same essential role in all normal globin chains. The identity and position of these amino acids cannot be changed without causing gross impairment to molecular function. Numbering according to primary sequence does not reveal the positional similarities of these so-called 'invariant amino acids', however.

Secondary structure of globin

The secondary structure of all globin chain types comprises nine non-helical sections joined by eight helical sections as shown in Figure 5.4. The helical sections are identified by the letters A–H while the non-helical sections are identified by a pair of letters corresponding to the adjacent helices, e.g. NA (N-terminal end to the start of A helix), AB (joins the A helix to the B helix) etc.

One complete turn of the helix requires between three and four amino acid residues. The amino acid side chains point outwards from the axis of the helix. This means that the side chains of amino acids which are in closest apposition, and therefore most likely to interact with each other, are not those of sequentially adjacent amino acids but of amino acids which are one turn of the helix apart. Individual amino acids can be identified according to their position in the secondary structure. This is a useful notation because invariant amino acids often appear in the same positions in all types of globin chain. For example, the α^{58} and β^{63} amino acids are both histidine residues, but their position in the primary structure provides no clue that their function may be related. However, both residues occupy the position E7 in the secondary structure of their respective globin chains. A histidine residue must always occupy this position because it is one of the two sites to which the haem group is bound.

Tertiary structure of globin

The tertiary folding of each globin chain forms an approximate sphere. The intramolecular bonds that give rise to the helical parts of the chain impart considerable structural rigidity, causing chain folding to occur in the non-helical parts. Tertiary folding gives rise to at least three functionally important characteristics of the haemoglobin molecule:

- Polar or charged side chains tend to be directed to the outside surface of the subunit and, conversely, non-polar structures tend to be directed inwards. The effect of this is to make the surface of the molecule hydrophilic and the interior hydrophobic.

- An open-topped cleft in the surface of the subunit known as the **haem pocket** is created. Each globin subunit has one haem pocket in which is bound a single haem group. Within this hydrophobic cleft, the ferrous ion of the haem group is protected from the oxidative effects of water, which would destroy its oxygen-binding capability.

- The amino acids which form the inter-subunit bonds responsible for maintaining the quaternary structure, and thus the function, of the haemoglobin molecule are brought into the correct spatial orientation to permit these bonds to form.

Quaternary structure of haemoglobin

The quaternary structure of haemoglobin has four subunits arranged tetrahedrally as shown in Figure 5.5. The structure of haemoglobin A is often written as $\alpha_2 \beta_2$ but the designation $(\alpha\beta)_2$ is preferred because this implies, correctly, that the molecule is made up of two equal and identical dimers. Each dimer is held together very firmly and inflexibly by strong inter-subunit bonds involving over 30 amino acid residues, which impart stability. The area of contact is known as the $\alpha_1 \beta_1$ or $\alpha_2 \beta_2$ junction. Dimers have a limited ability to exist separately and a small proportion of all normal haemoglobin exists in this dissociated form.

The $\alpha_1 \beta_2$ and $\alpha_2 \beta_1$ contact areas which hold the tetramer together are much less tight than the $\alpha_1 \beta_1$ and $\alpha_2 \beta_2$ contact areas. The $\alpha_1 \beta_2$ and $\alpha_2 \beta_1$ contact areas involve less than 20 amino acid residues each, and it is across these junctions that the sliding molecular movements which accompany oxygen uptake and release occur.

There are two other areas of contact between globin subunits in the haemoglobin tetramer, i.e. the $\alpha_1 \alpha_2$ and the $\beta_1 \beta_2$ contact areas. Bonding at these contact areas is, of necessity, considerably weaker than at the other contact areas. In deoxyhaemoglobin, the two β chains are too far apart for bonding to occur, and a functionally significant area, the **β cleft**, exists. On oxygenation, however, the whole molecule contracts and the β cleft disappears as the two

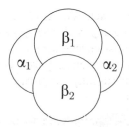

Figure 5.5 *The quaternary structure of haemoglobin*

chains move very close together. Weak interaction between the β chains is possible in this state. Strong bonding would interfere with oxygen release because deoxygenation involves the two β chains separating again. Conversely, the two α chains are some distance apart in the oxygenated state and move closer together on deoxygenation when weak interaction is possible: strong bonding between α chains would inhibit oxygenation.

Haemoglobin function

Haemoglobin–oxygen binding

Each haemoglobin molecule is capable of carrying four oxygen molecules, one for each haem group. The ferrous (Fe^{2+}) ions at the centre of each haem molecule are capable of forming six bonds using electrons in their outer shell. Four of these bonds bind to the nitrogen atoms of the four pyrrole groups and the remaining two bind to invariant histidine residues in the attached globin chain. The distal histidine (E7) residue binds closely but the distance between the proximal histidine (F8) and the ferrous ion is large enough to permit the insertion of a single oxygen molecule. It is important that the iron in the haem is maintained in the ferrous state. If it is oxidized to the ferric (Fe^{3+}) form, the ion can only form five bonds and oxygen cannot be bound. This form is known as **methaemoglobin**.

Oxygenation of haemoglobin is associated with considerable movement within the molecule. In the deoxygenated state, the central ferrous ions of the four haem groups are too large to fit into the plane of their porphyrin rings without causing severe distortion of the optimal ring structure. Oxygenation of the first haem group causes distortion of the electron cloud of the ferrous ion and facilitates the assumption of a truly planar configuration. Movement of the ferrous ion into the plane of the porphyrin ring pulls the attached α globin chain inwards, thereby reducing the width of the haem pocket and allowing the haem group to tilt from its upright, deoxygenated position.

Movement of the first α globin chain pulls on the other globin chains and causes a conformational change in the whole haemoglobin molecule which results in increased oxygen affinity. As each haem group is oxygenated, reduction in the size of its haem pocket induces further conformational change, which further increases the oxygen affinity of the molecule. This process, whereby the sequential oxygenation of haem groups has an effect on the subsequent oxygenation of the others is known as **haem–haem interaction**, and is an important feature of normal haemoglobin function.

In the process of complete oxygenation, the diameter of the haemoglobin molecule is reduced by about 10%. Molecular compaction makes the binding of an oxygen molecule to the fourth haem group difficult despite the high oxygen affinity of

Iron is a transition metal with atomic number 26. The electrons in an atom of iron are arranged as $1s^2\,2s^2\,2p^6\,3s^2\,3p^6\,3d^6\,4s^2$. The ferrous ion ($Fe^{2+}$) is formed by the loss of the two $4s$ electrons. This leaves six electrons in the outer shell that can form bonds. Thus the ferrous ion in haem can bond as described in the text and is capable of binding oxygen. Ferric ions (Fe^{3+}) are formed by loss of one of the $3d$ electrons, leaving only five electrons available for bonding. Thus the ferric ions in methaemoglobin bond with the four pyrrole nitrogen atoms and the distal histidine residue at E7. They cannot bind to the proximal histidine at F8 or to oxygen.

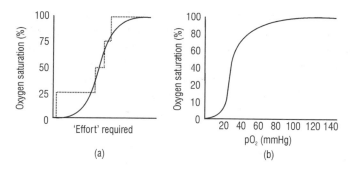

Figure 5.6 *(a) The effort required to sequentially oxygenate the four haem groups of a single molecule of haemoglobin. (b) The haemoglobin:oxygen dissociation curve*

this binding site. The 'effort' required to oxygenate the four haem groups of a typical haemoglobin molecule is depicted graphically in Figure 5.6a. Oxygenation of the first haem group requires the greatest effort but haem–haem interaction ensures that oxygenation of the second and third haem groups is made progressively easier. Steric hindrance caused by molecular compaction makes oxygenation of the last haem group more difficult than expected.

The derivation of Figure 5.6a is clearly hypothetical and simplistic. Oxygenation is an integrated process, involving all four subunits acting in concert. It is the whole molecule that oxygenates or releases oxygen, not the individual subunits. For this reason, each haemoglobin molecule exists only in the fully oxygenated or fully deoxygenated states. Based on the free energy required or generated as the transition between them occurs, the fully deoxygenated and fully oxygenated conformations are known as 'tense' (T) and 'relaxed' (R) forms of haemoglobin respectively.

Exposure of a haemoglobin solution to increasing partial pressures of oxygen results in an increasing proportion of haemoglobin molecules that exist in the fully oxygenated (R) form. The relationship between partial pressure of oxygen and the degree of oxygen saturation it causes is shown graphically in Figure 5.6b. This curve is known as the **haemoglobin:oxygen dissociation curve** and is characteristically sigmoidal in shape.

Oxygen delivery

The haemoglobin:oxygen dissociation curve shown in Figure 5.6b is of limited value as drawn because it is difficult to interpret in terms of oxygen carriage and delivery. The Y-axis can be recalibrated to show the volume of oxygen carried per 100 ml of blood. Under physiological conditions, 100 ml of normal adult blood is capable of carrying a theoretical maximum of about 20 ml of oxygen.

Although the mean alveolar pO_2 of 100 mmHg is sufficient to saturate the oxygen-binding capacity of haemoglobin, not all of the alveoli are equally well ventilated. This means that some of the blood that perfuses the lungs is exposed to a lower pO_2 and so

The oxygen-carrying protein of muscle, myoglobin consists of a single polypeptide chain with a single prosthetic haem group. Because it has no haem–haem interaction, the oxygen dissociation curve of myoglobin is hyperbolic rather than sigmoidal.

The theoretical maximum oxygen binding capacity of 'normal blood' assumes a haemoglobin concentration of 14.6 g/dl. Since 1 g of haemoglobin can bind up to 1.34 ml of oxygen, it follows that 100 ml of normal blood can bind up to 1.34×14.6 ml of oxygen, i.e. ~ 20 ml. Obviously, if the haemoglobin concentration is higher or lower, the maximum oxygen binding capacity alters proportionately.

Figure 5.7 *(a) Delivery of oxygen under normal physiological conditions. (b) Increased delivery of oxygen in response to decreased tissue* pO_2

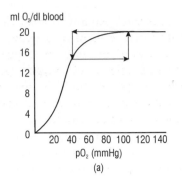

(a)

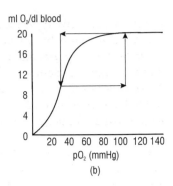

(b)

cannot saturate with oxygen. The result is that blood that enters the aorta typically carries only about 97% of the theoretical maximum quantity of oxygen, i.e. about 19.5 ml of oxygen per 100 ml of blood. When this oxygenated blood reaches the systemic capillaries where the pO_2 is typically about 40 mmHg, it is no longer in equilibrium with its environment and so releases about 4.5 ml of oxygen per 100 ml of blood to the tissues. This reduces the oxygen saturation of the haemoglobin to 75%. The partially deoxygenated blood is then transported back to the lungs where it will, again, encounter a mean pO_2 of 100 mmHg and start the cycle all over again with 19.5 ml of oxygen per 100 ml of blood. This chain of events is shown in Figure 5.7a.

The extra oxygen, which is apparently needlessly carried, acts as an instantly available reserve when oxygen demand increases. For example, when a muscle contracts, oxygen utilization increases, causing a localized fall in pO_2. When blood arrives at the capillaries supplying that muscle, it encounters a pO_2 of, for example, 30 mmHg and is forced to give up more oxygen as it equilibrates. Because of the sigmoidal shape of the haemoglobin:oxygen dissociation curve, a drop in partial pressure of oxygen causes a disproportionately large increase in oxygen donation. This chain of events is shown in Figure 5.7b.

As shown in Figure 5.7, a reduced alveolar pO_2 of 70 mmHg still results in about 90% haemoglobin saturation. It is extremely unlikely that, under normal atmospheric conditions, a sufficiently low alveolar pO_2 could ever arise so as to significantly reduce the oxygen saturation of blood leaving the lungs. Indeed, breathing could cease altogether for a considerable time before an alveolar pO_2 of 70 mmHg was reached and, even then, the oxygen saturation of the arterial blood would be sufficient to meet the demands of the tissues.

At rest, the typical cardiac output is about 5 litres of blood per minute. This is the minimum blood flow that meets the resting oxygen demand of the body. Since each 100 ml of blood delivers about 4.5 ml of oxygen, the resting, or basal, oxygen requirement is about 225 ml of oxygen per minute. Oxygen demand increases

Long distance runners often train at high altitude before an important race. Running in a reduced partial pressure of oxygen stimulates erythropoiesis which increases their oxygen carrying capacity and triggers a rise in red cell 2,3-DPG concentration which improves oxygen delivery to the tissues. These changes favour the prolonged effort required of distance runners, particularly when they return to lower altitudes.

rapidly when activity exceeds the basal level. Failure to meet this increased demand by an appropriate increase in oxygen delivery severely limits performance. The necessary increase in oxygen delivery can be achieved by increased release of oxygen per 100 ml of blood, by increasing cardiac output, or both. In normal individuals these and other mechanisms ensure that oxygen delivery to the tissues is adequate over a wide range of activity levels.

When severe anaemia is present, increases in oxygen demand may be difficult to meet. The value of 20 ml of oxygen carried per 100 ml of blood assumes a normal haemoglobin concentration of 14.6 g d/l. If the haemoglobin concentration falls to, for example, 7 g d/l, maximal oxygen carriage falls to less than 10 ml per 100 ml of blood. Greater proportional donation of oxygen by the mechanism described above can still meet basal oxygen demands in this case, but a greatly increased cardiac output and respiration rate are required when activity levels rise. This is manifest as a normal heart rate at rest, but an exaggerated cardiovascular response to exercise: the degree of exaggeration is directly related to the severity of the anaemia. This gives rise to the classical signs of anaemia, i.e. shortness of breath on exertion and palpitations.

Carbon dioxide transport

Carbon dioxide is excreted via the lungs in exhaled air. It is transported from the tissues to the lungs in the blood in three forms:

- Approximately 78% is transported in the form of bicarbonate ions (HCO_3^-), formed by the ionization of carbonic acid (H_2CO_3). Carbonic acid is formed by the reaction of carbon dioxide and water, a reaction catalysed by the red cell enzyme carbonic anhydrase. Haemoglobin, acting as a buffer, is an important acceptor of the H^+ ions produced along with the HCO_3^- ions.

- Approximately 13% is transported bound to proteins as carbaminoproteins. About half of the total is bound to plasma proteins, principally as carbaminoalbumin, and the other half is bound intracellularly to globin chains as carbaminoglobins. The mechanism of carbon dioxide binding to globin is completely different to that of oxygen binding to haem. Carbon dioxide is acidic and therefore binds to the basic groups which are present on all proteins at physiological pH.

- Approximately 9% is transported in solution in plasma and cell water.

Haemoglobin oxygen affinity

The haemoglobin molecule must achieve two apparently contradictory functions, i.e. it must have a high enough affinity for

Animals that live only at high altitude such as Andean llamas typically have haemoglobins that have a high affinity for oxygen. This adaptation ensures maximum uptake of oxygen in the lungs, even at the low partial pressures of oxygen found at altitude. Llamas do not develop the raised red cell count that typifies humans at altitude.

oxygen to load up fully in the lungs but have a low enough affinity to deoxygenate in the tissues. A number of substances help to solve this dilemma by modulating the oxygen affinity of haemoglobin, e.g. carbon dioxide, bicarbonate ions (HCO_3^-), H^+ and 2,3-DPG.

The oxygen affinity of haemoglobin is affected by the presence of carbon dioxide in two ways:

- H^+ ions formed by the ionization of carbonic acid within the red cell bind preferentially to deoxyhaemoglobin, thereby favouring the deoxygenated form of haemoglobin.

- Carbon dioxide binds to basic amino groups at the N-terminal ends of deoxygenated α and β globin chains, again favouring the deoxygenated form. The effect of pH on haemoglobin oxygen affinity is much more important and is known as the **Bohr effect**.

This is a physiologically appropriate response because the pCO_2 and H^+ concentration are relatively high in the tissues where pO_2 is relatively low, thereby maximizing oxygen donation to the tissues. In the lungs pO_2 is high and pCO_2 and H^+ concentration are relatively low, thereby promoting expulsion of CO_2 from the haemoglobin and uptake of oxygen as shown in Figure 5.8.

One of the products of red cell glycolysis is 2,3-diphosphoglyceric acid (2,3-DPG). This substance binds to the β globin chains of deoxygenated haemoglobin A $(\alpha\beta)_2$ and occupies the β cleft, thereby favouring the low oxygen affinity form. Thus, the relatively high concentration of 2,3-DPG found in red cells decreases the oxygen affinity of haemoglobin A and improves oxygen delivery to the tissues.

2,3-DPG binds avidly to β globin, but not to other non-α globins. This means that haemoglobins which lack β globin chains, such as haemoglobin F $(\alpha\gamma)_2$ have a higher oxygen affinity than haemoglobin A in the presence of 2,3-DPG. This increased oxygen affinity of haemoglobin F confers its ability to extract oxygen from maternal haemoglobin A at the placental barrier. However, the high oxygen affinity also means oxygen is released to the tissues somewhat less readily than in the adult. This does not present a problem because

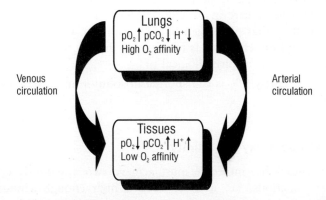

Figure 5.8 *Changes in oxygen affinity of haemoglobin in the lungs and tissues*

foetal activity levels necessarily are restricted and the excess oxygen demand that accompanies strenuous physical exercise does not arise.

Suggested further reading

Bunn, H.F. and Forget, B.G. (1985). *Haemoglobin: Molecular, Genetic and Clinical Aspects*. Philadelphia: W.B. Saunders.

Giardina, B., Messana, I., Scatena, R. and Castagnola, M. (1995). The multiple functions of hemoglobin. *Critical Reviews in Biochemistry and Molecular Biology* 30(3), 165–196.

Mallick, A. and Bodenham, A. (1996). Modified haemoglobins as oxygen-transporting blood substitutes. *British Journal of Hospital Medicine* 55(7), 443–448.

Ogden, J. and Macdonald, S. (1995). Ti:hemoglobin-based red-cell substitutes – current status. *Vox Sanguinis* 69(4), 302–308.

Self-assessment questions

1. What is the rate-limiting step in haem synthesis?
2. Where in the cell does haem synthesis occur?
3. Name three embryonic haemoglobins and define their globin content?
4. Why is it important that haem does not come into contact with water?
5. What is the normal alveolar pO_2?
6. Why is anaemia associated with shortness of breath on exertion?
7. Why is anaemia associated with pallor?

Key Concepts and Facts

Haemoglobin synthesis

- Haem and globin synthesis occur separately but in a carefully coordinated fashion.

- Globin synthesis is under the genetic control of eight functional genes arranged in two clusters – the α globin gene cluster on chromosome 16 and the β globin gene cluster on chromosome 11.

- The major haemoglobin in the foetus is HbF $(\alpha\gamma)_2$ and in adults HbA $(\alpha\beta)_2$.

Haemoglobin structure

- Primary structure refers to the amino acid sequence of globin; secondary structure comprises nine non-helical sections joined by eight helices; tertiary structure describes globin chain folding to form a sphere; and the quaternary structure of haemoglobin describes the tetrahedral arrangement of the four globin subunits.

- The external surface of each folded globin tends to be hydrophilic and the inner surface hydrophobic. This protects the haem from oxidation.

- The haem group of each chain sits in a protective hydrophobic pocket.

- In haemoglobin A, $\alpha\beta$ dimers are held together strongly at the $\alpha_1\beta_1$ or $\alpha_2\beta_2$ junction. The tetramer is held together much less tightly at the $\alpha_1\beta_2$ and $\alpha_2\beta_1$ contact areas.

Haemoglobin function

- Each haemoglobin molecule can carry four oxygen molecules.

- Oxygenation and deoxygenation are accompanied by molecular expansion and contraction via haem–haem interaction.

- The haemoglobin:oxygen dissociation curve is sigmoidal in shape.

- Under physiological conditions, blood in the aorta carries about 19.5 ml of oxygen per 100 ml of blood. Upon entering the tissues about 4.5 ml of oxygen are donated per 100 ml of blood.

- 2,3-DPG is an important modulator of haemoglobin A oxygen affinity in red cells.

Chapter 6
Haemoglobin disorders

Learning objectives

After studying this chapter you should confidently be able to:

Differentiate clearly between the thalassaemias and structural haemoglobinopathies.

Describe the geographic distribution of the thalassaemias.

Explain the classification of α and β thalassaemia.

Outline the molecular basis of α and β thalassaemias.

Describe the pathophysiology of α and β thalassaemias.

Outline the classification of the structural haemoglobinopathies and describe at least one example of each type.

Describe the pathophysiology of sickle cell disease.

Haemoglobin disorders, or **haemoglobinopathies**, fall into two main types:

- The **thalassaemias** involving disorders of the *rate* of globin synthesis. Globin structure is normal in thalassaemia.
- The **structural haemoglobinopathies** where globin *structure* is abnormal.

Classification is not always straightforward, however. Many structurally abnormal globins are synthesized at a reduced rate and so do not fit clearly into either category.

The thalassaemias

The thalassaemias are characterized by reduced or absent synthesis of one or more globin chain type. The resultant imbalance of globin chain synthesis leads to ineffective erythropoiesis and a shortened red cell lifespan.

The name thalassaemia was coined by the eminent haematologist George Whipple in 1932 as an alternative to the eponymous 'Cooley's anaemia'. He wanted a name that would convey the sense of an anaemia which is prevalent in the region of the Mediterranean Sea, since most of the early cases originated there. Thalassaemia is derived by contraction of thalassic anaemia (from the Greek *thalassa* – sea, *an* – none and *haima* – blood).

Figure 6.1 *The worldwide distribution of the thalassaemias. The shaded area represents areas where the disease is most common, but it is found in most populations of the world*

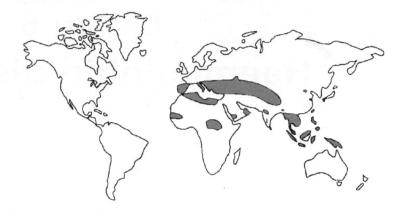

The geographic distribution of the thalassaemias overlaps with that of sickle cell disease and G6PD deficiency. This is because carriage of these abnormal genes affords some protection against malaria. Thus, being heterozygous for one of these conditions offers a selective survival advantage and increases the opportunity for these genes to be passed on.

Incidence and distribution

The thalassaemias are among the most common single gene disorders in the world. They are most common in parts of the world where malaria is endemic because the heterozygous state affords some protection against malaria (Figure 6.1). The incidence of thalassaemia is also high in immigrant populations that originate in these parts of the world. The distribution of the different forms of thalassaemia is not uniform:

- β thalassaemia is most common in people from the Mediterranean, Africa, India, South-East Asia and Indonesia. The incidence of β thalassaemia mutations is almost 10% in some parts of Greece.
- α^+ thalassaemia is most common in American blacks and in people from Indonesia, South-East Asia, the Middle East, India, the Mediterranean and the South Pacific islands. Thirty per cent of American blacks are 'silent' carriers of α^+ thalassaemia, while about 3% are homozygous. Homozygotes express minimal symptoms of disease.
- α° thalassaemia is most common in people from the Philippines, South-East Asia and Southern China. The population incidence of deletions that lead to this form of α thalassaemia reaches 25% in some parts of Thailand.

Classification

The thalassaemias are classified according to three criteria:

- The affected globin gene(s), e.g. α, β, δβ etc.
- Whether the reduction in the rate of synthesis of the affected globin is partial, e.g. β^+, or absolute, e.g. β°.
- The genotype, e.g. homozygous β°.

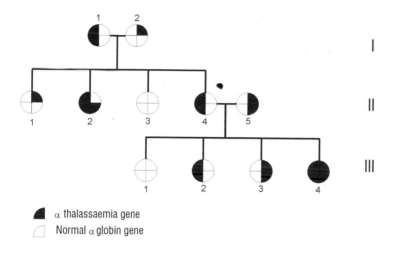

Figure 6.2 *Pedigree chart of a Thai family with α thalassaemia. The investigation was prompted by the stillbirth of baby III4. Patient II2 has inherited haemoglobin H disease. The dead baby had inherited haemoglobin Barts hydrops foetalis*

◣ α thalassaemia gene

◺ Normal α globin gene

α Thalassaemia

Normal individuals carry four α globin genes, two tandem pairs on the short arm of each chromosome 16. More than 95% of α thalassaemias result from the deletion of one or both of the tandem α globin genes. This gives rise to six possible genotypes:

Type type	Geno- type
Normal	$\alpha\alpha/\alpha\alpha$
α^+ heterozygote	$\alpha-/\alpha\alpha$
α^+ homozygote	$\alpha-/\alpha-$
α° heterozygote	$\alpha\alpha/---$
α° homozygote (Barts hydrops foetalis)	$---/---$
$\alpha^\circ\alpha^+$ double heterozygote (haemoglobin H disease)	$---/\alpha-$

Individuals are assigned to one of the above groups according to the results of simple laboratory tests. The tests are performed on as many family members as possible and a pedigree chart constructed (Figure 6.2).

The frequencies of the different deletions that give rise to α thalassaemia vary widely in different races. Deletion of both α globin genes on one chromosome 16 is relatively common in South-East Asia and the Philippines, leading to a high incidence of haemoglobin H disease and haemoglobin Barts hydrops foetalis. Conversely, the most common deletion in American blacks is of only one α globin gene: haemoglobin H disease is rare in this population and haemoglobin Barts hydrops foetalis exceedingly so.

β Thalassaemia

Normal individuals carry two β globin genes, one on the short arm of each chromosome 11. Most β thalassaemias result from a point mutation within or close to the β globin gene complex. Each mutation can result in a reduction or abolition of β globin gene

> Because there are two α globin genes on each chromosome 16, classification of the α thalassaemias relies on applying the synthesis rules to each *pair* of genes rather than each individual gene, e.g. deletion of one gene reduces but does not abolish α globin synthesis by that pair of genes and so α⁺ thalassaemia results.

function and so to β^+ or β° thalassaemia. Therefore, the classification of β thalassaemia is similar to that for α thalassaemia:

Type	Genotype
Normal	β/β
β^+ heterozygote	β^+/β
β^+ homozygote	β^+/β^+
β° heterozygote	β°/β
β° homozygote	β°/β°

Molecular basis

The classification scheme outlined above, although useful, greatly underestimates the complex nature of the relationship between genotype and phenotype in the thalassaemia syndromes. More than 100 different gene defects which cause thalassaemia have been described.

Gene deletion forms

α *Thalassaemia*

Most α thalassaemias result from gross deletions within the α gene complex. At least nine deletions that result in complete abolition of α globin synthesis have been described. Each is associated with a particular population and is denoted as such, e.g. the most common deletion in South-East Asia affects almost 20% of the population and is designated —^{SEA}: the —^{FIL} deletion accounts for about 30% of α thalassaemia genes in the Philippines and the —^{MED} deletion is most common in the Mediterranean region (Figure 6.3). All three deletions remove both α globin genes on one chromosome and so result in an α° haplotype. Haemoglobin Barts hydrops foetalis is most common in those parts of the world where such deletions are prevalent.

Deletions of only one α globin gene have been described in many populations and are the most common deletions in α thalassaemia.

> Crossing-over describes the reciprocal exchange of chromosomal material between homologous chromosome pairs during prophase I of meiosis. The exchange occurs when two chromatids align, break at corresponding locations, swap sides and rejoin. Unequal crossing-over occurs when the material swapped is of different length, and results in gene deletion on one chromosome and the acquisition of an extra gene on the other.
>
> Chromosomes with three α genes are relatively common in the populations in which these deletions are found. These represent the reciprocal $\alpha\alpha\alpha^{anti3.7}$ and the $\alpha\alpha\alpha^{anti4.2}$ formed during the process of unequal crossing-over. The extra α globin gene in these cases usually is functional.

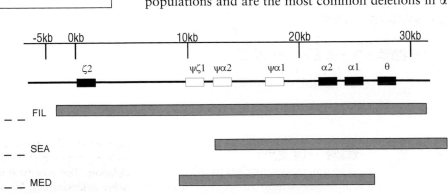

Figure 6.3 *Deletions which result in α° thalassaemia. Shaded regions denote areas of deletion*

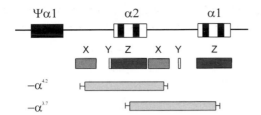

Figure 6.4 *Deletions which result in* α^+ *thalassaemia*

Such deletions are denoted according to their size as shown in Figure 6.4. These deletions arise from unequal crossing-over of two chromosomes 16 within the homologous α globin gene complexes as shown in Figure 6.5.

β Thalassaemia

Several deletions that affect only the β globin gene and result in β thalassaemia have been described but all except one are extremely rare. About one-third of β thalassaemias from the Indian sub-continent result from deletion of a large part of the 3′ end of the β

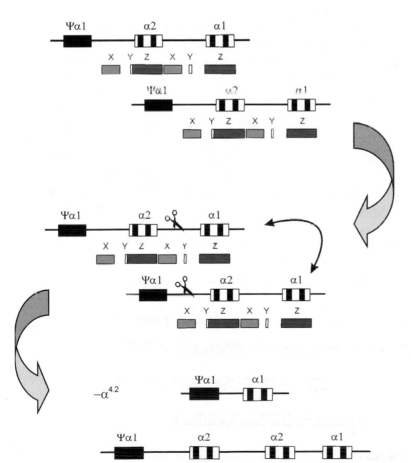

Figure 6.5 *The process of unequal crossing-over which results in the* $-\alpha^{4.2}$ *deletion. The process is identical for other deletions and for chain fusion variants such as haemoglobins Lepore and Kenya*

globin gene. This mutation is most common in the Gujurati and Sind peoples.

Non-deletion forms

Point mutations that result in thalassaemia are classified according to the stage of globin gene expression at which the defect is manifest. Examples of each of the following defects have been recognized in thalassaemia:

- **Inefficient transcription** of the gene into *m*RNA.
- **Defective processing** of the primary *m*RNA transcript. If the newly transcribed globin *m*RNA is not stabilized by capping and tailing it degrades quickly, leading to a reduction in protein synthesis.
- **Defective splicing** of the *m*RNA transcript. If the non-coding sequences of the globin *m*RNA transcript are not spliced out correctly, functional globin cannot be synthesized.
- **Improper translation** into protein. **Haemoglobin Constant Spring** results from deletion of the stop codon of the α2 globin gene and gives rise to a thalassaemic phenotype.
- **Post-translational instability**. If an extremely unstable globin chain is synthesized, it degrades almost immediately, resulting in a thalassaemic phenotype. **Haemoglobin Quong Sze** is an example of a such a hyperunstable haemoglobin variant.

Most β thalassaemias arise as a result of point mutations within or close to the β globin complex.

Pathophysiology

The thalassaemia syndromes encompass a wide spectrum of clinical severity. The heterogeneity is further increased by the frequency of coincident inheritance of a structural haemoglobinopathy such as haemoglobin S.

The myriad manifestations of this complex group of disorders can all be traced to a single cause: the imbalance of the synthesis of α-like and non-α-like globin chains. All normal mammalian haemoglobins are composed of two α-like and two non-α-like globin chains. Under normal circumstances, the rate of α globin synthesis is matched by the total synthesis of α, δ and γ globin chains. Impaired synthesis of α globin results in the accumulation of unpaired non-α globins within the developing erythroblast and *vice versa*. Unpaired globin chains are unstable; they form aggregates and precipitate within the cell, causing membrane damage and selective removal of the damaged cell by the reticuloendothelial system.

α Thalassaemia

Although α thalassaemia encompasses the complete spectrum of disease severity, affected individuals are considered to belong to one of four groups, according to the increasing severity of their symptoms:

- 'Silent' carriers
- α thalassaemia trait
- Haemoglobin H disease
- Haemoglobin Barts hydrops foetalis

The groups correspond approximately to the *functional equivalent* of the deletion of 1, 2, 3 or 4 α globin genes respectively. Thus, if a point mutation completely prevents expression of an α globin gene, the result is equivalent to deletion of that gene. Similarly, the presence of two point mutations, which reduce the output of their respective genes to about 50% of normal, approximates to deletion of a single gene.

Silent carriers

Deletion of a single α globin gene (heterozygous α^+ thalassaemia) has no significant effect on the well-being of the affected individual. In adults, no haematological abnormality can be demonstrated using standard laboratory techniques (i.e. excluding DNA analysis). Blood drawn from the umbilical cord of newborns contains 1% of haemoglobin Barts (γ_4). Such individuals are most often identified by deduction from a pedigree chart in the course of a family study. They can only be defined with complete reliability by DNA analysis.

α Thalassaemia trait

Individuals with the equivalent of two α globin genes deleted may be α^+ homozygotes ($\alpha-/\alpha-$) or α° heterozygotes ($--/\alpha\alpha$). It is important to know to which group a given individual belongs so that accurate genetic counselling may be offered. The two groups are clinically indistinguishable and present identical laboratory profiles using standard laboratory techniques.

Affected individuals show a mild microcytic, hypochromic anaemia but exhibit no significant symptoms of disease. Precipitated haemoglobin H (β_4) can be demonstrated by supravital staining in a small minority of red cells. Blood drawn from the umbilical cord can be shown to contain up to 10% of haemoglobin Barts.

Unpaired α globin chains are extremely insoluble and cause severe damage to developing erythroblasts. Unpaired β globin chains, on the other hand, form haemoglobin H, which is relatively stable and only precipitates as the red cell ages. Thus moderate impairment of β globin synthesis is associated with a greater degree of ineffective erythropoiesis and haemolysis than an equivalent impairment of α globin synthesis.

Different forms of haemoglobin can be separated from each other by electrophoresis. This method involves application of a blood lysate to a carrier such as a cellulose acetate strip soaked in buffer at pH 8.4. When a current is applied across the strip, the haemoglobins present migrate towards the cathode at a rate proportional to the charges present on the haemoglobin molecule, i.e. changes in the amino acid structure affect electrophoretic mobility and permit identification of abnormal forms. Not all haemoglobins are separated by this method, however. Supplementary tests are required to confirm the identity of any abnormal haemoglobins.

Haemoglobin H within red cells is demonstrated by incubation in a redox dye such as 1% brilliant cresyl blue at 37°C for 1 h, followed by microscopic examination. Precipitated HbH appears as multiple blue inclusions, giving a 'golf ball' appearance. This method can also be used, with a much shorter incubation time, to demonstrate reticulocytes.

An abnormal haemoglobin which travelled faster than haemoglobin A on electrophoresis was identified in the blood of a baby with haemoglobin H disease in 1958 by Ager and Lehmann. Since the letters of the alphabet had been exhausted by then, the new variant was called after the hospital where the baby was a patient – St Bartholomew's Hospital in London. Haemoglobin Barts subsequently was shown to be a γ globin tetramer.

Poikilocytosis is the term used to denote variation in red cell shape. Although the term describes all variations in red cell shape, its use is normally reserved to describe situations where the alteration is not characteristic, e.g. elliptocytes, spherocytes, sickle cells, target cells etc.

Anisocytosis denotes variation in red cell size while *polychromasia* is the term used to indicate the presence of reticulocytes on a Romanowsky stained blood film. Mature red cells stain pink with Romanowsky dyes but the residual RNA in reticulocytes causes them to stain varying shades of bluish-grey. Where a reticulocytosis is present, the red cells on a stained film will have many different shades, i.e. the film will be polychromatic.

Haemoglobin H disease

Haemoglobin H disease arises from the deletion of three α globin genes or the equivalent and is seen most commonly in South-East Asian populations. The most common genotype is that of a compound heterozygote for α^+ and α° thalassaemia ($\alpha-/—$).

Haemoglobin H disease is characterized by a moderately severe anaemia and hepatosplenomegaly. Typically, the haemoglobin level is maintained at around 8 g d/l and transfusion support is unnecessary. Characteristic findings on the peripheral blood film include microcytosis, hypochromasia, fragmented red cells, poikilocytosis, polychromasia and target cells. Multiple haemoglobin H inclusions are demonstrable in most of the red cells and are the main cause of the haemolytic anaemia that characterizes the condition. Adult blood contains between 5 and 35% of haemoglobin H and traces of haemoglobin Barts. Umbilical cord blood contains up to 40% haemoglobin Barts. The α : β globin chain synthesis ratio is typically reduced to between 0.2 and 0.4. Haemoglobin molecules that are composed of four identical globin chains such as haemoglobin H and haemoglobin Barts do not carry oxygen effectively.

Haemoglobin Barts hydrops foetalis

The most severe form of α thalassaemia results from the deletion of all four α globin genes and is seen most commonly in South-East Asia and the Mediterranean region. Because of the absence of α globin synthesis, no functionally normal haemoglobins are formed after the cessation of ζ globin synthesis at about 10 weeks' gestation. Instead, functionally useless tetrameric molecules such as haemoglobin Barts (γ_4) and haemoglobin H (β_4) are synthesized. Thus, although the haemoglobin concentration at delivery is typically about 6 g d/l, the *functional* anaemia is much more severe. The severity of the anaemia causes gross oedema secondary to congestive cardiac failure and massive hepatosplenomegaly. Pregnancy usually terminates in a third trimester stillbirth, often after a difficult delivery. The peripheral blood smear shows marked microcytosis, hypochromasia, poikilocytosis, fragmentation and numerous nucleated red cells. Haemoglobin electrophoresis confirms the presence of haemoglobin Barts and haemoglobin H.

β Thalassaemia

Because β thalassaemia usually results from point mutations within the β globin gene cluster, the relationship between genotype and phenotype is less straightforward than for α thalassaemia. It is still convenient, however, to group affected individuals according to the severity of their symptoms. Three groups are recognized:

- β thalassaemia minor (or trait)
- β thalassaemia major
- β thalassaemia intermedia

β Thalassaemia minor

The mildest form of β thalassaemia arises from the inheritance of a single abnormal β globin gene. Affected individuals exhibit no significant signs of disease, and may be unaware of their condition. Laboratory analysis reveals a mild microcytic, hypochromic anaemia, with target cells a prominent feature on the peripheral blood film. In most cases, the red cell count appears to be inappropriately high given the degree of anaemia. Most cases can be demonstrated to have raised levels of one or both of the minor haemoglobins A_2 and F. It is important to differentiate β thalassaemia minor from iron deficiency anaemia which produces superficially similar results. Iron deficiency causes a greater decrease in the level of Hb A_2 than Hb A, which may obscure the diagnosis of β thalassaemia minor when iron deficiency is also present.

β Thalassaemia major

β thalassaemia major results from the inheritance of two β thalassaemia genes. Affected individuals are thus either homozygous for a particular gene defect or doubly heterozygous for two distinct mutations. In the absence of treatment, the condition is characterized by severe anaemia, gross hepatosplenomegaly, failure to thrive and skeletal deformities such as bossing of the skull and maxillary prominence. The skeletal deformities are the result of marked erythroid hyperplasia with consequent expansion of the bone marrow volume, which causes outward pressure and marked thinning of the bones.

The peripheral blood film shows marked microcytosis, hypochromasia, numerous target cells and nucleated red cells. The prominent haemolytic component of the anaemia is manifest as teardrop poikilocytes, fragmented red cells and microspherocytes. Analysis of the haemoglobins present reveals a marked increase in the proportion of haemoglobin F, the precise value of which is dependent on the genetic defect(s) present. In homozygous $β°$ thalassaemia, for example, Hb F accounts for up to 98% of the total. Marked reduction in the synthesis of β globin is reflected in an $α:β$ globin synthetic ratio of greater than 2.5.

Bone marrow examination reveals extreme erythroid hyperplasia with marked ineffective erythropoiesis. The presence of precipitated aggregates of excess α globin chains promotes intramedullary death of developing erythroblasts and a reduced lifespan of circulating red cells.

The mainstay of current treatment is regular blood transfusion, aimed at maintaining the haemoglobin level above about 10–12 g d/l,

---

One approach to the discrimination between thalassaemia and iron deficiency anaemia is the use of a mathematical formula known as the discriminant function:

$$DF = MCV - ([5 \times Hb] - RBC - k)$$

where MCV = mean cell volume, Hb = haemoglobin concentration, RBC = red cell count and k is a locally determined constant. Using this formula, positive values of DF indicate iron deficiency and negative values indicate thalassaemia.

thereby effectively suppressing erythropoiesis and preventing skeletal changes and extramedullary haemopoiesis. However, such a programme of regular, lifelong transfusion leads to the accumulation of large amounts of iron within the body, which is severely toxic.

β Thalassaemia intermedia

Not all cases of homozygous or doubly heterozygous β thalassaemia have severe disease. Because of the diversity and high frequency of thalassaemic mutations, a complete spectrum of disease severity exists. Thalassaemia intermedia encompasses all cases of β thalassaemia with significant symptoms of disease which do not require regular transfusion to maintain their haemoglobin level above about 7 g d/l.

Typically, thalassaemia intermedia arises from one of three circumstances:

- Inheritance of 'mild' β thalassaemia mutation(s).
- Co-inheritance of a gene which increases the rate of γ globin synthesis.
- Co-inheritance of α thalassaemia. Reduction in α globin synthesis reduces the imbalance in the α : non-α globin synthetic ratio.

The laboratory and clinical features of thalassaemia intermedia mirror those of the more severe phenotype. Paradoxically, despite the absence of regular transfusion, iron overloading remains a major cause of morbidity.

The structural haemoglobinopathies

The structural haemoglobinopathies are characterized by the synthesis of structurally abnormal globin chains. These abnormal globins can exert a wide range of effects on the behaviour of the haemoglobin molecule. More than 500 different structurally abnormal haemoglobins have been described, but most are rare. The four most common examples are, in order of decreasing incidence, haemoglobins S, C, D and E. Haemoglobin S is by far the most common structural haemoglobinopathy and is most prevalent in Afro-Caribbeans but it is also relatively common in Central India, the Eastern Arabian peninsula and the Southern Mediterranean. About 30% of live births in Nigeria carry the abnormal gene. In common with thalassaemia, the carrier state for haemoglobin S confers selective resistance to the malarial parasite *Plasmodium falciparum*. Haemoglobin C is most common in West and Central Africa, particularly in Ghana. It frequently is co-inherited with haemoglobin S. Haemoglobin D is most common in the Punjab but is seen in a wide range of populations. Haemoglobin E is most common in South-East Asia.

In 1953 a standard nomenclature for haemoglobins was proposed. It was decided that normal Adult haemoglobin should be designated HbA, Foetal haemoglobin HbF and Sickle haemoglobin HbS. The two abnormal haemoglobins discovered by Itano in 1950 and 1953 were designated HbC and HbD respectively. There is no haemoglobin B because some workers had used this term to describe sickle haemoglobin. When the term HbS was adopted HbB was permanently abandoned.

Classification

The alteration in molecular function induced by structural abnormality is dependent upon the position of the mutation and on the properties of the amino acids involved. Functionally, the haemoglobin molecule can be considered to have a number of important areas:

- The exterior surface of the molecule, which confers water solubility.
- The $\alpha_1\beta_1$ and $\alpha_2\beta_2$ contact areas, which confer stability on the molecule.
- The $\alpha_1\beta_2$ and $\alpha_2\beta_1$ contact areas, which confer flexibility during oxygenation and deoxygenation.
- The $\alpha_1\alpha_2$ and $\beta_1\beta_2$ contact areas.
- The 2,3-DPG binding site, which affects the oxygen affinity of the molecule.
- The hydrophobic haem pockets, which protect the haem groups from oxidation.
- The C-terminal histidines of the β chains, which contribute to the Bohr effect.

Alterations to the amino acid sequence within these areas typically lead to predictable alterations in molecular behaviour. For example, changes in the $\alpha_1\beta_1$ and $\alpha_2\beta_2$ contact areas are likely to affect molecular stability, while changes in the $\alpha_1\beta_2$ and $\alpha_2\beta_1$ contact areas are likely to affect oxygen affinity. In general terms, the phenomena resulting from the presence of an abnormal haemoglobin will fall under one or more of the following headings:

- Clinically silent.
- Thalassaemia-like syndrome.
- Methaemoglobinaemia.
- Molecular instability.
- Altered oxygen affinity.
- Miscellaneous atypical effects, e.g. haemoglobin S.

Clinically silent haemoglobinopathies

Most structurally abnormal haemoglobins have no apparent effect. Over 200 such 'silent' abnormal haemoglobins have been described. Almost all are caused by alterations to amino acids on the external surface of the haemoglobin molecule, a position where change is readily tolerated; many involve the so-called 'variable' amino acid residues. Most of these silent haemoglobinopathies have been discovered by chance and are mainly of interest to population geneticists.

Medical workers in Northern Japan had been puzzled for some time about the origin of a familial disease, which they called *kuchikuru* or 'black mouth'. The mystery was solved when the abnormality was linked to haemoglobin M. The black discolouration of the mouth was due to the peripheral cyanosis which accompanies methaemoglobinaemia.

The thalassaemia-like syndromes

Any abnormality of globin that leads to *m*RNA instability is likely to lead to a thalassaemia-like syndrome. Abnormalities of this type are more common in β globin than in α globin, probably because severe abnormalities of α globin synthesis are more likely to be incompatible with life. Important examples of thalassaemic haemoglobinopathies include haemoglobin E and the chain fusion haemoglobins such as **haemoglobin Lepore** and **haemoglobin anti-Lepore** which are δ–β and β–δ fusions respectively, and **haemoglobin Kenya** which is a $^A\gamma$–β fusion. These haemoglobins result from unequal crossing-over during meiosis with the formation of hybrid globin genes.

Methaemoglobinaemia

Methaemoglobinaemia is the result of irreversible oxidation of the ferrous ion in haem to the ferric state. In all instances where this occurs, molecular instability also results. Similarly, in many cases where an amino acid change causes the formation of an unstable haemoglobin there is an increase in methaemoglobin formation. Whether the abnormal haemoglobin is classified as unstable or as a methaemoglobinaemia is to some extent arbitrary, but as a general rule it is classified according to which of the results predominates.

The four members of the **haemoglobin M** group are the most important of the abnormal haemoglobins that cause methaemoglobinaemia. All result from the substitution of the haem-binding histidine by tyrosine as shown in Table 6.1.

Haemoglobin Milwaukee originally was also classified as a haemoglobin M but the substitution involved is not of a haem-binding histidine, but of β67 (E11) valine by glutamic acid with resultant methaemoglobin formation. Similarly, **haemoglobin Zürich** (β63 (E7) distal His → Arg) was originally classified as a haemoglobin M because of the methaemoglobinaemia which results. However, the predominant effect of this substitution is molecular instability and haemoglobin Zürich is now classified as an unstable haemoglobin.

Table 6.1 *The M haemoglobins*

Haemoglobin	Mutation
Hb M Saskatoon	β63 (E7) distal His → Tyr
Hb M Hyde Park	β92 (F8) proximal His → Tyr
Hb M Boston	α58 (E7) distal His → Tyr
Hb M Iwate	α87 (E7) proximal His → Tyr

Unstable haemoglobins

More than 60 haemoglobin variants have been described where the principal defect is instability. Frequently the amino acid substitution involves the invariant amino acids. The reasons for the instability can be grouped under three main headings:

- Weakened haem–globin contact.
- Weakened tetrameric structure.
- Disruption of normal or helical structure.

Weakened haem–globin contact

The abnormalities leading to weak haem–globin contact usually involve amino acids in the haem pocket. In **haemoglobin Hammersmith**, the invariant β42 (CD1) phenylalanine is substituted by serine. Serine is a much smaller molecule than phenylalanine so the distance between the globin chain and the haem at this point is greater. The consequent weakening of the haem-β globin binding at this important position results in molecular instability. In addition, serine is hydrophilic and so encourages water to enter the haem pocket, leading to oxidation of the haem iron and methaemoglobinaemia.

Weakened tetrameric structure

The substitution of the β35 (C1) tyrosine by phenylalanine (which has no polar OH group) in **haemoglobin Philly** results in weakened $\alpha_1\beta_1$ bonding, monomer formation and precipitation of the haemoglobin as **Heinz bodies**.

Disruption of helical structure

Haemoglobin Genova results from substitution of the β28 (B10) leucine by the imino acid proline. The introduction of the relatively large ring structure in proline causes a 'kink' within the B helix with consequent molecular instability.

Insertion of a polar amino acid into the interior of the haemoglobin molecule also causes molecular instability. In **haemoglobin Wien** substitution of the tyrosine at β130 (H8) by aspartic acid causes the NA2 histidine to move closer to the −COO⁻ of the aspartic acid thereby disrupting the alignment of the A helix and leading to instability.

Altered oxygen affinity

Several mechanisms exist which result in altered oxygen affinity:

- Direct interference with oxygen binding, especially of α haem.

The earliest description of an unstable haemoglobin was made in 1952. It concerned a young boy with congenital haemolytic anaemia of unknown aetiology for whom splenectomy in early childhood had had no beneficial effect. The presence of Heinz bodies in his red cells suggested to the investigators that chemical poisoning was the most likely cause of the haemolysis but no culprit could be identified. It was not until 1970 that the presence of an unstable haemoglobin, Hb Bristol (β67 (E11) Val → Asp), was demonstrated.

The first unstable haemoglobin to be definitively identified was haemoglobin Zürich, which was identified in a young girl who developed acute haemolysis after ingestion of sulphonamide drugs.

The R groups of phenylalanine and tyrosine are identical apart from the tyrosine OH group. Phenylalanine is a non-polar (hydrophobic) amino acid while tyrosine is polar (hydrophilic).

Proline is designated an imino acid rather than an amino acid because it contains a secondary, not a primary, α amine group.

- Abnormality of the $\alpha_1\beta_2$ $(\alpha_2\beta_1)$ contact area.
- Alteration of $\alpha_1\alpha_2$ or $\beta_1\beta_2$ interaction.
- Changes in 2,3-DPG binding.
- Changes in Bohr effect H^+ binding.

Interference with oxygen binding

The unstable haemoglobin Hammersmith also has a reduced oxygen affinity because the CD1 phenylalanine helps to maintain the correct orientation of the haem group and is responsible for the tilt of the haem on oxygenation. In the absence of phenylalanine, the haem group remains in the upright, deoxygenated position, which lowers its oxygen affinity.

Abnormality of the $\alpha_1\beta_2$ $(\alpha_2\beta_1)$ contact

Interference with the $\alpha_1\beta_2$ $(\alpha_2\beta_1)$ contact is a common cause of altered oxygen affinity. For example, in **haemoglobin Chesapeake** the $\alpha92$ (FG4) arginine is substituted by leucine. The $\alpha92$ arginine normally is in Van der Waals' contact with the arginine at $\beta35$ (C2), stabilizing the deoxygenated conformation of haemoglobin. In haemoglobin Chesapeake, this interaction is absent and the deoxygenated conformation is no longer favoured.

Conversely, the oxygenated conformation normally is stabilized by a bond between the $\beta102$ (G4) asparagine and $\alpha94$ (G1) aspartic acid. In **haemoglobin Kansas**, formation of this stabilizing bond is precluded by the substitution of threonine for the $\beta102$ (G4) asparagine. This mutation therefore reduces the stability of the oxygenated conformation and results in reduced oxygen affinity.

Alteration of $\alpha_1\alpha_2$ and $\beta_1\beta_2$ interaction

Abnormalities affecting $\alpha_1\alpha_2$ are very rare. No mutations affecting $\beta_1\beta_2$ interaction have yet been reported.

In the deoxygenated form, the N-terminal ($\alpha1$) valine of each α chain bonds with C-terminal arginine ($\alpha141$) and aspartic acid ($\alpha126$) on the opposite α chain. These bonds stabilize the deoxygenated conformation, since they must be broken during oxygenation. In **haemoglobin Suresnes** the $\alpha141$ arginine is replaced by histidine, which precludes bonding with the $\alpha1$ valine on the opposite α chain and results in increased oxygen affinity.

Changes in 2,3-DPG binding

There are three amino acid residues on the β globin chain which are responsible for the binding of 2,3-DPG: the $\beta1$ (NA1) valine, the $\beta82$ (EF6) lysine and the $\beta143$ (H21) histidine. One of the sequence differences between β and γ globin is at H21 where the histidine is replaced by serine. This explains the inability of γ globin to bind 2,3-DPG and the resultant elevated oxygen affinity of haemoglobin F ($\alpha_2\gamma_2$).

Altered H$^+$ binding

Hydrogen ions (H$^+$) are bound in the process of deoxygenation, but must be released for association of oxygen to occur. The shift in the position of the haemoglobin:oxygen dissociation curve that results from changes in pH is called the **Bohr effect**. Half of the H$^+$ binding is due to the interaction of the C-terminal histidines of the β chains (β146, HC3), via their side chains, to the aspartic acid at β94 (FG1) of their own chains. Mutations that remove the β146 (HC3) histidine therefore affect H$^+$ binding and the oxygen affinity of the molecule. For example, the increased oxygen affinity of **haemoglobin York** is explained by the substitution of the β146 (HC3) histidine by proline.

Miscellaneous effects

Polymerization

The most clinically significant structural haemoglobinopathy is **haemoglobin S**. The clinical consequences of the presence of this abnormal haemoglobin all stem from its tendency to polymerize, causing contortion of the red cell into elongated and poorly deformable sickle shapes. Haemoglobin S results from a substitution of the glutamic acid in the external position β6 (A3) by valine. Substitution of the same amino acid by lysine gives rise to **haemoglobin C** which is the second most common of the structural haemoglobinopathies.

Heterozygotes for haemoglobin S are said to have **sickle cell trait**, while homozygotes have **sickle cell anaemia**. Typically, individuals with sickle cell trait are clinically normal and may be unaware of their condition. Laboratory analysis reveals the presences of about 40% HbS. Sickle cell crises are extremely rare in heterozygotes but affected individuals should be warned of the potential dangers of severe hypothermia or hypoxia.

Sickle cell anaemia follows a highly variable clinical course; some patients die in infancy from the disabling effects of recurrent crises or overwhelming infection, while others may live for a normal lifespan. The precise causes of this variability are poorly understood but the physical and social environment plays a large part. Symptoms of sickle cell anaemia are seldom manifest before the age of about 6 months when the level of circulating foetal haemoglobin falls to the adult level. Between crises, the condition is characterized by a chronic haemolytic state with jaundice and a relatively constant haemoglobin level of 7–8 g/dl. The anaemia may

James Herrick published the first description of a case of sickle cell anaemia in 1910 (*Archives of Internal Medicine* **6**, 517–521). The patient described was a young West Indian student who demonstrated many of the classical clinical features of this condition recognized today.

Repeated sickling crises within the microcirculation of the spleen cause cumulative damage, which ultimately leads to the loss of a functional spleen. This condition is relatively common in adults with sickle cell disease and is known as **autosplenectomy**.

be exacerbated by the presence of folate deficiency. This quiescent state is punctuated by crises of four main types:

- **Vaso-occlusive sickling crises** are the most common manifestation and occur when poorly deformable sickle cells occlude small blood vessels, e.g. in the spleen, leading to downstream tissue hypoxia and infarction. Repeated sickling crises cause cumulative tissue damage.

- **Aplastic crises** are manifest as a sudden fall in haemoglobin concentration with no compensatory reticulocytosis and are usually secondary to infection, most commonly with parvovirus.

- **Acute splenic sequestration** where a large proportion of the circulating red cell mass suddenly is sequestered by the spleen is a major cause of infant mortality in sickle cell anaemia.

- **Susceptibility to bacterial infection** is a hallmark of sickle cell anaemia, and a common cause of infant mortality. The most common infections are pneumococcal and staphylococcal.

Co-inheritance of other haemoglobinopathies can influence the clinical course of sickle cell trait or anaemia. For example, HbS homozygotes that also inherit a thalassaemia trait typically have higher haemoglobin levels and a less severe clinical picture. On the other hand, compound heterozygotes for HbS and β° thalassaemia have relatively severe disease. One particularly important example of such an interaction is where sickle cell anaemia is co-inherited with the benign condition hereditary persistence of foetal haemoglobin (HPFH) in which levels of haemoglobin F do not fall. The presence of significant amounts of haemoglobin F has a protective effect against sickling and such individuals have relatively mild disease.

Suggested further reading

Griffin, J.P. (1997). Methaemoglobinaemia. *Adverse Drug Reactions and Toxicological Reviews* **16**, 45–63.

IHIC Variants List (1995). *Hemoglobin* **19(1–2)**, 39–124.

Petrou, M. and Modell, B. (1995). Prenatal screening for haemoglobin disorders. *Prenatal Diagnosis* **15(13)**, 1275–1295.

Roath, S. and Huisman, T. (1992). *Current Views on Thalassaemia*. Reading: Harwood Academic.

Young, N.S. (1995). B19 parvovirus. *Baillieres' Clinical Haematology* **8(1)**, 25–56.

Self-assessment questions

1. Do you think that δ° thalassaemia would be a severe disease?
2. How would heterozygous γ° thalassaemia be manifest in an

affected newborn? How would you expect the disease to change as the child grows?

3. Why is haemoglobin Barts hydrops foetalis rare in American blacks? α^+

4. What effect would coincident inheritance of heterozygous α° thalassaemia have on the severity of a moderately severe β thalassaemia?

5. Why are haemoglobins M associated with peripheral cyanosis?

6. Why should patients with sickle cell disease avoid flying in unpressurized aircraft?

Key Concepts and Facts

- The thalassaemias are disorders of the *rate* of globin synthesis; structural haemoglobinopathies are disorders of globin structure.

- The thalassaemias are most common in parts of the world where malaria is endemic.

- The thalassaemias are classified according to the globin gene affected, the severity of the effect and the genotype.

- Most α thalassaemias result from gross gene deletions whereas most β thalassaemias result from point mutations.

- The clinical abnormalities seen in thalassaemia result from the imbalance of globin chain synthesis within developing red cells. Free α globin chains are severely toxic to the cell. Free β globin chains can form the relatively stable but useless haemoglobin H.

- The structural haemoglobinopathies can be classified according to the predominant effect they exert, e.g. clinically silent, thalassaemic phenotype, methaemoglobinaemia, molecular instability, altered oxygen affinity or miscellaneous effects.

- Most structural haemoglobinopathies are clinically silent.

- The most common structural haemoglobinopathy is haemoglobin S.

- Haemoglobin S crystallizes and polymerizes in hypoxic conditions, forcing the red cell into a poorly deformable sickle cell.

Chapter 7
The red cell membrane

Learning objectives

After studying this chapter you should confidently be able to:

List the main functions of the red cell membrane.

Outline the composition of the red cell membrane.

Differentiate between integral and peripheral proteins in the red cell membrane.

Describe the function of some important red cell membrane integral proteins.

Describe the structure and composition of the red cell cytoskeleton.

Outline the ABO and Rh blood group systems.

The primary function of the mature red cell is the transport of respiratory gases to and from the tissues. The effective performance of this task requires that the cell should be capable of traversing the microvascular system without mechanical damage and that the cell should normally retain a shape which facilitates gaseous exchange. These demands require the red cell membrane to be extremely tough yet highly flexible. The secret of the success of the red cell membrane in meeting the conflicting demands of strength and flexibility lies in the design of its **protein cytoskeleton** and the way in which the cytoskeleton interacts with the membrane **lipid bilayer**.

The main functions of the red cell membrane may be summarized as follows:

- To separate the contents of the cell from the plasma.
- To maintain the characteristic shape of the red cell.
- To regulate intracellular cation concentrations.
- To act as the interface between the cell and its environment via membrane surface receptors.

The role of the membrane in separating the contents of the cell from the plasma allows the red cell to control its own internal

During its 120 day lifespan, a red cell travels about 300 miles along blood vessels with a diameter of as little as 3 μm and is subjected to the extreme stresses of passage through the heart at least 500 000 times.

environment. For example, a constant supply of glucose from the plasma is required by the red cell to supply its energy needs and requirement for reducing potential. A specific transport protein in the membrane facilitates the transport of glucose into the red cell. Conversely, it is important that, once inside the cell, the phosphorylated intermediates of glycolysis are retained or the glycolytic pathway would fail in its purpose. Retention is assured because the red cell membrane is impermeable to phosphorylated sugars. This property of controlling which substances can cross the membrane is called **selective permeability** and is vital to the economy of the cell.

Mature red cells are biconcave discs with an average diameter of 7.2 μm, a volume of ~ 85 fl and a surface area of ~ 140 μm^2. This unusual shape maximizes the surface area:volume ratio (a sphere of the same volume has a surface area of 95 μm^2) and so facilitates gaseous exchange across the membrane. Biconcave discs are also readily deformable, assuming an 'arrowhead' conformation to allow passage through narrow capillaries.

The red cell membrane contains channels that facilitate the rapid passage across the membrane of water and monovalent anions such as Cl^- and HCO_3^-. In contrast, the passage of monovalent cations such as Na^+ and K^+ across the membrane is relatively slow. Large plasma:cell concentration gradients exist for these cations. The intracellular Na^+ concentration is relatively low (~ 8 mmol/l) while the plasma Na^+ concentration is relatively high (~ 140 mmol/l). This results in a slow translocation of Na^+ from the plasma into the cell. On the other hand, the intracellular K^+ concentration is relatively high (~ 100 mmol/l) while the plasma concentration is relatively low (~ 5 mmol/l). Thus, there is a slow leakage of K^+ from the cell into the plasma. In the absence of some mechanism to counter the leakage of monovalent cations, their concentrations would gradually equalize. However, the red cell membrane contains a protein which acts as a 'cation pump', i.e. it actively pumps Na^+ from the cell into the plasma and pumps K^+ in the opposite direction. The energy required to drive the pump is derived from the conversion of ATP to ADP by a membrane ATPase. The ADP thus formed is utilized by the Embden–Meyerhof pathway of glycolysis and so is reconverted to ATP (see Chapter 9). The activity of the pump is stimulated by extracellular K^+ or by a rise in the intracellular Na^+ concentration. The activity rate of the cation pump is controlled in such a way that it precisely balances the rate of leakage of cations across the membrane. Thus, the intracellular Na^+ and K^+ concentrations are maintained within very narrow limits.

Composition of the red cell membrane

The approximate composition of the red cell membrane is shown in Table 7.1.

Table 7.1 *Composition of the red cell membrane*

50% Protein		
10% Carbohydrate	(Glycoproteins and glycolipids)	
40% Lipid	30% Free unesterified cholesterol	
	10% Glycerides and free fatty acids	
	60% Phospholipid	30% Phosphatidyl choline
		30% Phosphatidyl ethanolamine
		25% Sphingomyelin
		15% Phosphatidyl serine

Lipids

All of the lipid associated with red cells is present in the cell membrane. The mature red cell has no capacity to synthesize lipid: alterations in membrane lipid content can only occur by exchange with plasma lipids.

As shown in Table 7.1, about 60% of the red cell membrane lipid is composed of one of four different phospholipids: **phosphatidyl choline, phosphatidyl ethanolamine, sphingomyelin** and **phosphatidyl serine**. Phospholipid molecules are characterized by a polar head group attached to a non-polar fatty acid tail. The polar head group is hydrophilic (water-loving) while the fatty acid tail is hydrophobic (water-fearing) or lipophilic (fat-loving). Thus, the phospholipid molecules in the cell membrane tend to arrange themselves in a bilayer with their hydrophilic heads pointing towards the inner and outer aqueous phases (the cytoplasm and plasma respectively) while the hydrophobic tails point towards each other as shown in Figure 7.1.

The distribution of the different phospholipids between the two leaflets of the bilayer is not symmetrical. The choline phospholipids phosphatidyl choline and sphingomyelin are mainly present in the plasma layer while the amino phospholipids phosphatidyl ethanolamine and phosphatidyl serine are restricted to the cytoplasmic layer.

The membrane **cholesterol** is unesterified and lies between the two layers of the lipid bilayer. The concentration of cholesterol in the membrane is an important determinant of membrane surface area and fluidity: an increase in membrane cholesterol leads to an increased surface area and decreased deformability. Red cell membrane cholesterol is in rapid exchange with the unesterified cholesterol of plasma lipoproteins. Plasma lipoproteins contain cholesterol in the free and esterified states in a ratio of about 1 : 3. The ratio of free to esterified cholesterol is controlled by the action of the enzyme **lecithin : cholesterol acyl transferase (LCAT)**. A decrease in LCAT activity leads to an increased plasma concentration of free cholesterol and thus, indirectly, to an increased concentration of cholesterol levels in the red cell membrane. In

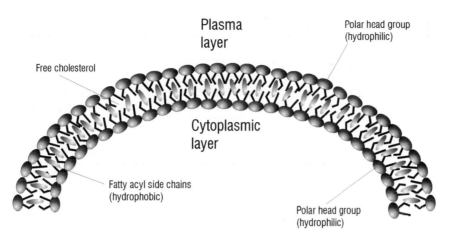

Figure 7.1 *Arrangements of phospholipids and cholesterol in the red cell lipid bilayer*

extreme circumstances, the decreased deformability that results can lead to premature destruction of the red cell.

Red cell lysophosphatidyl choline, phosphatidyl choline and sphingomyelin also are in exchange with their plasma lipoprotein counterparts. The rate of exchange of phosphatidyl choline and sphingomyelin is slow (less than 1% is exchanged per hour). The phospholipids of the cytoplasmic layer cannot exchange with the plasma.

> The lysophospholipids such as lysophosphatidyl choline (lysolecithin) differ from their phospholipid cousins in that they have only one fatty acid attached to their glycerol backbone instead of two. The *'lyso'* prefix alludes to their pronounced detergent-like properties, which can induce red cell haemolysis if they accumulate within the red cell membrane.

Proteins

Most red cell membrane proteins are tightly associated with the lipid bilayer, and require treatment with powerful detergents such as sodium dodecyl sulphate (SDS) to extract them for analysis by polyacrylamide gel electrophoresis (PAGE). This technique separates substances according to their molecular weight, the lightest travelling the furthest from the origin. Red cell membrane proteins have been named according to their relative positions on SDS-PAGE electrophoresis, as shown in Figure 7.2. Some of the better characterized proteins also have trivial names, as shown in Table 7.2.

Red cell membrane proteins can be grouped into two types:

- **Integral proteins**, which penetrate the lipid bilayer and are firmly anchored within it via interactions with the hydrophobic core. Only a relatively small portion of an integral protein molecule is exposed to the inner and outer aqueous phases. About 60–80% of red cell membrane proteins are of this type. Examples of important integral proteins include **band 3** and the **glycophorins**. Band 3 acts as the anion transport channel while the glycophorins are associated with the MNSs blood group system.

Figure 7.2 *Red cell membrane proteins separated by SDS-PAGE electrophoresis. Coomassie blue is a protein stain. Periodic acid Schiff stains carbohydrate and therefore reveals the glycophorins*

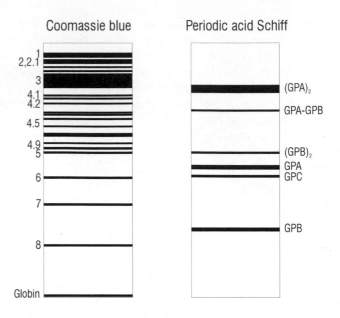

Table 7.2 *Red cell membrane proteins*

Protein	Trivial name	Mol. Wt
Band 1	Spectrin	240 000
Band 2	Spectrin	220 000
Bands 2.1–2.6	Ankyrin	200 000
Band 3	Anion exchange channel	95 000
Band 4.1		80 000
Band 5	Actin	42 000
Band 6	Glyceraldehyde-3-phosphate dehydrogenase	35 000
Band 7		29 000
PAS-1	Glycophorin A	29 000

- **Peripheral proteins,** which are in contact with the lipid bilayer but are not strongly attached to it. About 20–40% of red cell membrane proteins are peripheral proteins. Examples of important peripheral proteins include haemoglobin, the enzyme glyceraldehyde-3-phosphate dehydrogenase and the cytoskeletal proteins **spectrin** and **actin**.

Red cell membrane integral proteins

Band 3

Band 3 is a single chain molecule with a molecular weight of about 95 000. It accounts for close to 25% of the total protein content of the red cell membrane. Band 3 has two major functions within the red cell membrane, each associated with a distinct functional domain. Its primary function is to facilitate anion transport across the membrane but it also acts as an important binding site for cytoskeletal and other red cell proteins.

The central portion of the band 3 molecule consists of a series of hydrophobic helices that traverse the lipid bilayer. These helices are linked by short hydrophilic sequences which are exposed to the inner and outer aqueous phases. This arrangement forms a transmembrane channel, which facilitates the rapid transport of Cl^- and HCO_3^- anions. Band 3 is not particularly selective because SO_4^{2-} and PO_4^{3-} anions are also transported, albeit much more slowly, via this channel. A large carbohydrate side chain that carries the Ii blood group antigens is attached to one of the external hydrophilic linking sequences.

The N-terminal portion of band 3 is hydrophilic and projects into the cytoplasm of the cell. This functional domain has a molecular weight of about 43 000 and contains binding sites for haemoglobin, the glycolytic enzymes glyceraldehyde-3-phosphate dehydrogenase, aldolase and phosphoglycerate kinase, and the cytoskeletal proteins ankyrin, band 4.1 and band 4.2.

Glycophorins

The three members of the red cell glycophorin family are known as glycophorins A, B and C. Glycophorin A accounts for close to 2% of the mass of the red cell membrane. The glycophorin A molecule has been shown to consist of three distinct domains: a hydrophilic receptor domain, which projects into the outer aqueous phase, a hydrophobic transmembrane domain, which spans the lipid bilayer and anchors the molecule in the membrane, and a hydrophilic interior domain, which projects into the cytoplasm of the cell.

Red cell membrane glycophorin A is thought to exist as a dimer coupled at the transmembrane domains. The glycophorins are thought to act as transmembrane signal transducers. Glycophorins A, B and C have been shown to act as receptors for the malarial parasite *Plasmodium falciparum*.

Glycophorins B and C are similar in gross structure to glycophorin A. The N, Ss and U blood group antigens are located on the receptor domain of glycophorin B.

Na⁺/K⁺ ATPase

The Na^+/K^+ ATPase enzyme exists as an oligomer containing two large α subunits of molecular weight 110 000 and two smaller glycoprotein β subunits of molecular weight 55 000. The α subunits span the lipid bilayer while the β subunits project into the outer aqueous phase. This enzyme catalyses the hydrolysis of ATP to ADP, liberating energy in the process. Each ATP molecule hydrolysed via this system results in the ejection of three Na^+ ions from

The haematocrit of venous blood is normally greater than that of arterial blood. This interesting phenomenon is explained by changes in anion concentrations within the red cell as it passes from the arterial to the venous system.

Deoxyhaemoglobin is a weaker acid than oxyhaemoglobin and so has a lower net polyvalent anionic charge. Thus, deoxygenation is accompanied by a reduction in the net negative charge within the red cell. Electrochemical neutrality is restored by the rapid uptake of Cl^- ions via the band 3 anion exchange channel and water, leading to a slight swelling of the cell. Venous blood largely is deoxygenated and so the mean red cell volume and haematocrit is increased with respect to fully oxygenated arterial blood.

Phosphorylation and pumping out of 3Na$^+$

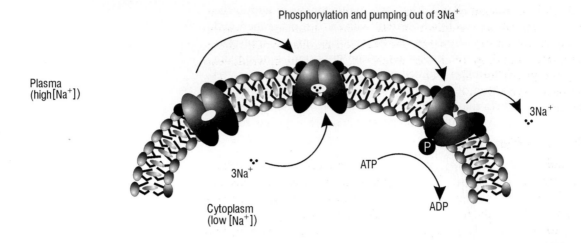

Plasma
(high[Na$^+$])

3Na$^+$

Cytoplasm
(low [Na$^+$])

ATP

ADP

3Na$^+$

Dephosphorylation and pumping in of 2K$^+$

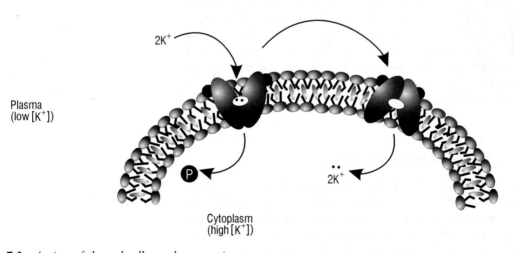

2K$^+$

Plasma
(low [K$^+$])

2K$^+$

Cytoplasm
(high [K$^+$])

Figure 7.3 *Action of the red cell membrane cation pump*

the cell and the transport of two K$^+$ ions into the cell. This mechanism is present in all mammalian cells and accounts for about one-third of all ATP hydrolysis at rest. The action of the red cell cation pump is shown schematically in Figure 7.3.

Glucose transport protein

The glucose transport protein has a molecular weight of 60 000 and shows some structural similarity to band 3, the anion transport protein. The motive force for transport of plasma glucose into the red cell is derived from the electrochemical gradient of Na$^+$ ions across the cell membrane. ATP hydrolysis is not required for glucose transport. Each molecule of glucose transported into the red cell is accompanied by a Na^+ ion, leading to a net reduction in the transmembrane gradient of Na^+ ions. Failure of the cation pump to constantly regenerate the Na^+ ion gradient would, therefore, result in failure of glucose transport. This, in turn, would lead to glycolytic failure and a consequent lack of ATP generation. The net result would be a rapid downward spiral leading to the death of the cell.

Surface receptors

Physiologically, the most important surface receptor of red cells is the **transferrin receptor**. This membrane protein has a molecular weight of 85 000 and consists of a short N-terminal interior domain, a lipophilic transmembrane domain and a large C-terminal receptor domain. The receptor domain is capable of binding two transferrin molecules. Following binding of plasma transferrin to its receptor, the receptor:transferrin complexes are internalized, the iron is released from the transferrin and the apotransferrin:receptor complex is recycled to the cell surface. The transferrin receptor has a relatively low affinity for apotransferrin at plasma pH, causing the release of the binding protein into the plasma to rejoin the iron transport cycle. Transferrin receptors are present on the surface of most cells but are present at particularly high concentration on the red cell surface. The concentration of transferrin receptors is highest on intermediate normoblasts when haemoglobin synthesis is maximal.

Red cell membrane peripheral proteins

The red cell membrane peripheral proteins interact to form a **cytoskeleton** which acts as a tough supporting framework for the lipid bilayer. Four proteins play a key role in the structure of the red cell cytoskeleton: spectrin, ankyrin, band 4.1 and actin, although many others play ancillary roles in this complex structure.

Spectrin (bands 1 and 2)

Spectrin constitutes about two-thirds of the total weight of the cytoskeleton. This protein is a heterodimer composed of two subunits designated α and β which have molecular weights of 240 000 and 220 000 respectively. These subunits are bound together in an antiparallel ('head to tail') configuration. Further, the two subunits are twisted around one another as shown in Figure 7.4. Spectrin heterodimers can associate head to head to form heterotetramers or can form higher oligomers in a branching, radial structure. *In vivo*, red cell membrane spectrin is thought to be composed of a mixture of these three forms, with the heterotetrameric form predominating. Spectrin also associates with ankyrin, band 4.1, actin and anionic phospholipids.

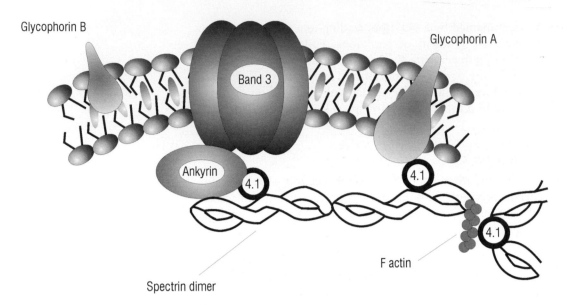

Figure 7.4 *Structure of the red cell membrane*

Ankyrin (bands 2.1–2.3 and 2.6)

Ankyrin has a molecular weight of 210 000 and serves to anchor assembled spectrin molecules to the lipid bilayer. This is accomplished by binding simultaneously to spectrin tetramers and to the interior domain of the integral protein, band 3.

Actin

Actin is synthesized as a globular protein, a form known as **G actin**. The assembly of G actin molecules 'head to tail' into double helical filaments forms an alternative configuration, **F actin**. Assembly and disassembly of actin filaments is an important process in neutrophil locomotion. Red cell membrane actin takes the form of relatively short F actin filaments. These filaments bind weakly to the tail end of both α and β spectrin. The result is a two-dimensional lattice of spectrin tetramers held together by actin filaments. The lipid bilayer is attached to this lattice via band 3.

Band 4.1

Band 4.1 is a globular protein of molecular weight 80 000 which serves two distinct functions in the red cell membrane. It binds to spectrin close to the actin binding site, thereby strengthening and stabilizing the cytoskeletal lattice. It also binds directly to glycophorins A and C, band 3 and phosphatidyl serine, and therefore strengthens the links between the lipid bilayer and the protein cytoskeleton.

Red cell blood group antigens

Study of red cell blood group antigens has provided important insights into such diverse fields as population genetics, mechanisms of gene expression, blood transfusion, forensic pathology and organ transplantation. There are 19 different blood group systems and nine collections recognized in humans, encompassing well over 200 different antigens. Only the clinically most important blood group systems are described in this chapter: an exhaustive review is beyond the scope of this book.

The following conventions are used to describe blood group antigens, antibodies and genes:

- The location of a gene which encodes a blood group antigen is called its **locus**.
- The various forms of the gene which encode the different antigens of the blood group system are **alleles** and are mutually exclusive.
- The genes present in an individual constitute the **genotype** irrespective of expression.
- The expressed blood group antigens constitute the **phenotype** of the individual.
- To differentiate between genes and antigens, genes are written in italics, i.e. A is an antigen whereas *A* refers to the gene which encodes A.

The ABO blood group system

The ABO blood group system was the first to be discovered and is by far the most important. Transfusion of ABO-incompatible blood results in an acute haemolytic reaction which may be life-threatening.

The ABO blood group system is controlled by the allelic genes *A*, *B*, *H* and *h*, which are inherited in a simple Mendelian fashion. The dominant *H* allele encodes a transferase enzyme (α2-L-fucosyltransferase) which converts a precursor substance in the red cell membrane to **H substance**.

The *A* and *B* alleles also encode transferase enzymes which are called α3-N-acetyl-galactosaminyltransferase (A-transferase) and α3-D-galactosyltransferase (B-transferase) respectively. These enzymes add specific sugar molecules to the terminal galactose of H substance, forming A or B substance on the cell surface. In the case of A-transferase the added sugar is N-acetylgalactosamine; in the case of B-transferase the added sugar is galactose. It is these terminal sugars which determine the ABO specificity. The development of A, B and H antigens is shown schematically in Figure 7.5.

Because ABO-like polysaccharides are widespread in nature, exposure to A and B substance with subsequent immunization occurs early in life. This means that neonates typically do not have ABO antibodies in their plasma but that, in the first months

In 1900, Karl Landsteiner performed a series of mixing experiments with the blood of 22 colleagues in which the red cells of each individual were mixed with the serum of each of the others. On the basis of the patterns of agglutination observed, Landsteiner could discern three groups of individuals, which he named A, B and C. The red cells of group A individuals were agglutinated by the serum of group B and C individuals. The red cells of group B individuals were agglutinated by the serum of group A and C individuals. The red cells of group C individuals were not agglutinated by serum from any individual.

It is easy to see that Landsteiner's groups A, B and C equate with the blood groups A, B and O recognized today. The fourth ABO blood group, AB, was not recognized until 2 years later when the experiment was repeated with a much larger sample.

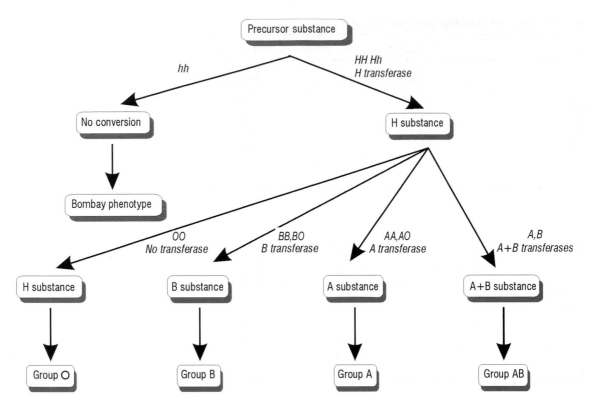

Figure 7.5 *Synthesis of ABH blood group antigens*

Table 7.3 *The ABO blood group system*

Blood group	Genotype	Phenotype	Red cell antigens	Plasma antibodies	Frequency
A	AA	A	A	Anti-B	0.44
	AO				
B	BB	B	B	Anti-A	0.08
	BO				
O	OO	O	H	Anti-A + B	0.45
AB	AB	AB	A + B	None	0.03

of life, exposure to A and B substance elicits the formation of IgM immunoglobulins with ABO specificity complementary to the host ABO type. The ABO blood group system is summarized in Table 7.3.

The Rh blood group system

The Rhesus or Rh blood group system is clinically the most important after the ABO system because Rh antigens are highly immunogenic and frequently are associated with haemolytic transfusion reactions and severe haemolytic disease of the newborn. The

---

In the absence of the *H* gene, the individual has the genotype *hh* and α2-L-fucosyltransferase is not synthesized. This means that the conversion of precursor substance into H substance cannot occur and the result is a complete absence of ABH antigens. This rare abnormality is known as the **Bombay phenotype**.

Table 7.4 *Frequency of Rh haplotypes in UK whites*

Haplotype	Designation	Frequency
CDE	R^z	Rare
CDe	R^1	0.41
CdE	r^y	Rare
Cde	r'	0.01
cDE	R^2	0.14
cDe	R^0	0.03
cdE	r''	0.01
cde	r	0.39

Table 7.5 *Frequency of most common Rh genotypes in UK whites*

Genotype	Designation	Phenotype	Frequency
CDe/cde	R_1r	CcDe	0.31
CDe/CDe	R_1R_1	CDe	0.16
Cde/cde	rr	ce	0.15
CDe/cDE	R_1R_2	CcDEe	0.13
CDE/cde	R_2r	cDEe	0.13
CDE/cDE	R_2R_2	cDE	0.03

Rh system is highly polymorphic with more than 40 different antigens described although, in practice, only five antigens (C, c, D, E and e) are clinically important.

The genetics of the Rh system are complex and still not fully understood. For all practical purposes, however, the system can be considered to be the product of three closely linked alleles, namely C and c, D and d and E and e, which are inherited *en bloc*. This arrangement gives rise to eight possible haplotype combinations: CDE, CDe, CdE, Cde, cDE, cDe, cdE and cde. The d allele is thought to be amorphic: no red cell antigen with d specificity has ever been described. For this reason, the 'd antigen' can be thought of as an absence of D antigen and homozygotes are said to be Rh negative. Conversely, individuals who possess at least one D gene are said to be Rh positive. The frequency of the different haplotypes and the most common genotypes in UK whites are shown in Tables 7.4 and 7.5.

Most Rh antibodies are IgG immunoglobulins that are produced in response to contact with foreign Rh antigens as a result of blood transfusion or pregnancy. Because the most immunogenic of the Rh antigens is the D antigen, antibodies with anti-D specificity are particularly common. Antibodies with anti-C, anti-E or anti-c specificity are also relatively commonly encountered in clinical practice.

In 1940, Landsteiner and Wiener were immunizing rabbits with the blood of rhesus monkeys. The antibody obtained was named anti-rhesus and was shown to agglutinate the red cells of 85% of Caucasians. These individuals were said to possess the Rhesus factor or to be Rhesus positive. Rhesus negative individuals were assumed to lack the Rhesus factor on their red cells.

Although this discovery formed the basis of the Rh blood group system, it was subsequently discovered that the antigen involved did not belong to the Rh system and so was renamed the LW antigen in honour of its discoverers.

Suggested further reading

Gilham, B., Papachristodoulou, D.K. and Thomas, J.H. (1997). Roles of extracellular and intracellular membranes: membrane structure and membrane transport. In *Wills' Biochemical Basis of Medicine* 3rd edn. Oxford: Butterworth-Heinemann.

Hollan, S. (1996). Membrane fluidity of blood cells. *Haematologia* **27**(3), 109–127.

Palek, J. and Lambert, S. (1990). Genetics of the red cell membrane skeleton. *Seminars in Hematology* **27**, 290.

Tanner, M.J.A. (1997). The structure and function of band 3 (AE1): recent developments. *Molecular Membrane Biology* **14**(4), 155–165.

Self-assessment questions

1. Which of the following statements are true?
   (a) The red cell membrane is rich in esterified cholesterol.
   (b) Phosphatidyl serine is concentrated in the outer leaflet of the lipid bilayer in red cells.
   (c) Red cell membrane sphingomyelin is in rapid exchange with the plasma.
   (d) Lysolecithin is present at high concentration in normal red cell membranes.
   (e) Spectrin is a red cell membrane integral protein.
   (f) Band 3 acts as an exchange channel for negatively charged ions.
   (g) Ankyrin binds to both spectrin and band 3.
   (h) Red cell membrane actin is mainly in the globular form.

2. A group O Rh R_1r woman has given birth to a Group O Rh R_1R_2 baby. Which of the following could be the father?
   (a) Steve, who is group O and Rh R_1r.
   (b) Phil, who is group A and Rh R_1R_2.
   (c) Chris, who is group AB and Rh R_1R_2.
   (d) Mike, who is group B and Rh rr.
   (e) Richard, who is group A and Rh R_1r.
   (f) Glynn, who is group B and Rh R_2r.
   (g) Malcolm, who is group O and Rh R_2r.

Key Concepts and Facts

- The red cell membrane consists of a protein cytoskeleton and an attached lipid bilayer.

- The red cell membrane is selectively permeable.

- The red cell membrane consists of 50% protein, 40% lipid and 10% carbohydrate.

- The lipid content of the red cell membrane is mainly phospholipid and free cholesterol.

- The phospholipid content of the red cell membrane consists of 30% phosphatidyl choline, 30% phosphatidyl ethanolamine, 25% sphingomyelin and 15% phosphatidyl serine.

- Because phospholipid molecules are characterized by a hydrophilic head group attached to a hydrophobic tail, they arrange themselves in a bilayer with their heads pointing outwards.

- Phosphatidyl choline and sphingomyelin are mainly present in the plasma layer while phosphatidyl ethanolamine and phosphatidyl serine are restricted to the cytoplasmic layer.

- Red cell membrane cholesterol lies between the two leaflets of the lipid bilayer.

- Red cell membrane proteins are of two types: integral proteins, which penetrate the lipid bilayer and are firmly anchored, and peripheral proteins, which are not strongly attached.

- Important red cell membrane integral proteins include band 3, the anion transporter, Na^+/K^+ ATPase which functions as a cation pump and the glucose transport protein.

- The red cell membrane peripheral proteins form the cytoskeleton.

- Important red cell membrane peripheral proteins include spectrin, ankyrin, actin and band 4.1.

- The ABO blood group system is the most important clinically and comprises groups A, B, O and AB.

- Normally, people carry antibodies in their plasma complementary to the ABH antigens they carry.

- The Rh blood group system is clinically the most important after ABO and comprises the antigens C, c, D, E and e.

- If an individual carries the D antigen, they are said to be 'Rh positive'.

Chapter 8
Disorders of red cell survival

Learning objectives

After studying this chapter you should confidently be able to:

Differentiate between the terms haemolytic disorder, haemolytic anaemia and haemolytic component.

Outline the difficulties associated with the classification of haemolytic disorders.

Demonstrate a detailed knowledge of the pathogenesis of hereditary spherocytosis and hereditary elliptocytosis.

Outline the pathogenesis of other inherited primary red cell membrane disorders.

Demonstrate a detailed knowledge of selected autoimmune and alloimmune haemolytic disorders.

List the triggers and outline the pathogenetic mechanisms of selected non-immune haemolytic disorders.

Outline the pathophysiology of the haemolytic disorders.

Hawkins and Whipple performed the earliest reliable determination of red cell lifespan in 1938. They created an opening in the bile ducts of dogs to enable the measurement of the amount of bile excreted daily. A number of experimental animals were rendered acutely anaemic by the administration of acetylphenylhydrazine, thereby eliciting a marked reticulocytosis. About 120 days after the reticulocyte response was noted, a peak of bile pigment production was observed. This was interpreted to be due to the destruction of the reticulocyte response cohort, suggesting that newly released red cells survive in the circulation for 120 days.

A normal, mature red cell survives in the circulation for about 120 days. The ageing process within red cells is associated with a reduction in glycolytic activity, reduced concentrations of 2,3-DPG and ATP, accumulation of Na^+ and Ca^{2+} ions, and increased rigidity due to loss of membrane lipid and changes in the cytoskeleton. These changes promote the sequestration and destruction of senescent cells in the spleen. Normally, the rate of destruction of senescent cells is balanced by the rate of synthesis and release of juvenile cells from the bone marrow.

Any condition which leads to a reduction in the mean lifespan of the red cell is a **haemolytic disorder**. Any reduction in red cell lifespan requires a balancing increase in the rate of erythropoiesis if anaemia is to be avoided. The reserve erythropoietic capacity of normal bone marrow is usually sufficient to prevent the development of anaemia until the mean red cell lifespan falls to about 15 days, when **haemolytic anaemia** ensues. The onset of anaemia is often accelerated by the presence of a haematinic deficiency or by another complicating pathological condition. Such conditions are said to have a **haemolytic component** in their pathogenesis but typically are not considered to be haemolytic disorders.

The haemolytic disorders can be classified in several different ways:

- **Site of haemolysis.** Most haemolytic disorders result from the premature destruction of red cells by the macrophages of the reticuloendothelial system. These are **extravascular haemolytic disorders.** Conversely, where haemolysis occurs mainly within the circulatory system, an **intravascular haemolytic disorder** is said to exist. This scheme groups together some highly disparate disorders and says little about the pathogenesis of particular disorders.

- **Site of the defect.** Haemolytic disorders can be divided into those caused by a structural or functional defect within the red cell (i.e. an **intrinsic defect**) and those caused by an abnormality in the red cell environment (i.e. an **extrinsic defect**). Knowledge of the site of the defect is useful in that transfused blood normally survives where the defect is intrinsic but may be rapidly destroyed in the presence of an extrinsic defect.

- **Nature of the defect.** Grouping haemolytic disorders according to the mechanism involved can aid understanding of underlying processes but can lead to confusion between hereditary and acquired types and unnecessary investigation of blood relations.

- **Inherited or acquired.** Typically, inherited haemolytic disorders are caused by an intrinsic defect whereas acquired haemolytic disorders are caused by an extrinsic defect. However, there are several exceptions to this rule, e.g. paroxysmal nocturnal haemoglobinuria (PNH) is an acquired intrinsic defect and severe hereditary G-6-PD deficiency typically requires the presence of an extrinsic trigger such as an antimalarial drug for this intrinsic defect to be manifest. Recognition that a disorder is hereditary can facilitate diagnosis in blood relations.

None of these classification schemes is universally applicable and, in practice, an amalgam of all four schemes is used.

Inherited haemolytic disorders

The inherited haemolytic disorders can be subclassified into three main groups according to the nature of the defect:

- Disorders of globin synthesis and/or structure.
- Enzyme disorders.
- Primary membrane disorders.

The disorders of globin synthesis and/or structure are described in

The earliest description of a case of HS was published in 1871 by two Belgian physicians, Vanlair and Masius. The index case presented with the classical symptoms of an aplastic crisis, jaundice, splenomegaly, abdominal pain and collapse. Microscopic evaluation of the blood of this patient revealed numerous microspherocytes which remained after the apparent remission of the crisis. Similar symptoms were noted in her sister and mother. Vanlair and Masius, who named this hitherto unknown condition *'microcythemie'*, thought it was caused by an overproduction of the spherocytes by the spleen coupled with a deficiency in their removal by the liver.

Chapter 6 and disorders of red cell metabolism are described in Chapter 10. The inherited membrane defects are described below.

Primary membrane disorders

Primary red cell membrane disorders are associated with alterations of cell shape and are classified according to the shape of the abnormal red cells.

Hereditary spherocytosis

Hereditary spherocytosis (HS) has an incidence of at least 1 in 5000 in North European populations. The condition is transmitted as an autosomal dominant characteristic although a less common autosomal recessive variant exists. No homozygotes for the autosomal dominant form have been described, suggesting that this state is incompatible with life. HS is caused by a deficiency or defect of the cytoskeletal proteins spectrin, band 4.1 or ankyrin. The most common abnormality is spectrin deficiency.

The principal features of HS include congenital haemolytic anaemia with variable spherocytosis, increased red cell osmotic fragility, episodic jaundice and variable splenomegaly. The haemolysis in HS is episodic and highly variable: it is not uncommon for the diagnosis to be missed until adulthood. Less common manifestations of HS include pigment gallstones (cholelithiasis), often at an unusually young age, and aplastic crises in which erythropoiesis is almost completely suppressed for up to 72 h, leading to severe but self-limiting anaemia. Aplastic crises commonly follow infection with human parvovirus type B19.

The major site of haemolysis in HS is the spleen. Two routes through the spleen exist: the faster, open circulation and the slower and more challenging closed circulation. Red cells which take the closed route face an inhospitable environment which tests to the limit the deformability and metabolic competence of the cell. The defective red cells in HS have an increased flux of Na^+ ions into the cell leading to greatly increased activity of the cation pump and necessitating an increased rate of glycolysis. Because of this, HS red cells find passage through the spleen particularly hazardous. Detention in the glucose-poor environment of the splenic cords rapidly leads to metabolic exhaustion in HS red cells and causes the loss of intact portions of membrane. The cell which results has a reduced surface area : volume ratio and so is less readily deformable. Reduced deformability of the cell causes an increase in subsequent splenic transit times. HS reticulocytes have a normal biconcave discoid shape and normal deformability but, with each passage through the spleen, they become progressively spherocytic and rigid. This vicious circle leads inevitably to the early death of the spherocyte within the splenic circulation. HS red cells survive an average of 30 passages through the spleen before they succumb.

The clinical severity of HS is highly variable. In mild cases, increased erythropoiesis compensates for the shortened red cell lifespan and the haemoglobin concentration remains within normal limits. A common consequence of chronic erythroid hyperplasia such as this is depletion of body folate stores. Oral folate supplementation may be required to prevent the development of megaloblastic anaemia. Where haemolysis is troublesome, the only effective treatment is splenectomy. Although this procedure does not affect the red cell defect, removal of the main site of haemolysis effectively 'cures' the condition and returns the mean red cell lifespan to normal.

Hereditary elliptocytosis

Hereditary elliptocytosis (HE) encompasses a disparate group of primary red cell membrane disorders characterized by the presence of a large proportion of oval or elliptical red cells. The frequency of HE may be as high as 1 in 1000. The condition typically is transmitted as an autosomal dominant characteristic. Homozygous HE presents as severe, transfusion-dependent haemolytic anaemia. An unusual autosomal recessive variant of HE exists but appears to be restricted to Melanesian aborigines and Filipinos.

The clinical severity of HE ranges from clinical silence to severe, life-threatening haemolysis. Broadly, HE can be divided into four major forms:

- **Common HE** has been described in virtually all races of the world and is a mild, compensated haemolytic disorder. Homozygotes have a severe, transfusion-dependent haemolytic anaemia which is characterized by marked poikilocytosis, microelliptocytosis and red cell fragmentation.

- **HE with infantile poikilocytosis** is almost restricted to blacks and presents as a moderately severe congenital haemolytic disorder with neonatal jaundice, elliptocytosis, marked poikilocytosis, red cell fragmentation and susceptibility of the red cells to heat damage. This condition progressively moderates until, by the age of 1 year, it is indistinguishable from common HE.

- **HE with spherocytosis** has mainly been described in Caucasians and is characterized by rounded elliptocytes, microspherocytes, microelliptocytes and a mild, incompletely compensated haemolytic state. About one in five cases of HE in Caucasians are of this type.

- **HE with stomatocytosis** is characterized by elliptocytes which show slit-like areas of pallor, an autosomal recessive mode of inheritance and mild or absent haemolysis. The condition is most common in Melanesian aborigines but has also been described in Filipinos.

The earliest published description of hereditary elliptocytosis is attributed to M. Dresbach, a physiology lecturer at Ohio State University. The abnormality first came to his attention during a student practical class in which students were examining their own blood. The hereditary nature of the condition was not established until 1929 when W.C. Hunter demonstrated transmission of HE through three generations of a white US family.

A wide range of cytoskeletal defects has been described in association with HE, but the most common are structural abnormalities of spectrin. Heterozygotes synthesize an abnormal spectrin which forms heterodimers but cannot self-associate to form tetramers and higher oligomers, resulting in a clinically mild form of HE. Deficiency of band 4.1 is a common cause of HE in Southern France and Northern Africa, accounting for more than one-third of cases in this area. Heterozygotes have a partial deficiency of band 4.1 and mild HE with spherocytosis whereas homozygotes have a complete absence of this protein and severe haemolytic anaemia. Abnormal binding of the integral protein band 3 to ankyrin has been described in association with HE with moderately severe haemolysis. The molecular basis for this abnormality remains obscure.

HE reticulocytes are normal in shape but become progressively elliptocytic with age. Elliptocytes are poorly deformable and so are sequestered in the spleen. In most cases of HE, haemolysis is so mild that clinical intervention is unnecessary. Where haemolysis is troublesome, splenectomy typically provides a functional cure.

Hereditary pyropoikilocytosis

Hereditary pyropoikilocytosis (HPP) is characterized by moderately severe haemolysis, microspherocytosis, micropoikilocytosis and an unusual susceptibility of the red cells to heat damage. The condition is inherited as an autosomal recessive characteristic and is most common in blacks. HPP is caused by defective spectrin synthesis and self-association. Splenectomy ameliorates the haemolysis in most cases of HPP but does not provide the 'cure' seen in HS or HE with haemolysis.

Hereditary stomatocytosis

Hereditary stomatocytosis (HSt) is characterized by the presence of bowl-shaped red cells which on dried films have a slit-like area of central pallor. These stomatocytes result from increased sodium transport into the cell which cannot be compensated for by increased cation pump activity, resulting in the ingress of water and cellular deformation. HSt is inherited in an autosomal dominant fashion and presents as congenital haemolytic anaemia of variable severity which is incompletely resolved by splenectomy. The molecular defect responsible for this disorder remains obscure.

Hereditary xerocytosis

The red cells of hereditary xerocytosis (HX) are characterized by excessive leakage of K^+ from the cell, leading to progressive water depletion. Xerocytes are thus dehydrated cells which are irregularly contracted and have an abnormally high mean cellular haemoglobin concentration (MCHC). Haemolysis is usually mild and compensated. Splenectomy has no clinical effect. Hereditary xerocytosis is inherited as an autosomal dominant characteristic. The molecular defect which causes this condition remains obscure.

Acquired haemolytic disorders

The acquired haemolytic disorders can be subclassified into four groups, according to the nature of the defect:

- Haemolysis secondary to immune mechanisms.
- Haemolysis secondary to the action of chemicals, drugs or toxins.
- Haemolysis secondary to infection.
- Haemolysis secondary to physical damage.

Haemolysis secondary to immune mechanisms

Immune haemolysis results from the binding of antibodies to the red cell surface with consequent complement activation. The antibodies concerned may be synthesized by the host immune system and be directed against host red cell antigens leading to **autoimmune haemolysis** or they may be derived from exogenous sources or be directed against foreign antigens leading to **alloimmune haemolysis**. Therapy with certain drugs can also stimulate immune haemolysis.

Autoimmune haemolysis

The autoimmune haemolytic anaemias (AIHAs) can be divided into three types:

- Warm-reactive antibody AIHA where the offending autoantibody reacts most strongly above 32°C.
- Cold-reactive antibody AIHA where the offending autoantibody reacts most strongly below 32°C.
- Drug-induced AIHA where immune haemolysis is triggered by the presence of a drug.

Warm-reactive antibody AIHA

Warm-reactive antibody AIHA is a relatively common condition affecting all ages and races, commonly in association with viral infections, lymphoproliferative disorders, immunodeficiency states or autoimmune disorders such as systemic lupus erythematosus (SLE). Typically, the autoantibody in warm-reactive antibody

The earliest clear description of a cold-reactive antibody AIHA was published in 1873 by R. Druitt. In this paper, he described two cases of haematinuria, one of which was a fellow doctor who had suffered from acrocyanosis with haematinuria and loss of sensation in the hands and feet for several years. Apparently miraculously, these distressing symptoms disappeared completely when the patient moved to the warmer climate of India.

PCH has been well recognized for over a century. The first description of this condition was published in 1854 and involved a young boy who probably had congenital syphilis. In the years that followed, several reports appeared of an association between inclement weather and haemoglobinuria. The relationship between cold and haemolysis in affected individuals was clearly demonstrated by Ehrlich 27 years later. His experiment involved the isolation of blood flow in a single finger of an affected individual by tying a cord tightly around its base. The finger was then held in iced water for some time. Serum obtained from the chilled finger was tinged red due to haemolysis whereas serum from a similarly isolated but unchilled finger remained unchanged.

AIHA is a polyclonal IgG_1 immunoglobulin, which activates complement via the classical pathway and triggers extravascular haemolysis. Treatment of this condition involves immunosuppressive drug therapy or splenectomy to remove the major site of red cell destruction.

Cold-reactive antibody AIHA

Cold-reactive antibody AIHA can be divided into two main types: **cold agglutinin syndrome** and **paroxysmal cold haemoglobinuria (PCH)**. Cold agglutinin syndrome is a disease of old age with a peak incidence over the age of 70 years. It is associated with *Mycoplasma pneumoniae*, Epstein–Barr virus and cytomegalovirus infection, where the autoantibody is polyclonal, and also with lymphoproliferative disorders where monoclonal antibodies are produced. The autoantibody is an IgM immunoglobulin with anti-I, anti-i or anti-Pr specificity. The temperature of capillary blood in the body extremities can be as low as 25°C, allowing the cold-reactive antibody to agglutinate red cells and activate complement and thus leading to intravascular and, more importantly, extravascular haemolysis and obstruction of capillary blood flow. Capillary obstruction is reversible on warming but, over a period of time, necrotic tissue damage and even gangrene can result. The most important measure in the treatment of cold agglutinin syndrome is the avoidance of cold. Immunosuppressive therapy is usually ineffective.

Classically, paroxysmal cold haemoglobinuria (PCH) is a chronic haemolytic condition which is characterized by intravascular haemolysis following exposure to cold, and is found in association with syphilis and viral illnesses such as measles or mumps. It is caused by a unique haemolytic IgG antibody called the **Donath–Landsteiner antibody**, which has anti-P blood group specificity. Haemolysis in PCH is biphasic, requiring both exposure to cold and subsequent warming. **The Donath–Landsteiner antibody** binds to red cells most strongly at temperatures below 15°C, so exposure to cold triggers antibody binding but no haemolysis because complement is inactive at these temperatures. However, following warming, rapid complement-mediated intravascular haemolysis ensues.

Alloimmune haemolysis

Alloimmune haemolysis results from the immunization of the host to transplanted foreign antigen or the action of foreign antibody to normal host antigen. Broadly speaking, there are two circumstances where this can occur:

- Haemolytic transfusion reactions.
- Haemolytic disease of the newborn.

Haemolytic transfusion reactions

Transfusion of blood from one individual to another is fraught with dangers. Chief among these is the risk of antibody-mediated haemolysis of donor or recipient red cells, a condition that can be life-threatening. The most severe haemolytic transfusion reactions are seen when ABO-incompatible blood is transfused. For example, if group A blood is transfused into a group O individual the IgM anti-A in the recipient plasma will immediately bind to the donor cells and activate the complement cascade. The resultant acute intravascular destruction of the donor cells can cause renal failure, hypotension and disseminated intravascular coagulation, and may be fatal. Transfusion of red cells that carry an antigen to which the recipient has previously been sensitized also causes an immediate haemolytic transfusion reaction.

Less commonly, haemolytic transfusion reactions can be delayed, often for several days following transfusion. In these cases, the recipient usually has previously been sensitized to donor red cell antigen, but the titre of the immune antibody is very low. Transfusion of red cells that carry the offending antigen stimulates a vigorous synthesis of antibody and, after a variable delay of up to several days, haemolysis ensues.

Haemolytic disease of the newborn

During pregnancy, the mother supplies nutrients to the developing foetus via the placenta and umbilical cord and foetal waste products are transported in the opposite direction for excretion by the mother. In the placenta, the foetal and maternal circulation are separated by a single layer of endothelium. Given this, it is inevitable that minor bleeds occur, even in normal pregnancy, allowing small amounts of foetal blood to enter the maternal circulation. At delivery, compression of the placenta can result in the injection of much larger amounts of foetal blood into the maternal circulation. If these foetal red cells carry paternal antigens, which are foreign to the mother, she may respond by producing antibody directed against the offending antigen. For example, a Rh negative mother (rr) carrying a Rh positive foetus (e.g. R_1r) is likely to respond to the presence of foetal red cells in her circulation by synthesizing an antibody with anti-D specificity. In subsequent pregnancies, further stimulation by foetal R_1r red cells can provoke the synthesis of a high titre IgG anti-D, which can cross the placental barrier and trigger the premature destruction of foetal red cells.

In severe cases, acute haemolysis in the foetus results in profound anaemia, hepatosplenomegaly, oedema secondary to cardiac failure and portal hypertension. This full-blown manifestation of HDN is known as **hydrops foetalis**, and was a relatively common cause of stillbirth in the first half of this century. In less severe cases, the baby is born alive but haemolysis continues after birth, causing progres-

Although Dr P. Levine is credited with the first unequivocal demonstration that most cases of HDN could be attributed to maternal immunization against a shared foeto-paternal Rh factor, a much less well-known figure deserves much of the credit. In 1938, a year before Levine's seminal observation, Dr Ruth Darrow published a theoretical account of the pathogenesis of HDN in which she speculated that the most likely cause was maternal immunization against a hitherto unrecognized foetal antigen.

sive anaemia and hyperbilirubinaemia as a result of haemoglobin catabolism. Unless treated by exchange transfusion, the hyperbilirubinaemia may cause severe neurological damage leading to spasticity, deafness and mental retardation. This condition is known as **bilirubin encephalopathy** or **kernicterus** and is irreversible once established.

Prior to 1970, the most common cause of severe HDN was maternal antibodies with anti-D specificity. The incidence of this form of HDN has been greatly reduced by the routine injection of IgG anti-D into all Rh negative mothers immediately following delivery. This procedure elicits the rapid destruction of any Rh positive foetal red cells which may be present, thereby minimizing the risk of maternal sensitization.

The most common cause of HDN today is ABO incompatibility of maternal and foetal blood. This form of HDN is almost always associated with group O mothers and group A or B babies. It is caused by the presence of naturally occurring IgG antibodies with anti-A or anti-B specificity in maternal plasma crossing the placental barrier and eliciting the destruction of foetal red cells which carry the A or B antigen. Typically, ABO incompatibility produces mild, self-limiting HDN: kernicterus and hydrops foetalis are rarely observed.

Drug-induced immune haemolysis

Treatment with a wide range of drugs can stimulate immune haemolysis by one of three mechanisms:

- **Penicillin-type immune haemolysis** in which the drug binds non-specifically to the red cell surface where it acts like a foreign antigen stimulating the production of IgG anti-drug antibodies. These antibodies bind to the surface-bound drug, leading to the selective removal of affected cells by the reticuloendothelial system. This type of immune haemolysis is most commonly associated with high-dose intravenous penicillin therapy.

- **α-Methyldopa-type immune haemolysis.** A minority of patients on long-term treatment with this antihypertensive drug produce a warm-reactive autoantibody which, in most cases, has anti-Rh specificity. Other drugs implicated in this form of immune haemolysis include levodopa and mefenamic acid.

- **Rifampicin-type immune haemolysis** in which the drug forms a stable complex with plasma protein and induces the synthesis of IgG and IgM anti-drug antibodies which form large immune complexes. These are adsorbed onto the surface of red cells and trigger complement-mediated intravascular haemolysis. Because the red cells are not directly the subject of the antibody attack, this mechanism is sometimes known as **'innocent bystander' immune haemolysis.** Withdrawal of the drug typically resolves the problem.

Table 8.1 *Drugs and chemicals commonly implicated as triggers of non-immune haemolysis*

Substance	Comment
Sulphonamides and sulphones Sulphadiazine Sulphanilamide Sulphapyridine	Antimicrobial drugs less used nowadays because of bacterial resistance and side-effects
Antimalarials Chloroquine Primaquine Quinine Maloprim	Used in the treatment and prevention of malaria
Nitrofurans Nitrofurantoin	Antimicrobials used for urinary tract infections
Others Salazopyrin *p*-Aminosalicylic acid	Used in treament of Crohn's disease and ulcerative colitis
Vitamin K derivatives	Used for treatment of vitamin K deficiency (especially in neonates)
Chemicals Potassium chlorate	Widely used as a weedkiller
Naphthalene	Used in mothballs
Arsine	AsH_3 encountered in extraction and refining of metal ores

Haemolysis secondary to the action of chemicals, drugs or toxins

Immune-mediated haemolysis is not the only mechanism whereby drug therapy can promote premature destruction of red cells. Free oxygen radicals and peroxides generated by the action or metabolism of a wide range of drugs can inflict severe oxidative damage on haemoglobin and red cell membrane components and lead to early cell death. Some drugs are powerful oxidizing agents in their own right, and directly inflict oxidative damage to the red cell. The drugs most commonly associated with haemolysis are shown in Table 8.1.

The bite of a number of venomous spiders and snakes can cause acute intravascular haemolysis, e.g. bites from the brown recluse spider *Loxosceles reclusa*, the king cobra *Ophiophagus hannah*, the Indian cobra *Naja naja* and the Egyptian cobra *Naja haje*. In extreme cases, even multiple honeybee (*Apis mellifera*) stings have caused acute haemolysis in children.

Haemolysis secondary to infection

A wide range of infections is associated with secondary haemolysis. By far the most common culprits are the *Plasmodia* parasites that cause malaria. Other parasitic diseases also are associated with haemolysis, e.g. toxoplasmosis, trypanosomiasis, leishmaniasis and babesiosis.

Oroya fever is caused by infection with *Bartonella bacilliformis*. The infection is transmitted by the bite of the *Phlebotomus* sandfly and is found most commonly in Peru and surrounding countries. The acute phase of the disease is frequently accompanied by severe, acute extravascular haemolysis.

Infections with the anaerobic bacterium *Clostridium perfringens* are most commonly seen in poorly treated or contaminated wounds. This organism secretes a substance called phospholipase C that causes severe, acute intravascular haemolysis, which commonly results in death.

Haemolysis secondary to physical damage

Haemolysis secondary to physical damage to red cells is characterized by the presence of fragmented red cells (**schistocytes**), in the peripheral blood. Physical damage may be inflicted by abnormalities within the circulatory system or by external changes such as thermal injury or repeated physical trauma.

The classical cause of haemolysis secondary to physical damage to red cells occurs in a minority of patients who have undergone surgery to replace diseased aortic or mitral valves. In most cases, haemolysis is associated with extreme turbulence due to regurgitation of blood around an improperly fitted or faulty prosthesis. Local shear stresses in such circumstances may be sufficient to tear the red cell apart, resulting in intravascular haemolysis. The presence of non-physiological material in the prosthesis is almost certainly an important contributor to the promotion of red cell fragmentation. Recent improvements in surgical technique and the design of implants have made this form of haemolysis much less common.

Disorders of the microvasculature are frequently associated with intravascular deposition of fibrin, thrombocytopenia and intravascular haemolysis secondary to physical trauma. This clinical syndrome is termed **microangiopathic haemolytic anaemia** and encompasses a number of important disease states including **haemolytic uraemic syndrome (HUS)**, **thrombotic thrombocytopenic purpura (TTP)**, **disseminated intravascular coagulation (DIC)** and **eclampsia of pregnancy**. These disorders are described in Chapter 18. All are characterized by the deposition of fibrin within the microvasculature which acts like a cheese-wire, 'slicing' passing red cells to form schistocytes.

Prolonged and repeated physical trauma, especially to the hands and feet, can cause transient intravascular haemolysis. This condition was first described following prolonged marching and was termed **march haemoglobinuria**. The haemolysis results from the crushing action on red cells in surface capillaries caused by repeatedly striking a hard surface. March haemoglobinuria has also been described in long distance runners, in bongo drum players and in karate practitioners.

Severe and extensive burns are frequently accompanied by intravascular haemolysis induced by thermal injury to the red cells. Subjecting red cells to temperatures above 49°C, even for relatively short periods, causes irreversible denaturation of spectrin and membrane disruption. In most cases, the haemolysis is acute and self-limiting, resolving within 48 h of the initial injury. The intravascular haemolysis is made worse by the sequestration of minimally heat-damaged red cells in the spleen.

Pathophysiology of haemolytic disorders

The signs and symptoms produced by the various haemolytic disorders are very similar. A haemolytic state is defined by the presence of a shortened red cell lifespan and a compensatory increase in the rate of erythropoiesis. These two features are responsible for the characteristic physiological changes that permit the recognition of haemolytic disorders on clinical grounds:

- **Anaemia** frequently is absent because of the compensatory increase in the rate of erythropoiesis. Severe, decompensated haemolysis can lead to severe anaemia, particularly where folate deficiency also is present.
- **Jaundice.** Haemolysis is accompanied by increased breakdown of the liberated haem. The primary breakdown product, **bilirubin**, is a bright yellow pigment and is responsible for the characteristic yellow discolouration of jaundice.
- **Pigment gallstones** are composed of precipitated bilirubin crystals and are found in relatively young people with chronic congenital haemolysis.
- **Splenomegaly** is a common feature of haemolysis but typically is slight. Marked splenomegaly may indicate the presence of an underlying condition such as lymphoma as the cause of the haemolysis.
- **Haemoglobinuria.** The passage of dark red or even black urine is strongly indicative of intravascular haemolysis.
- **Intractable leg ulcers** are relatively common in chronic haemolytic states such as HS and sickle cell disease.
- **Aplastic crisis.** Acute arrest of erythropoiesis accompanied by a dramatic fall in circulating red cell count following parvovirus infection is associated with chronic haemolytic disorders such as HS.
- **Growth retardation and delayed puberty** are seen in association with severe congenital haemolytic disorders such as homozygous β thalassaemia.

The form of bilirubin that predominates in haemolytic jaundice is unconjugated and circulates tightly bound to albumin. Because unconjugated bilirubin is not excreted into the urine, an increase in this form of bilirubin leads to jaundice but no increase in bilirubin excretion in urine, i.e. *acholuric jaundice*.

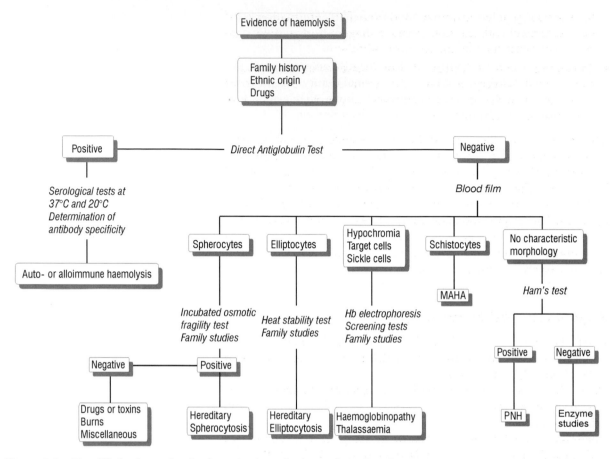

Figure 8.1 *Simplified schema for the investigation of a haemolytic disorder*

- **Hypertrophic skeletal changes** due to expansion of erythropoietic marrow are only seen in severe congenital haemolytic disorders.

Once a haemolytic disorder is suspected on clinical grounds, further enquiry may provide useful indicators of the mechanism or cause of the haemolysis:

- **Family history**. If the disorder is present in other family members, especially if several generations are involved, a hereditary condition may be suspected. Construction of a pedigree chart can sometimes provide information about the possible mode of inheritance of the disorder.

- **Ethnic origin**. Some inherited haemolytic disorders are associated with particular ethnic groups. For example, G-6-PD deficiency is most common in Mediterranean and Chinese populations. However, such associations cannot be used to *exclude* any possible cause of haemolysis.

- **Patient history**. Neonatal jaundice may be indicative of congenital conditions such as HS or G-6-PD deficiency whereas a late age of onset suggests an acquired condition. This information must be interpreted with caution because diagnosis of a mild congenital disorder may be missed until adulthood.

- **Triggering events.** A history of drug ingestion, infection, exposure to cold, surgery or some other event which appears to be associated with the onset of haemolysis may provide evidence of the cause of an acquired condition.

Clinical findings seldom are sufficient to enable a definitive diagnosis of a particular haemolytic condition to be made; laboratory investigation plays a central role in the accurate diagnosis of haemolysis. The various laboratory features of the different haemolytic disorders can all be grouped under two headings: signs of increased haemolysis and signs of an increased rate of erythropoiesis. A detailed consideration of the laboratory investigation of haemolysis is beyond the scope of this book, but a summary of a typical schema is shown in Figure 8.1.

Suggested further reading

Bossi, D. and Russo, M. (1996). Hemolytic anemias due to disorders of red cell membrane skeleton. *Molecular Aspects of Medicine* **17**(2), 171–188.

Dacie, J.V. (1992). *The Haemolytic Anaemias. Volume 3: The Auto-immune Haemolytic Anaemias.* Edinburgh: Churchill Livingstone.

Delaunay, J. (1995). Genetic disorders of the red cell membrane. *Critical Reviews in Oncology/Hematology* **19**(2), 79–110.

Delaunay, J., Alloisio, N., Morle, L. *et al.* (1996). Molecular genetics of hereditary elliptocytosis and hereditary spherocytosis. *Annales de Genetique* **39**(4), 209–221.

Iolascon, A., delGiudice, E.M., Perrotta, S. *et al.* (1998). Hereditary spherocytosis: from clinical to molecular defects. *Haematologica* **83**(3), 240–257.

Mollison, P.L., Engelfriet, C.P. and Contreras, M. (1997). *Blood Transfusion in Clinical Medicine.* Oxford: Blackwell Science.

Self-assessment questions

1. Define the terms **haemolytic disorder, haemolytic anaemia** and **haemolytic component.**
2. Why is splenectomy an effective measure in hereditary spherocytosis? Does this manoeuvre constitute a cure?
3. Name the four major forms of hereditary elliptocytosis.
4. What is the reason for progressive erythrocyte water depletion in hereditary xerocytosis?
5. Outline the mechanism of haemolysis in paroxysmal cold haemoglobinuria.

6. Why is IgG anti-D routinely administered to all Rh negative mothers immediately following delivery?
7. Outline the three mechanisms involved in drug-induced immune-mediated haemolysis.

Key Concepts and Facts

- Any condition that leads to a reduction in the mean lifespan of the red cell is a haemolytic disorder.

- If the increased haemolysis is not compensated by a balancing increase in the rate of erythropoiesis a haemolytic anaemia ensues.

- Many haematological conditions due to other causes have a haemolytic component.

- Hereditary spherocytosis (HS) is the most common of the inherited primary red cell membrane abnormalities.

- HS is caused by a deficiency or defect of the cytoskeletal proteins spectrin, band 4.1 or ankyrin.

- The major site of haemolysis in HS is the spleen.

- Hereditary elliptocytosis (HE) can be divided into four major forms: common HE, HE with infantile poikilocytosis, HE with spherocytosis and HE with stomatocytosis.

- A wide range of cytoskeletal defects has been described in HE, but the most common are structural abnormalities of spectrin.

- Hereditary pyropoikilocytosis, hereditary stomatocytosis and hereditary xerocytosis are all inherited primary red cell membrane disorders.

- The autoimmune haemolytic anaemias (AIHAs) can be divided into three types: warm AIHA, cold AIHA and drug-induced AIHA.

- Alloimmune haemolysis results from immunization to transplanted foreign antigen or the reaction of foreign antibody to normal host antigen and is manifest as haemolytic transfusion reactions or haemolytic disease of the newborn.

- Treatment with a wide range of drugs can stimulate immune haemolysis by one of three mechanisms: penicillin-type, α-methyldopa-type and rifampicin-type or 'innocent bystander' immune haemolysis.

- Haemolysis can also be triggered by a wide range of chemicals, drugs, toxins, infections or direct physical damage.

Chapter 9
Red cell metabolism

Learning objectives

After studying this chapter you should confidently be able to:

Describe the requirements for energy and reducing power in mature red cells.

Differentiate between the primary functions of the Embden–Meyerhof pathway, hexose monophosphate pathway and glutathione cycle.

Describe the physiological importance of the Rappaport–Luebering shunt.

Explain how the net effect of the Embden–Meyerhof pathway is the production of 2 moles of ATP per mole of glucose metabolized.

As red cells mature they lose their nucleus, mitochondria and ribosomes. Absence of the nucleus and ribosomes makes the mature red cell incapable of protein synthesis and the lack of mitochondria deprives the cell of the most efficient means of energy production, oxidative phosphorylation. The cell is thus entirely dependent upon the relatively inefficient mechanism of anaerobic glycolysis via the **Embden–Meyerhof pathway** (Figure 9.1) to provide its energy requirement. Protection of the red cell against oxidative stresses is provided mainly via the **hexose monophosphate pathway** (Figure 9.1). Because of the dependence of the red cell upon the proper functioning of these two pathways, defects in the enzymes which catalyse them can be catastrophic.

The glucose that is used by the red cell in the two glycolytic pathways is derived from plasma via a specific transport protein in the red cell membrane. Normally, about 95% of red cell glucose is metabolized via the Embden–Meyerhof pathway while the remainder enters the hexose monophosphate pathway.

The Embden–Meyerhof pathway

The primary role of the Embden–Meyerhof pathway in the economy of the mature red cell is the generation of ATP.

The ability of cells to extract energy anaerobically from glucose in the form of ATP represents an extremely important survival mechanism. Anaerobic glycolysis can provide a short-term energy reserve for vital organs when oxygen supply is cut off and aerobic glycolysis ceases. For example, at birth, changes in the foetal blood circulation temporarily starve all of the major organs except the brain of oxygenated blood. During this period, the energy demands of the foetal organs are met via anaerobic glycolysis. In other words, if anaerobic glycolysis did not exist, nor could we!

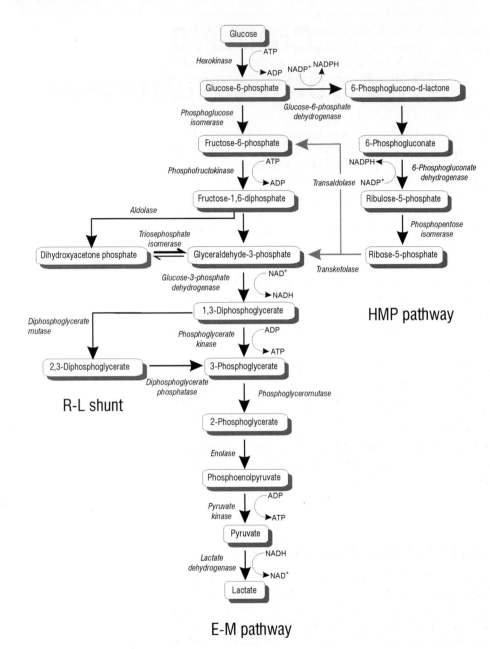

Figure 9.1 *Glycolytic pathways within the mature red cell*

Large quantities of energy are released from ATP during its conversion to ADP. Thus, ATP can be thought of as an energy store for use by the cell. The Embden–Meyerhof pathway is also a source of nicotinamide adenine dinucleotide (NADH) which acts as a cofactor for the enzyme methaemoglobin reductase in the conversion of methaemoglobin to functional haemoglobin.

2,3-Diphosphoglycerate (2,3-DPG) is formed via a diversion from the main pathway known as the **Rappaport–Luebering shunt** (Figure 9.1). This molecule functions to increase oxygen delivery to the tissues by altering the oxygen affinity of haemoglobin as described in Chapter 5. There are three main requirements for energy within normal red cells:

- **Maintenance of intracellular cation balance.** The intracellular concentrations of Na^+ and K^+ differ markedly from those of the surrounding plasma. This difference is maintained by an active process, which pumps Na^+ from the cell into the plasma and K^+ into the cell from the plasma. The energy required to drive this process is provided via the conversion of ATP to ADP by a membrane-bound ATPase. Failure of the cation pump results in rapid loss of K^+ and water and leads to the premature death of the red cell.

- **Maintenance of cell shape.** Maintenance of the characteristic biconcave shape and deformability of the red cell is an energy-consuming process. Failure of energy production results in loss of deformability and shape changes, which shorten the lifespan of the cell.

- **Phosphorylation of glucose and fructose-6-phosphate.** The early stages of the Embden–Meyerhof pathway involve the phosphorylation of glucose to glucose-6-phosphate and fructose-6-phosphate to fructose-1,6-diphosphate. Failure of these steps results in failure of the pathway and a consequent reduction in ATP synthesis. Low levels of ATP lead to failure of these early phosphorylation steps, thus establishing a vicious circle which culminates in the death of the cell.

Reaction steps of the Embden–Meyerhof pathway

The first reaction of the Embden–Meyerhof pathway involves the **phosphorylation** of glucose to form glucose-6-phosphate (G-6-P). This reaction consumes a mole of ATP for every mole of glucose phosphorylated and is catalysed by the enzyme hexokinase in the presence of divalent metal ions such as Mg^{2+}. The catalytic action of hexokinase is inhibited by the product of the reaction, G-6-P, thus providing an important control mechanism on the rate of glycolysis. An important effect of this reaction is to 'lock' the intermediates of glycolysis within the red cell: the red cell membrane is impermeable to phosphorylated sugars.

G-6-P is subsequently converted to fructose-6-phosphate (F-6-P) in a reaction called an **isomerization**. This reaction is catalysed by the enzyme phosphoglucose isomerase.

F-6-P is further phosphorylated, again at the expense of ATP, to form fructose-1,6-diphosphate (F-1,6-DP), a reaction catalysed by

Strictly speaking, phosphorylated intermediates such as fructose-1,6-diphosphate (F-1,6-DP) and 2,3-diphosphoglycerate (2,3-DPG) should be called fructose-1,6-bisphosphate (F-1,6-BP) and 2,3-bisphosphoglycerate (2,3-BPG) because the two phosphate groups are located on separate carbon atoms. However, the abbreviations F-1,6-DP and 2,3-DPG have been used so extensively that to replace them with the correct forms would be confusing. The diphosphate nomenclature has therefore been retained in this book.

the enzyme phosphofructokinase. High levels of ATP inhibit the catalytic function of phosphofructokinase. Thus, in the presence of adequate levels of ATP, glycolysis is inhibited and, conversely, when the supply of energy falls, glycolysis is stimulated. This mechanism provides the most important regulator of the rate of glycolysis.

The **cleavage** of F-1,6-DP into dihydroxyacetone phosphate and glyceraldehyde-3-phosphate (G-3-P) is catalysed by the enzyme aldolase. These two products are isomers and are interconvertible under the influence of the enzyme triose phosphate isomerase. Because G-3-P is constantly consumed in the next step of the pathway, the dynamic equilibrium that exists between dihydroxyacetone phosphate and G-3-P is shifted to the right. Thus, in effect, 1 mole of F-1,6-DP is cleaved to form 2 moles of G-3-P.

The next reaction involves the conversion of G-3-P to 1,3-diphosphoglycerate (1,3-DPG). This reaction is catalysed by the enzyme glyceraldehyde-3-phosphate dehydrogenase and also results in the formation of NADH.

At this stage of the Embden–Meyerhof pathway, 2 moles of ATP have been consumed and none generated. However, everything is now in place to commence production of ATP. 1,3-DPG has a high potential to donate one of its phosphoryl groups to ADP thus forming 3-phosphoglycerate (3-PG) and ATP. This reaction is catalysed by the enzyme phosphoglycerate kinase. However, remember that 1 mole of glucose has been converted into 2 moles of 1,3-DPG. Thus, for each mole of glucose that enters the Embden–Meyerhof pathway, 2 moles of ATP are generated by this reaction. This balances the energy equation of the pathway: 2 moles of ATP have been expended and 2 moles have been generated.

The final stages of the Embden–Meyerhof pathway are designed to generate a further 2 moles of ATP in the conversion of 3-PG to lactate. This outcome requires the synthesis of a molecule which, like 1,3-DPG, has a high phosphoryl group transfer potential. The first step towards achieving this goal occurs under the influence of the enzyme phosphoglyceromutase and involves the rearrangement of 3-PG to form 2-phosphoglycerate (2-PG). 2-PG is converted into phosphoenolpyruvate (PEP) in the presence of the enzyme enolase. Enol phosphates such as PEP have a high phosphoryl group transfer potential. In the presence of the enzyme pyruvate kinase, PEP donates its phosphoryl group to ADP, resulting in the formation of 2 moles of ATP and 2 moles of pyruvate per mole of glucose metabolized. Thus, although 2 moles of ATP have been consumed by the early reactions of the Embden–Meyerhof pathway, 4 moles of ATP are generated by subsequent reactions, resulting in a net gain of 2 moles of ATP per mole of glucose metabolized. Pyruvate is subsequently converted into lactate under the influence of the enzyme lactate dehydrogenase.

The Rappaport–Luebering shunt

1,3-DPG, in addition to its direct conversion to 3-PG, can be converted in the presence of the enzyme diphosphoglycerate mutase into 2,3-diphosphoglycerate (2,3-DPG). This diversion from the main Embden–Meyerhof pathway is called the Rappaport–Luebering shunt and is of prime physiological importance because of the role that 2,3-DPG plays in controlling the oxygen affinity of haemoglobin. The unique role of 2,3-DPG in red cells is underlined by its high concentration within these cells. Most other cells of the body contain only traces of the substance.

   2,3-DPG can be converted to 3-PG under the influence of the enzyme 2,3-diphosphoglycerate phosphatase, thus completing the shunt. However, the coproduct of this reaction is free phosphate rather than ATP.

The hexose monophosphate pathway

The hexose monophosphate pathway generates reducing potential for the red cell in the form of nicotinamide adenine dinucleotide phosphate (NADPH) which is an essential component of the glutathione cycle as shown in Figure 9.2. Reduced glutathione (GSH) is the most important antioxidant within red cells. Under normal circumstances, hexose monophosphate pathway activity consumes about 5% of the glucose-6-phosphate formed as the first step of glycolysis. However, the rate of activity can be increased when required to deal with an increased level of oxidants.

   Reducing power is required by the red cell for three main reasons:

- **Combating membrane lipid oxidation.** Oxidation and peroxidation of membrane lipids would cause an increase in membrane rigidity and permeability and so render the red cell liable to destruction in the spleen.

- **Reduction of methaemoglobin.** Oxidation of the ferrous (Fe^{2+}) ion in haem to the ferric (Fe^{3+}) form results in the formation of methaemoglobin, which is incapable of oxygen transport. Small quantities of methaemoglobin are constantly formed within the red cell. It is essential that accumulation of methaemoglobin is prevented by its rapid reduction to functional haemoglobin.

- **Detoxification of oxidants.** In the process of methaemoglobin formation, highly reactive oxygen radicals such as superoxide and hydroxyl radical are formed which lead to the generation of the powerful oxidant, hydrogen peroxide. Ingestion of oxidant drugs such as primaquine also results in the formation of hydrogen peroxide. Detoxification of these substances via the glutathione cycle is essential if severe oxidant damage to the cell is to be avoided.

Enzymes are classified into six major classes, each with several subclasses.

Class 1: Oxidoreductases catalyse redox reactions and include **dehydrogenases**, **oxidases** and **peroxidases**.

Class 2: Transferases catalyse the transfer of functional groups such as amino groups (**aminotransferases**) and phosphoryl groups (**kinases**).

Class 3: Hydrolases catalyse the transfer of functional groups to water and include **peptidases**, **esterases** and **deaminases**.

Class 4: Lyases catalyse the addition or removal of the elements of water, ammonia or carbon dioxide and include the **decarboxylases** and the **dehydratases**.

Class 5: Isomerases catalyse isomerization reactions and include the **epimerases**, the **racemases** and the **mutases**.

Class 6: Ligases catalyse synthetic reactions where two molecules are joined together and include the **synthetases** and **carboxylases**.

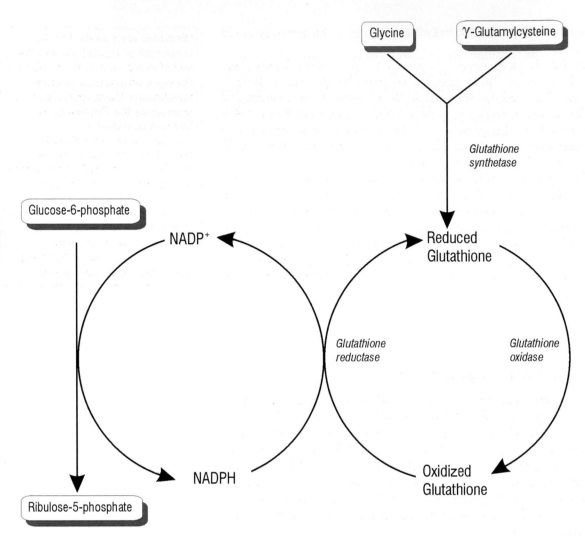

Figure 9.2 *The glutathione cycle*

Reaction steps of the hexose monophosphate pathway

The first reaction of the hexose monophosphate pathway involves the **dehydrogenation** of G-6-P to form 6-phosphogluconate (6-PG) via an intermediate called 6-phosphoglucono-δ-lactone. The conversion of G-6-P into 6-phosphoglucono-δ-lactone is the rate-determining step of the hexose monophosphate pathway and is catalysed by the enzyme glucose-6-phosphate dehydrogenase (G-6-PD). This reaction is accompanied by the generation of NADPH.

6-PG is then **decarboxylated** in the presence of the enzyme 6-phosphogluconate dehydrogenase to form ribulose-5-phosphate (Ru-5-P) and, in the process, another mole of NADPH is formed. Thus, for each mole of glucose that enters the hexose monophosphate pathway, 2 moles of NADPH are generated. NADPH formation is the physiologically relevant role of this pathway in red cells.

Ru-5-P is subsequently converted into ribose-5-phosphate (R-5-P) under the influence of the enzyme phosphopentose isomerase. R-5-P is used by other cells in the synthesis of nucleotides and nucleic acids. In red cells, however, R-5-P is converted into F-6-P and G-3-P in the presence of the enzymes transaldolase and transketolase respectively. These substances are then metabolized via the Embden–Meyerhof pathway.

The conversion of G-6-P to R-5-P constantly consumes $NADP^+$ and generates NADPH. The NADPH thus formed acts as a reducing agent in the reduction of oxidized glutathione (GSSG) in the presence of the enzyme glutathione reductase. In this process, $NADP^+$ is formed which is then utilized in the generation of more R-5-P. Reduced glutathione (GSH) is required for the detoxification of oxidants as described above. In this process, GSH is cycled back to GSSG.

> Otto Meyerhof worked at the University of Heidelberg and was awarded a Nobel Prize in 1922 for his work on anaerobic muscle metabolism. Gustav Embden was Director of the Physiological Institute at Frankfurt Sachsenhausen and shared Meyerhof's interest in muscle metabolism, although the two men did not collaborate. The full Embden–Meyerhof pathway was not elucidated until 1949, 16 years after Embden's premature death. Rappaport and Luebering described the mode of 2,3-DPG formation the following year.

The purine salvage pathway

Red cells are incapable of *de novo* synthesis of purines because the enzyme 5′-phosphoribosyl-1-pyrophosphate (PRPP) amidotransferase is absent. However, an active purine salvage pathway exists which can generate ATP from preformed bases. Adenine can penetrate red cells where, in the presence of PRPP and the enzyme adenine phosphoribosyl transferase, it is converted to adenosine monophosphate (AMP). AMP can then be phosphorylated to form first ADP and then ATP in the presence of the enzyme adenylate kinase.

The existence of the purine salvage pathway in red cells is exploited in the storage of blood for transfusion. The addition of adenine to the storage medium provides a supplementary source of fuel for ATP synthesis and so prolongs the useful life of the stored red cells. However, purine salvage is of doubtful physiological significance.

Suggested further reading

Devlin, T.M. (ed.) (1992). *Textbook of Biochemistry with Clinical Correlations* 3rd edn. New York: Wiley-Liss.

Gilham, B., Papachristodoulou, D.K. and Thomas, J.H. (1997). *Wills' Biochemical Basis of Medicine* 3rd edn. Oxford: Butterworth-Heinemann.

Self-assessment questions

1. Why are mature red cells particularly vulnerable to disorders of their glycolytic enzymes?
2. Why are red cells unable to derive energy via oxidative phosphorylation?
3. What chemical reaction is responsible for the liberation of energy in red cells?
4. Why do red cells require energy?
5. Why is 2,3-DPG physiologically important?
6. Why do red cells require reducing power?

Key Concepts and Facts

- Mature red cells normally contain no nucleus, mitochondria or ribosomes and so are incapable of protein synthesis or energy production via oxidative phosphorylation.

- Red cell energy production is accomplished by anaerobic glycolysis via the Embden–Meyerhof pathway.

- The red cell needs energy to maintain its shape, intracellular cation balance and to drive the early stages of anaerobic glycolysis.

- Each mole of glucose metabolized via the Embden–Meyerhof pathway results in the net production of 2 moles of ATP.

- 2,3-DPG is synthesized via the Rappaport–Luebering shunt and plays a major role in modulating the oxygen affinity of haemoglobin A.

- Reducing power is provided primarily via the hexose monophosphate pathway.

- The red cell requires a reducing capacity to combat oxidation of membrane lipids, for reduction of Fe^{3+} to Fe^{2+} in haem and for detoxification of oxidants.

- Normally, about 95% of glucose is metabolized via the Embden–Meyerhof pathway and the remainder via the hexose monophosphate pathway.

- A purine salvage pathway exists in red cells but is probably of limited physiological significance.

Chapter 10

The red cell enzymopathies

Learning objectives

After studying this chapter you should confidently be able to:

Name the most common defects of the Embden–Meyerhof and hexose monophosphate pathways.

Explain the importance of the Rappaport–Luebering shunt in determining the clinical severity of defects of the Embden–Meyerhof pathway.

Outline the pathophysiology of pyruvate kinase deficiency.

Differentiate clearly between the G-6-PD variants Gd^{A+}, Gd^{A-} and Gd^{B}.

List some common triggers of acute haemolysis in G-6-PD deficiency.

Explain the phenomenon of episodic haemolysis in G-6-PD deficiency.

The mature red cell has lost its nucleus and mitochondria and so depends almost completely upon glycolysis via the Embden–Meyerhof pathway for the fulfilment of its energy requirement and on the hexose monophosphate pathway for its reducing power. Thus, a defect or a deficiency of any of the enzymes which catalyse these pathways can have serious deleterious effects on the overall economy of the cell and may lead to a shortening of red cell lifespan. By common agreement, the definition of an enzyme deficiency relates to suboptimal activity of the enzyme, both quantitative and qualitative enzyme disorders are encompassed by this term.

Disorders of the Embden–Meyerhof pathway

Failure of the Embden–Meyerhof pathway is associated with deficiency of ATP within the red cell and a consequent collapse of energy-dependent processes such as cation pump activity. The

Red cell disorders that are characterized by an enzyme deficiency are known as the *red cell enzymopathies*. This name is derived from the Greek word for disease – *pathos*. Thus, enzymopathies are disorders of enzymes. Similarly, the disorders that are characterized by abnormal haemoglobin synthesis are known as the *haemoglobinopathies*. Learning the meaning of word fragments like this is a useful way of working out what haematological terms mean.

Congenital means present at birth. Congenital conditions are not necessarily inherited and inherited conditions are not necessarily congenital. For example, spina bifida is present at birth but is not inherited and Huntington's chorea is an autosomal dominant inherited disorder that usually does not appear until middle age.

result, in most cases, is a shortening of red cell lifespan. Defects of the Embden–Meyerhof pathway are manifest as a **congenital non-spherocytic haemolytic anaemia (CNSHA)** of highly variable severity. This clinical heterogeneity arises partly because of the great variety of mutations that are encountered but, as explained later in this chapter, it is also related to the position of the affected enzyme relative to the Rappaport–Luebering shunt.

Abnormalities of all of the enzymes of the Embden–Meyerhof pathway have been described, although most are extremely rare. The most common defect, pyruvate kinase deficiency, accounts for more than 90% of cases of glycolytic enzyme deficiency that are associated with haemolysis.

Pyruvate kinase deficiency

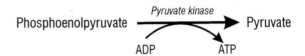

Pyruvate kinase (PK) catalyses the conversion of phosphoenol pyruvate (PEP) to pyruvate and exists in several isoenzyme forms in different tissues of the body. Because of this, a deficiency of red cell PK is not reflected in white cells and platelets. PK deficiency is inherited as an autosomal recessive trait, being expressed only in homozygotes and compound heterozygotes. Many different mutant forms of PK exist: most individuals who express disease are compound heterozygotes for two different variant enzymes. It is this genetic heterogeneity which is the major determinant of the clinical variability of this disorder.

Pyruvate kinase deficiency was first recognized in 1960 by Dr William Valentine and colleagues at the University of California in Los Angeles. Detailed investigation of several families with congenital non-spherocytic haemolytic anaemia pointed to a deficiency of this enzyme as the most likely cause of their condition. Amazingly, the original paper describing this important discovery was submitted for publication in *Science* but was rejected as being of limited interest!

Pathophysiology

The clinical severity of pyruvate kinase deficiency is highly variable, ranging from a severe CNSHA to a clinically silent, compensated form. In most cases, there is a moderate reduction in haemoglobin concentration to 6–10 g/dl. The haemoglobin concentration is usually stable but can fall suddenly during an infection. Some degree of jaundice and splenomegaly is usually present. Neonatal jaundice is relatively common and, occasionally, may be severe enough to require an exchange transfusion. The continuous presence of excess bilirubin in the plasma can result in the formation of pigment gallstones at a relatively young age. In common with other chronic haemolytic conditions, there is an increased incidence of folate deficiency in affected individuals.

Although most individuals with PK deficiency are moderately anaemic, clinical symptoms of anaemia may be minimal or absent.

This anomaly is explained by the position of PK in the Embden–Meyerhof pathway. Deficiency of PK causes an accumulation of PEP and other intermediates from higher up the E-M pathway. Most importantly, the concentration of red cell 2,3-DPG may treble. As explained in Chapter 5, 2,3-DPG binds to β globin chains, thereby stabilizing the haemoglobin A molecule in the low oxygen affinity configuration. Thus, although the haemoglobin concentration is reduced in PK deficiency, the capacity for oxygen delivery to the tissues is increased and the effects of the anaemia are minimized. There have been a number of reports of PK deficient individuals with haemoglobin concentrations of 8 g/dl or less who regularly indulge in middle distance running!

There are no characteristic features of red cell morphology associated with pyruvate kinase deficiency. Moderate reticulocytosis is usually present and irregularly contracted red cells (pyknocytes) may be seen, but these are not diagnostic. The severity of the anaemia is diminished by splenectomy.

> Splenomegaly means an enlarged spleen and is a relatively common finding in haematological disease. Similarly, hepatomegaly means enlargement of the liver and hepatosplenomegaly means enlargement of both.

Hexokinase deficiency

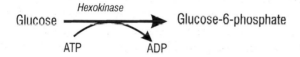

Hexokinase catalyses the phosphorylation of glucose to form glucose-6-phosphate (G-6-P) in the presence of divalent metal ions such as Mg^{2+}. The inhibition of hexokinase activity by the product of this reaction provides an important mechanism for the control of the rate of glycolysis. Hexokinase deficiency has no clinically significant effect on platelet or white cell function. Hexokinase activity diminishes rapidly with increasing red cell age. This phenomenon leads to a reduction in glycolytic activity and a relative lack of ATP within senescent red cells and contributes to their demise.

Hexokinase deficiency is extremely rare but most reported cases have shown an autosomal recessive mode of inheritance. Occasional examples of autosomal dominant inheritance have also been reported.

The sequelae of hexokinase deficiency are similar to those for PK deficiency in most respects. However, because hexokinase acts above the Rappaport–Luebering shunt, deficiency leads to an increased haemoglobin oxygen affinity due to lack of 2,3-DPG. This is manifest as severe symptoms of anaemia in the presence of a moderately reduced haemoglobin concentration.

Disorders of the hexose monophosphate pathway

Defects of the hexose monophosphate pathway result in an increased susceptibility of the red cell to oxidant stress. All are rare except deficiency of glucose-6-phosphate dehydrogenase (G-6-PD) which is by far the most common red cell enzymopathy, affecting almost 1% of the world's population.

Glucose-6-phosphate dehydrogenase deficiency

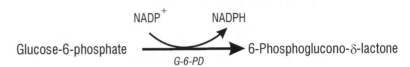

G-6-PD catalyses the dehydrogenation of glucose-6-phosphate (G-6-P) to form 6-phosphoglucono-δ-lactone with the simultaneous reduction of nicotinamide adenine dinucleotide phosphate (NADP) to form reduced nicotinamide adenine dinucleotide phosphate (NADPH). Deficiency of G-6-PD has been reported in most populations of the world but is most commonly seen in Western and Central Africa, the Mediterranean region, the Middle East and South-East Asia. For example, in some parts of Saudi Arabia, almost one-third of the population carry an abnormal G-6-PD gene. In common with thalassaemia and sickle cell disease, G-6-PD deficiency is associated with malarial areas because female carriers have increased resistance to malarial infection.

The gene that encodes G-6-PD is located on the tip of the q arm of the X chromosome, close to the factor VIII gene. The normal form of G-6-PD is designated G-6-PDB or Gd^B and the normal gene is denoted Gd^B. This form of G-6-PD is present in 99% of Caucasians and in about 70% of blacks. A functionally normal variant G-6-PD isoenzyme, Gd^A, is found in about 20% of blacks.

G-6-PD deficiency results from the synthesis of structurally abnormal enzyme variants that have impaired stability or catalytic activity. More than 350 different G-6-PD variants have been described but only a few are associated with clinically severe disease. The most common variant of G-6-PD is found in about 10% of blacks and is designated Gd^{A-}. All other abnormal G-6-PD variants are designated by their area of greatest incidence, e.g. Gd^{MED} is most prevalent in the Mediterranean region, India and South-East Asia while Gd^{CANTON} is most prevalent in Chinese populations.

G-6-PD deficiency is inherited in a sex-linked recessive manner, i.e. it is transmitted by symptomless female heterozygotes to affected male **hemizygotes**. Because of the relatively high incidence

The widespread use of antimalarial prophylactic drugs in US soldiers in World War II led to the observation that pamaquine triggered an acute and severe, but self-limited haemolytic anaemia in about one in ten blacks. US military-funded studies of a group of 'volunteers' from the Stateville Penitentiary, Illinois showed that this phenomenon was caused by an intracellular red cell defect. However, it was not until 1956 that Dr Paul Carson and colleagues traced this form of drug-induced haemolysis to a deficiency of G-6-PD.

The self-limited nature of the haemolysis is explained by the higher concentration of G-6-PD present in reticulocytes. The marked reticulocyte response that follows the primary haemolytic episode effectively raises the circulating G-6-PD level and thereby reduces the sensitivity of the circulating red cells to oxidant stress.

of aberrant genes in some populations, female homozygotes are not uncommon.

Pathophysiology

The red cell is protected from oxidative damage by the constant regeneration of reduced glutathione (GSH) via the glutathione cycle. The hexose monophosphate pathway provides the continuous supply of NADPH required to drive the glutathione cycle. Thus, red cells that are deficient in G-6-PD develop a secondary deficiency of GSH and are highly susceptible to oxidative damage. This can lead to a reduction in red cell lifespan in three ways:

- Cross-linking and aggregation of membrane cytoskeletal proteins causes a decrease in red cell deformability thereby promoting sequestration in the liver and spleen.
- Peroxidation of membrane lipids also causes a loss of deformability and intravascular haemolysis.
- Oxidation of thiol and other groups in globin chains leads to the aggregation and precipitation of denatured globin within the cell, forming **Heinz bodies**. These inclusion bodies bind to the inner aspect of the red cell membrane and are 'pitted' from the cell during its passage through the spleen, resulting in the formation of 'bite' cells and premature haemolysis.

Despite the large number of G-6-PD variants, individuals with G-6-PD deficiency typically exhibit one of two patterns of haemolysis: chronic non spherocytic haemolytic anaemia (CNSHA) or episodic haemolysis.

Chronic non-spherocytic haemolytic anaemia

CNSHA is associated with extremely unstable or severely dysfunctional G-6-PD variants. A large number of such variants exist but all are rare; many have only been described in a single family. This form of G-6-PD deficiency presents as lifelong haemolytic anaemia of variable severity which does not respond to splenectomy. The condition may be complicated by sporadic haemolytic or aplastic crises, which may be triggered by infection or ingestion of oxidant drugs.

Episodic haemolysis

The most common G-6-PD variants are characterized by episodes of acute haemolysis induced by increased oxidant stress. In the vast majority of cases of G-6-PD deficiency, red cell enzyme activity is sufficient to combat the oxidative stresses imposed by everyday life and red cell survival is almost normal. However, exposure to increased oxidant stress exposes the inability of the red cell to respond by increasing hexose monophosphate pathway activity and leads to acute intravascular haemolysis. Broadly speaking, three

Heinz bodies appear on Romanowsky stained blood films as small, purple, irregular bodies in the cytoplasm of red cells. They are seen in cases of G-6-PD deficiency, particularly after the administration of oxidant drugs such as primaquine, in the presence of unstable haemoglobin variants such as Hb Hammersmith and after removal of the spleen (splenectomy).

Heinz bodies are named after Dr R. Heinz, who was director of the Institute of Pharmacology at Erlanger, as he described the appearance of these inclusion bodies in guinea-pig blood following the administration of acetylphenylhydrazine. Heinz bodies are removed during passage of the red cell through the spleen. This process damages the red cell and leads to the formation of red cells that appear on the blood film to have been nibbled by mice! These are known as 'bite' cells.

Table 10.1   *Drugs commonly implicated as triggers of acute haemolysis in G-6-PD deficiency*

Drug family	Drug examples	Uses
Antimalarials	Chloroquine	Malaria prophylaxis and treatment
	Mefloquine	Malaria prophylaxis
	Amodiaquine	Malaria treatment
	Primaquine	Malaria prophylaxis and treatment
Sulphonamides and sulphones*	Sulphamethoxazole	Antibacterial (bladder and some GI infections)
	Sulphasalazine	Ulcerative colitis, Crohn's disease
	Cotrimoxazole	Antibacterial (urinary, respiratory, otitis media)
	Dapsone	Leprosy, dermatitis herpetiformis
Cardiovascular	Procainamide	Anti-arrhythmic
	Quinidine	Anti-arrhythmic
Cytotoxic/antibacterial	Chloramphenicol	Eye infections
	Nalidixic acid	Antibacterial (urinary tract)
	Nitrofurantoin	Antibacterial (urinary tract)
Miscellaneous	Aspirin	Non-narcotic analgesic and anti-inflammatory
	Probenicid	Gout
	α-Methyldopa	Antihypertensive
	Dimercaprol	Treatment of heavy metal poisoning
	Hydralazine	Antihypertensive
	Mestranol	Oral contraceptive
	Phenylhydrazine	Polycythaemia (no longer used)
	Vitamin K	Haemorrhagic disease of the newborn

*Most members of this group of antibacterials have been implicated as triggers of acute haemolysis in G-6-PD deficient individuals but, other than those listed, they have been superseded and are little used nowadays.

sets of triggers of acute haemolysis in G-6-PD deficient individuals have been identified:

- **Ingestion of oxidant drugs** can trigger acute intravascular haemolysis in G-6-PD deficient individuals. A wide range of drugs has been implicated as shown in Table 10.1. Most of the offending drugs are taken up by the red cell, where they mediate the transfer of electrons from intracellular reducing agents such as NADPH and GSH to molecular oxygen, thereby forming superoxide, hydrogen peroxide and hydroxyl radicals within the red cell. The inability of G-6-PD deficient red cells to detoxify these powerful oxidants leads to acute intravascular haemolysis.

- **Ingestion of the common broad bean,** *Vicia fava,* may trigger acute intravascular haemolysis in individuals with some types of G-6-PD deficiency. This form of haemolysis is known as **favism** and is associated particularly with the Gd^{MED} variant of G-6-PD. The Gd^{A-} variant is not associated with favism. The substance present in broad beans that elicits the haemolysis is thought to be **divicine**. Haemolysis is most common following ingestion of fresh, raw broad beans but has been reported following ingestion of cooked, dried and frozen beans. At least one report exists of haemolysis in a breast-fed infant following maternal ingestion of broad beans.

- **Infection** is a relatively common trigger of acute intravascular haemolysis in G-6-PD deficient individuals. Haemolysis is seen most commonly following pneumococcal infection or viral hepatitis. The exact mechanisms which trigger haemolysis remain obscure but release of oxidants from activated neutrophils, ingestion of antimicrobial drugs, hyperthermia and acidosis probably all contribute.

In the absence of acute haemolysis, the blood of a G-6-PD deficient individual appears essentially normal. During a haemolytic crisis, however, moderate anisocytosis, bite cells and occasional spherocytes are typically present. Heinz bodies may be present in acute drug-induced haemolysis or favism but are seldom seen otherwise. Methaemoglobinaemia may be present but is seldom severe.

G-6-PD deficiency is the most common cause of neonatal jaundice worldwide. Normal neonatal red cells typically have suboptimal activity of the glutathione cycle and so, when a deficiency of G-6-PD is superimposed upon this, are highly susceptible to oxidant-induced haemolysis. However, the degree of jaundice observed is frequently more severe than expected, due to the relative inability of the neonatal liver to conjugate bilirubin and, possibly, to a deficiency of hepatic G-6-PD. In some cases, the cause of acute haemolysis in a G-6-PD deficient neonate can be traced to an oxidant drug used by the mother during labour or to the use of sulphonamides to combat neonatal infection. In most cases, however, no trigger can be identified.

> *Anisocytosis* means variation in red cell size. *Poikilocytosis* means variation in red cell shape. If both phenomena are present together, the result is described as *anisopoikilocytosis*.

Suggested further reading

Arya, R., Layton, D.M. and Bellingham, A.J. (1995). Hereditary red cell enzymopathies. *Blood Reviews* **9**(3), 165–175.

Beutler, E. (1996). G6PD: Population genetics and clinical manifestations. *Blood Reviews* **10**(1), 45–52.

Jacobasch, G. and Rapoport, S.M. (1996). Hemolytic anemias due to erythrocyte enzyme deficiencies. *Molecular Aspects of Medicine* **17**(2), 143–170.

http://rialto.com/g6pd/

http://rialto.com/favism/index.htm.

Self-assessment questions

1. Name the most common enzyme defects of the Embden–Meyerhof and hexose monophosphate pathways.
2. Why is hexokinase deficiency clinically more severe than pyruvate kinase deficiency?

3. Why are the clinical manifestations of G-6-PD deficiency so variable?
4. Name the two normal variants of G-6-PD and the populations with which they are associated.
5. List three common triggers of acute haemolysis in G-6-PD deficiency.
6. What is favism?

Key Concepts and Facts

- A defect or deficiency of any of the enzymes of the Embden–Meyerhof or hexose monophosphate pathways can lead to a shortening of red cell lifespan.

- Defects of the Embden–Meyerhof pathway are manifest as a congenital non-spherocytic haemolytic anaemia (CNSHA) of highly variable severity. This clinical heterogeneity is related to the position of the affected enzyme relative to the Rappaport–Luebering shunt.

- The most common defect of the Embden–Meyerhof pathway, pyruvate kinase deficiency, accounts for more than 90% of cases of glycolytic enzyme deficiency that are associated with haemolysis.

- Although most individuals with PK deficiency are moderately anaemic, clinical symptoms of anaemia may be minimal or absent because of the low oxygen affinity which accompanies accumulation of 2,3-DPG.

- There are no characteristic features of red cell morphology associated with pyruvate kinase deficiency.

- Because hexokinase acts above the Rappaport–Luebering shunt, deficiency leads to severe symptoms of anaemia in the presence of a moderately reduced haemoglobin concentration.

- Defects of the hexose monophosphate pathway result in increased red cell susceptibility to oxidant stress. All are rare except G-6-PD deficiency which affects almost 1% of the world's population.

- The normal form of G-6-PD is designated Gd^B and is present in 99% of Caucasians and in about 70% of blacks. A functionally normal G-6-PD isoenzyme, Gd^A, is found in about 20% of blacks.

- G-6-PD deficiency is a sex-linked recessive condition. However, because of the high incidence of aberrant genes in some populations, female homozygotes are not uncommon.

- Despite the large number of G-6-PD variants, individuals with G-6-PD deficiency typically exhibit one of two patterns of haemolysis: chronic non-spherocytic haemolytic anaemia (CNSHA) or episodic haemolysis.

- Three sets of triggers of acute haemolysis in G-6-PD deficient individuals have been identified: ingestion of oxidant drugs, ingestion of broad beans and infection.

- G-6-PD deficiency is the most common cause of neonatal jaundice worldwide.

Chapter 11
Malignant disorders of the blood

Learning objectives

After studying this chapter you should confidently be able to:

List the various categories of haemopoietic malignancy and some examples of each.

Define the nature of epidemiological studies.

Demonstrate knowledge of the epidemiology of the malignant disorders of the blood.

Outline current understanding of the aetiology of the malignant disorders of the blood.

Explain the role of oncogenes in the development of selected malignant blood disorders.

Malignant disorders of the blood are characterized by an uncontrolled clonal proliferation of haemopoietic cells. Numerous classification schemes exist for this group of disorders. In this book, the different haemopoietic malignancies are grouped under one of the following headings:

- Acute leukaemias
- Chronic leukaemias
- Myelodysplastic syndromes
- Non-leukaemic lymphoproliferative disorders
- Non-leukaemic myeloproliferative disorders

The specific characteristics of each group are considered in detail in the following chapters. This chapter concentrates on topics that are important across the spectrum of haemopoietic malignancy.

General characteristics

Acute leukaemias

Acute leukaemias are characterized by an uncontrolled proliferation of poorly differentiated cells (blasts). The acute leukaemias are divided on the basis of the predominant haemopoietic lineage involved into **acute lymphoblastic leukaemia (ALL)** and **acute non-lymphoblastic leukaemia (ANLL)**. The most widely used system of classification of the acute leukaemias is the French-American-British or **FAB system**. The FAB system classifies individual cases of acute leukaemia according to their morphological appearance on Romanowsky-stained bone marrow smears and is described in detail in the next chapter.

Chronic leukaemias

Chronic leukaemias differ from acute types in that the predominant cell type shows some characteristics of maturity. The need for a standardized system of classification for the chronic leukaemias is not so great since they are usually easily recognizable on the basis of cell morphology and cytochemistry. There are four subtypes of chronic leukaemia: **chronic lymphocytic leukaemia (CLL)**, **prolymphocytic leukaemia (PLL)**, **hairy cell leukaemia (HCL)** and **chronic myeloid leukaemia (CML)**. A fifth type, chronic myelomonocytic leukaemia (CMML), is considered with the myelodysplastic syndromes.

Myelodysplastic syndromes

The myelodysplastic syndromes can be thought of as preleukaemic conditions. They are classified according to FAB criteria into **refractory anaemia (RA)**, **refractory anaemia with sideroblasts (RAS)**, **refractory anaemia with excess of blasts (RAEB)**, **refractory anaemia with excess of blasts in transformation (RAEB-t)** and **chronic myelomonocytic leukaemia (CMML)**. The classification criteria are described in Chapter 14.

Non-leukaemic lymphoproliferative disorders

This diverse group of conditions includes **multiple myeloma (MM)** and related plasma cell disorders, **Hodgkin's disease (HD)** and the **non-Hodgkin's lymphomas (NHL)**. These conditions and their classification are considered in Chapter 15.

Non-leukaemic myeloproliferative disorders

There are three different non-leukaemic myeloproliferative disorders: **primary proliferative polycythaemia (PPP)**, **primary thrombo-**

The division of the leukaemias into acute and chronic types describes the natural history of the diseases in the absence of treatment. In these circumstances, acute leukaemia typically is fatal within weeks or months of diagnosis. In contrast, survival in chronic leukaemia is measured in years. Modern treatment methods have made the distinction in survival time between acute and chronic leukaemias much less clear, however. In general, the acute leukaemias have proved to be more amenable to treatment than the chronic types. For example, acute lymphoblastic leukaemia of childhood is now considered to be a curable disease whereas conventional cytotoxic chemotherapy for chronic myeloid leukaemia is palliative and does not significantly influence survival time.

cythaemia and **myelofibrosis**. These conditions are considered in Chapter 15.

Epidemiology of haemopoietic malignancy

Epidemiology is a statistical approach to the study of disease incidence, distribution and aetiology. It involves surveys of defined populations to determine the incidence of the disease under study and factors such as age, sex, race, occupation and socio-economic status, which may influence the disease incidence. **Descriptive studies** such as this are designed to discern statistically significant *associations* between the disease and one or more of the factors under study. For example, suppose that a descriptive study revealed a higher incidence of acute leukaemia in those exposed to an imaginary pesticide, DPD. Although tempting, it cannot be concluded that exposure to DPD *causes* acute leukaemia. Evidence for causal relationships is derived from **analytical studies**.

Analytical studies in this case would attempt to quantify the risk of developing acute leukaemia in those exposed to DPD and to determine whether the association can be considered to be cause and effect. This is accomplished using both **retrospective case control studies** and **prospective cohort studies**. Retrospective case control studies compare the incidence of exposure to DPD in confirmed cases of acute leukaemia with that in a carefully matched, disease-free control group. Prospective cohort studies follow a disease-free group to determine the incidence of acute leukaemia so that the incidence in those exposed to DPD can then be compared to the incidence in those not so exposed. Similarly, failure to develop acute leukaemia following exposure to DPD can be determined. Definitive evidence that DPD is a cause of acute leukaemia would ideally include a statistically significant excess of the disease in those exposed in both retrospective and prospective studies, evidence of a dose effect, evidence that removal of exposure diminishes the incidence of the disease and evidence that the disease can be induced experimentally in animals by exposing them to DPD. Such complete evidence is difficult to obtain in many cases.

Epidemiological studies of the haemopoietic malignancies have always been difficult to perform because of the relative rarity of the conditions and the problems of misdiagnosis and misclassification. However, the use of objective classification regimes such as the FAB system for the acute leukaemias and myelodysplastic syndromes has increased concordance between investigators sufficiently to permit the gathering of reliable international data.

Acute leukaemia

ALL is most common in childhood with a peak incidence at age 4 or 5 years. Childhood ALL is more common in the developed

---

It is important not to confuse association with cause and effect. For example, a 1984 Government Committee of Inquiry concluded that there was an excess incidence (a cluster) of childhood ALL in the village of Seascale in Cumbria, which lies close to the nuclear reprocessing plant at Sellafield. The obvious and tempting conclusion is to blame Sellafield for these cases. However, there is no convincing evidence for such a conclusion.

An alternative explanation for this phenomenon implicates the pattern of common childhood infections. The suggestion is that the children of the developed world are overprotected from infections in the early months of life and that this leads to an abnormally restricted immunological repertoire, which responds abnormally to challenge. Thus, when a small, stable community suddenly experiences a major influx of population, the established spectrum of infections is disrupted and this may result in an excess of childhood ALL. This theory fits well with the observed temporary increases in the incidence of childhood ALL in several of the new towns that were created in the 1960s as urban overspill centres. Furthermore, the characteristic peak incidence of ALL in children aged 0–5 years has only been seen in the UK since the 1920s.

countries of the world whereas in relatively underdeveloped countries lymphoma predominates in this age group. For example, in Uganda, lymphoma is about 15–20 times more common in the under 14s than leukaemia. The incidence of ANLL is greatest in middle to old age, being most common in males over the age of 65. Although ALL predominates in young children, ANLL also shows a minor peak incidence in children under the age of 5 years.

Chronic leukaemia

CLL is very rare below the age of 30 years but then increases sharply with increasing age. There is little difference in the overall incidence of CLL in white and black populations but the disease has a much lower frequency in Asians over the age of 55 years. For example, in Canada and Scandinavia CLL accounts for about one-third of all leukaemias whereas in Japan this figure is less than 5% of the total. CLL is more common in men than in women with most countries having a male:female ratio of between 1.5 and 2.5. The excess of CLL is most remarkable in Australia where the male:female ratio is as high as 4.7.

CML is primarily a disease of middle to old age. Variation of CML incidence with ethnic background is much less impressive than for CLL although the disease appears to be more common in young blacks than whites. CML is slightly more common in men than in women. Most studies have shown a male:female ratio for CML of between 1.0 and 2.0.

The incidence of both CML and CLL and the median survival times have stayed remarkably stable over the last 20 years or so. Studies that show an increased incidence of either disease are thought to reflect improved diagnosis and increased access to health care.

Non-leukaemic lymphoproliferative disorders

Socio-economic status is an important risk factor in all forms of lymphoma (HD and NHL), with higher socio-economic status being associated with an increased incidence. This is the probable explanation for the excess of lymphomas in whites compared to blacks in developed countries. The incidence of the lymphomas is rising in the developed countries of the world.

Hodgkin's disease (HD) has a bimodal age distribution, with peaks of incidence occurring during the third decade of life and after the age of 55 years. A different age distribution is seen in developing countries, where the highest incidence of HD occurs in children and a second, smaller peak occurs in the elderly. HD is a rare condition in young adults in developing countries. Overall, HD is slightly more common in males with most studies showing a male:female ratio of about 1.5.

Epidemiological studies of non-Hodgkin's lymphoma (NHL) have been greatly hampered by confusion over the classification of this heterogeneous group of disorders. Reliable data are available for most developed countries but the picture in developing countries is much less clear. Overall, NHL is about four times more common than HD. The incidence of NHL rises with age, most obviously after the age of 40 years; these disorders are rare in children.

Multiple myeloma (MM) is predominantly a disease of old age, with a median age at diagnosis of 70 years. The disorder is more common in men with a male : female ratio of about 1.5. In contrast to HD and NHL, MM is much more common in blacks than whites and socio-economic status does not appear to be an important factor.

Aetiology of haemopoietic malignancy

Much of our current understanding of the aetiology of haemopoietic malignancy has been derived from epidemiological studies. Such studies are notoriously difficult to perform, bedevilled as they are by the rarity of the conditions under study, by lack of reliable historical data and by the confounding influences of socio-economic factors such as access to health care. The results of such studies must always be interpreted with caution.

Although exposure to certain environmental conditions, drugs and chemicals has been shown to be associated with the development of haematological malignancy, proof that this is cause and effect often is lacking. In addition, only a relatively small proportion of individuals exposed to these carcinogenic factors actually develop a malignant condition, suggesting that other factors such as genetic constitution may be operating.

The following factors are widely regarded as being involved in the aetiology of haemopoietic malignancy:

- Ionizing radiation.
- Therapeutic drugs.
- Chemicals.
- Viruses.
- Familial and genetic factors.

Ionizing radiation

The atomic bombs which were dropped on Hiroshima and Nagasaki have provided incontrovertible evidence that exposure to doses of ionizing radiation in excess of 1 gray is leukaemogenic. An increased incidence of CML, ALL, ANLL and MM in survivors of these horrific events was identified in 1948. The frequency of these malignant diseases continued to increase for a further 10 years, after which the incidence of CML returned to normal. ANLL

Confirmatory evidence that the observed excess of leukaemia was attributable to the effects of the atomic bombs was provided by the dual observations that the leukaemia risk was inversely related to the distance from the hypocentre of the explosion and that survivors of the Hiroshima bomb, which emitted a greater level of neutron radiation than that dropped on Nagasaki, were more likely to develop leukaemia.

and ALL are still more common in this unfortunate group of people than in those not exposed. The excess risk is greater in males and increases with increasing age at the time of exposure. There was no observable increase in the incidence of CLL or lymphoma observed in either group of survivors. Both of these conditions are relatively rare in Japan.

Chronic exposure to therapeutic X irradiation also has been associated with an increased incidence of leukaemia, aplastic anaemia and solid tumours in heavily exposed tissue. Retrospective studies of cause of death in medical staff showed an excess of fatal leukaemia in radiologists prior to 1940. This excess disappeared following the introduction of adequate shielding and dosage monitoring in such staff. Foetal exposure to X-rays in the first trimester of pregnancy has also been shown to be associated with an increased incidence of ALL in infancy.

> The biological damage inflicted by ionizing radiation is largely determined by the dosage, which is defined in terms of the amount of energy transferred to the irradiated tissue. Dosage is expressed in gray (Gy) where 1 gray is equivalent to the absorption of 1 joule of energy per kilogram of irradiated tissue. The older unit of dosage was the rad (1 Gy = 100 rad).

Therapeutic drugs

Treatment of established malignancy involves the administration of cytotoxic drugs. The use of **alkylating agents** is strongly associated with an increased incidence of secondary (therapy-induced) ANLL. The median time from initiation of therapy to the development of ANLL is 4 years. Epipodophyllotoxin has also been implicated in the development of secondary ANLL.

Therapy-induced ANLL differs from *de novo* ANLL in a number of important respects:

- At least 90% of therapy-induced ANLL cases have cytogenetic abnormalities, most commonly monosomy 5, 5q−, monosomy 7 and 7q−. Less than 60% of *de novo* cases bear cytogenetic abnormalities and chromosomes 5 and 7 are less commonly involved.

- A preleukaemic phase occurs in more than 65% of cases of therapy-induced ANLL but in less than 25% of *de novo* cases.

- Therapy-induced ANLL is refractory to treatment – the mean survival time from diagnosis is 4 months compared to 20 months for *de novo* cases.

The most likely explanation for the induction of ANLL by alkylating agents lies with their known mutagenic properties. Alkylating agents are capable of alkylating the nitrogen and oxygen molecules of all four DNA bases, phosphodiester bonds and the 2′ oxygen atom of ribose, resulting in inappropriate base-pairing, strand breaks, complex rearrangements and the deletion of part or all of a chromosome. Mutations that alter the expression of normal cellular oncogenes can result in malignant change.

> Alkylating agents are polyfunctional molecules with highly reactive alkyl groups which form crosslinks between the side chains of proteins and nucleic acids. These crosslinks interfere with the function of cellular enzymes and the replicative function of DNA. Attempts to repair the damage to DNA caused by these drugs result in their mutagenic potential.
>
> The alkylating agents affect only dividing cells. Toxic side-effects are therefore manifest most severely in rapidly dividing tissue, leading to pancytopenia, alopecia and ulceration of mucous membranes.
>
> Commonly prescribed alkylating agents include cyclophosphamide, chlorambucil, busulfan, melphalan, procarbazine and cisplatin.

Chemicals

A large number of different chemicals has been suggested as possible inducers or promoters of haemopoietic malignancy but, in most cases, the evidence is unconvincing. The exception is benzene: chronic exposure to benzene and its derivatives is associated with an increased incidence of hypoplastic anaemia and ANLL. Most cases have resulted from prolonged occupational exposure to relatively high concentrations of benzene. However, recent reports of an excess of ANLL in male cigarette smokers have raised the possibility that chronic exposure to the low levels of aromatic compounds found in tobacco smoke may be leukaemogenic.

Epidemiological studies of rates of haemopoietic malignancy in different occupations have revealed a slight excess incidence of myeloma, NHL, ANLL and CML in agricultural workers, possibly related to increased exposure to insecticides and herbicides. Similar studies have shown an excess of CLL and NHL in rubber industry workers, ALL in the children of nuclear industry workers, CML in welders and NHL in anaesthetists and those exposed to halomethane compounds. None of these associations is universally accepted as proven cases of cause and effect.

Viruses

There is a wealth of evidence for viral induction of leukaemia and solid tumours in animals including higher primates. These oncogenic viruses can be divided into two types: the DNA viruses (papovaviruses, adenoviruses and herpesviruses) and the RNA viruses including **retroviruses**. Examples of the involvement of DNA viruses in the induction of human tumours include **human papillomavirus (HPV)** in cervical neoplasia, **Epstein–Barr virus (EBV)** in Burkitt's lymphoma, Hodgkin's disease and nasopharyngeal carcinoma and **hepatitis B virus (HBV)** in primary hepatoma. The only convincing evidence for retroviral induction of neoplasia in humans comes from studies of the retrovirus **human T lymphotropic virus I (HTLV-I)**. The accumulated evidence for the role of this virus in the aetiology of an unusual form of acute T cell leukaemia/lymphoma (ATL) in Southern Japan and the Caribbean is compelling.

Viruses can induce malignant transformation of host cells in three ways:

- Retroviruses that contain an oncogene can induce malignant transformation in host cells by insertion of the viral oncogene into the host cell genome. This mechanism, known as **direct mutagenesis** typically leads to an acute and rapidly progressive tumour.

- Insertion of viral DNA at a specific point in the host DNA can

---

The earliest demonstration that leukaemia could be transmitted between animals was performed in 1908 at the Royal Veterinary School in Copenhagen by V. Ellermann and O. Bang. They showed that injecting leukaemic cells from chickens with avian myeloblastosis into healthy birds caused the development of the condition in the healthy birds. Further experiments showed that the same effect could be obtained by injecting carefully filtered, cell-free extracts. Three years later, P. Rous showed that solid tumours could be induced in chickens by the injection of cell-free extracts from similarly afflicted birds. These observations were not extended to mammals until 1936 when J.J. Bittner demonstrated the transmission of murine mammary carcinoma through maternal milk. The earliest clear demonstration of leukaemia induction by the injection of cell-free extracts was made in 1951 by L. Gross in New York who used newborn mice. Attempts to induce leukaemia in adult mice were unsuccessful.

enable the viral regulatory sequences to influence the expression of host cellular proliferation genes. This mechanism, known as **insertional mutagenesis**, is associated with a relatively long latency period and only a minority of infected animals develop neoplasia.

- HTLV-I differs in that the point of insertion of viral DNA into host DNA varies widely. HTLV-I is thought to be capable of transforming host T lymphocytes by a process known as **transactivation**. A viral protein designated TAX has been shown to transactivate the genes which encode the IL-2 receptor, IL-3, IL-4, GM-CSF and the oncogene *fos*.

Numerous epidemiological studies have suggested a possible role for infectious agents in human haemopoietic malignancy. The observation of an increased incidence of myeloma, NHL, ANLL and CML in agricultural workers raises the possibility that contact with oncogenic animal viruses may be involved. However, exhaustive studies of pet owners, slaughterhouse workers and children bitten by animals have failed to provide consistent confirmation of this observation.

Burkitt's lymphoma (BL) is a NHL which is endemic to tropical Africa and Papua New Guinea and is manifest as tumours of the jaw and abdomen with extensive extranodal involvement. Virtually all cases of African BL have definitive evidence of Epstein–Barr virus (EBV) infection and one of three chromosomal translocations: t(8;14); t(8;22) or t(2;8). EBV is a very common virus worldwide but infection in developed countries causes the self-limiting condition **infectious mononucleosis**. This relatively mild illness is associated with EBV infection during adolescence, which is common in developed countries. In Africa, primary infection with EBV usually occurs in the first year of life. It is suggested that EBV is implicated in the development of African BL via a multistep route:

- Primary EBV infection occurs and 'immortalizes' infected B lymphocytes. This occurs in all infected individuals.

- An immortalized B lymphocyte is stimulated to proliferate by some immunological challenge such as malaria infection, resulting in the formation of an immortalized B cell clone. The variety and frequency of infectious diseases in tropical Africa makes this step more likely.

- In the process of cell proliferation, a single cell in the immortalized clone develops one of the three chromosomal translocations that induce malignant transformation. The result is Burkitt's lymphoma.

Hodgkin's disease is a heterogeneous condition which has been suspected of having an infectious aetiology since it was first described in 1832. Recent evidence has suggested that EBV is implicated in the pathogenesis of HD in a large proportion of cases in children and adults over the age of 50 years. A multistep aetiology similar to that for African BL is also proposed for HD.

Host factors

The concept of 'built-in susceptibility' to haemopoietic malignancy remains unproved, except in particular, well-defined circumstances. Numerous case reports exist of families with several cases of leukaemia or lymphoma, but it is difficult to discern whether these are the result of genetic predisposition or shared exposure to a leukaemogen. There is a clearly increased risk of acute leukaemia in certain inherited and congenital conditions such as Down's syndrome, Bloom's syndrome and Fanconi's anaemia. Lymphoid malignancy is more common in inherited immunodeficiency states such as Bruton's agammaglobulinaemia and ataxia telangiectasia. Whether, in the absence of inherited states such as these, the blood relations of an individual with a haemopoietic malignancy are at increased risk of developing the same condition is highly contentious. Epidemiological studies have revealed a slight excess of CLL, ALL and ANLL, but no increased risk of CML, in blood relations of confirmed leukaemics.

The greatly increased risk of ALL in an identical twin of a confirmed case is well established. The risk of coincident development of ALL is highest in infancy. The most likely explanation for this phenomenon is the transmission of malignant cells from one twin, in whom the disease arose, to the other via the shared placental circulation *in utero*.

The role of oncogenes in haemopoietic malignancy

Cellular **proto-oncogenes** are highly conserved constituents of the normal human genome which act as controllers of cell growth, division and differentiation. They encode proteins that act as growth factors, growth factor receptors, signal transducers or nuclear transcription factors. Disruption of proto-oncogene function can lead to malignant transformation. Four types of chromosomal aberration that can lead to oncogene activation are commonly found in haemopoietic malignancies:

- **Translocations and inversions** which involve sections of chromosome breaking off and relocating either elsewhere on the same chromosome or onto another chromosome altogether. Translocation of a proto-oncogene can disrupt its function by bringing it under the influence of its new neighbours, by removing it from the influence of its old neighbours or by altering the biochemical action of the gene product.
- **Deletions and numerical changes** which involve the loss or gain of

part or all of a chromosome. Chromosomal trisomy can lead to increased expression of proto-oncogene products and may contribute to the early stages of malignant transformation. Equally, certain deletions remove proto-oncogenes, leading to the production of cells that are impervious to normal growth control mechanisms.

- **Point mutations** in proto-oncogenes which can cause the function of the gene product to be altered. For example, the products of the *ras* oncogenes are involved in cellular signal transduction pathways. Point mutations in *ras* are found in at least 50% of cases of ANLL, resulting in disturbed signal transduction and deranged cell growth.

- **Gene amplification** which involves the repeated replication of short segments of DNA to produce as many as 100 copies and leading to a gene dosage effect. For example, the c-*myc* proto-oncogene commonly is amplified in M3 ANLL.

There is a very close association between certain cytogenetic abnormalities and the types of haemopoietic malignancy in which they are found. In many of these abnormalities, there is clear evidence that the function of a proto-oncogene has been disturbed and that the altered gene is implicated in the malignant process. In these circumstances, the gene is said to be an **oncogene** (cancer-promoting gene).

t(8;14)(q24;q32) and Burkitt's lymphoma

The cytogenetic designation t(8;14)(q24;q32) indicates that chromosomes 8 and 14 have broken at positions 24 and 32 on their respective q arms and the fragments have been swapped, i.e. translocated. This translocation is associated with Burkitt's lymphoma. The proto-oncogene c-*myc* is located at 8q24 and in this translocation it moves close to the immunoglobulin heavy chain genes at 14q32. In this new position, c-*myc* comes under the influence of the promoter sequences of the immunoglobulin heavy chain genes and c-*myc* expression is greatly enhanced. The protein product of c-*myc* is a nuclear transcription factor. The ultimate consequence of increased production of this protein is neoplastic growth of B lymphoid cells. The t(8;14)(q24;q32) translocation is depicted in Figure 11.1.

The variant translocations t(2;8)(p12;q24) and t(8;22)(q24;q11) also are found in Burkitt's lymphoma. In these translocations, c-*myc* is juxtaposed with either the immunoglobulin light chain κ genes at 2p12 or the immunoglobulin light chain λ genes at 22q11. Both result in enhanced c-*myc* expression. No other translocations have consistently been found in Burkitt's lymphoma.

Normal human cells, other than gametes, contain 46 chromosomes: 22 pairs of **autosomes** and two **sex chromosomes**. Males carry dissimilar sex chromosomes (46XY) whereas females are designated 46XX. Normal chromosomes are divided into a long **q arm** and a short **p arm** by a **centromere**. Staining of chromosome preparations with Giemsa or quinacrine dyes reveals a characteristic pattern of bands which can be used to describe quite small areas of the chromosome, e.g. 8q22 refers to sub-band number 2 on region 2 on the long arm of chromosome number 8

Figure 11.1 *Molecular events in the t(8;4)(q24;q32) translocation. IgHCμ, immunoglobin heavy chain constant region genes; IgHV, immunoglobin heavy chain variable region genes*

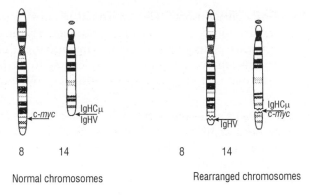

Normal chromosomes   Rearranged chromosomes

Cytogenetic abnormalities are expressed according to the International System for Human Cytogenetic Nomenclature. The total number of chromosomes is indicated first, followed by the sex chromosome constitution and then by the gains, losses or rearrangements of the autosomes. A prefix '+', e.g. +21, indicates trisomy of that chromosome while a prefix '−', e.g. −7, indicates monosomy. A suffix '+' or '−', e.g. 5q−, indicates loss of the named part of that chromosome.

Chromosomal rearrangements are indicated by an abbreviation which denotes the type of rearrangement, followed by the chromosome(s) involved in parentheses and then the bands in which the chromosomal breaks occurred in a second set of parentheses, e.g. t(8;21)(q22;q22) indicates translocation of material between chromosomes 8 and 21 with both breakpoints occurring in band 2 of region 2 of the q arm of the respective chromosomes. An inversion is designated with the prefix 'inv', e.g. inv(16)(p13;q32), and an isochromosome with the prefix 'i', e.g. i(17)q.

t(15;17)(q22;q21) or (q22;q11–12) and M3 ANLL

The t(15;17) translocation is specific for M3 ANLL; it has not been described in any other malignancy. Almost all patients with M3 ANLL have this translocation which is associated with a good prognosis. This translocation disrupts the *pml* gene on chromosome 15 and the retinoic acid receptor gene (*rar* α) on chromosome 17, resulting in the formation of two novel fusion genes, both of which are functional. Synthesis of the novel *pml/rar* α fusion protein leads to the development of M3 ANLL.

t(9;22)(q34;q11) and CML

At least 90% of cases of CML display a minute chromosome 22 which results from the reciprocal translocation t(9;22)(q34;q11). This abnormal chromosome 22 is known as the Philadelphia chromosome after the city of its discovery. Molecular analysis of many apparently Philadelphia negative cases of CML reveal similar but variant chromosomal rearrangements. The Philadelphia chromosome is also observed in a minority of cases of ALL and ANLL. The breakpoint on chromosome 9 (9q34) involves the *abl* gene, which is translocated to chromosome 22. The function of the normal ABL protein ($p145^{abl}$) is poorly understood but it is known to be important in the regulation of myelopoiesis. The chromosome 22 breakpoint (22q11) in CML always lies within a 5.8 kb region of the *bcr* gene called the **breakpoint cluster region**. The normal BCR protein ($p160^{bcr}$) is involved in the activation of cell signalling proteins within cells.

In the Philadelphia chromosome, the severed end of the *bcr* gene is joined to the translocated *abl* gene, forming a novel *bcr-abl* fusion gene. The unique product of this fusion gene, $p210^{bcr-abl}$ has a much more powerful activity than $p145^{abl}$ and has been shown to interact with its substrates in an altered manner. Although the way in which $p210^{bcr-abl}$ brings about malignant change is poorly characterized, there is little doubt that this protein is implicated in the causation of CML.

Suggested further reading

Cartwright, R.A., Alexander, F.E., McKinney, P.A. *et al.* (1990). *Leukaemia and Lymphoma: An Atlas of Distribution with Areas of England and Wales 1984–88.*

Elefanty, A.G., Robb, L. and Begley, C.G. (1997). Factors involved in leukaemogenesis and haemopoiesis. *Bailliere's Clinical Haematology* **10**(3), 589–614.

Linet, M.S. (1985). *The Leukemias: Epidemiological Aspects.* New York: Oxford University Press. London: Leukaemia Research Fund.

Wiernik, P.H., Canellos, G.P., Kyle, R.A. and Schiffer, C.A. (1991). *Neoplastic Diseases of the Blood* 2nd edn. Edinburgh: Churchill Livingstone.

http://www.pathology.washington.edu/Cytogallery/

Self-assessment questions

1. Name two types of acute leukaemia, chronic leukaemia, myelodysplastic syndrome, non-leukaemic lymphoproliferative disorder and non-leukaemic myeloproliferative disorder.
2. Outline the main distinguishing features of descriptive and analytical epidemiological studies.
3. Name one example of a haemopoietic malignancy that has a peak incidence in childhood and one that is almost restricted to the elderly.
4. What evidence exists for the leukaemogenic potential of high dose ionizing radiation?
5. Name the retrovirus that is implicated in the aetiology of acute T cell leukaemia/lymphoma (ATL) in Southern Japan and the Caribbean.
6. What is the difference between a proto-oncogene and an oncogene?

Key Concepts and Facts

- Malignant disorders of the blood are characterized by an uncontrolled clonal proliferation of haemopoietic cells.

- Haemopoietic malignancies can be grouped into acute leukaemias, chronic leukaemias, myelodysplastic syndromes, non-leukaemic lymphoproliferative disorders and non-leukaemic myeloproliferative disorders.

- Epidemiology is the statistical approach to the study of disease incidence, distribution and aetiology.

- The following factors are widely regarded as being involved in the aetiology of haemopoietic malignancy: ionizing radiation; certain drugs, chemicals and viruses; and familial and genetic factors.

- Cellular **proto-oncogenes** encode controllers of cell growth, division and differentiation.

- Mutation of a proto-oncogene to form an oncogene can contribute to malignant transformation.

Chapter 12
Acute leukaemias

Learning objectives

After studying this chapter you should confidently be able to:

Describe in detail the FAB classification system for the acute leukaemias.

Outline the immunological and genetic approach to the classification of the acute leukaemias.

Outline the pathophysiology of the acute leukaemias.

Identify characteristic features of the different forms of acute leukaemia.

Outline the approaches to treatment of the acute leukaemias.

The acute leukaemias are a heterogeneous group of malignant disorders which are characterized by the uncontrolled clonal proliferation and accumulation of poorly differentiated blast cells in the bone marrow and other body tissues.

Recognition and classification of the acute leukaemias

Recognition of acute leukaemia requires the examination of appropriately stained blood and bone marrow smears. The presence of more than 30% blast cells in the bone marrow at clinical presentation is an objective criterion for defining acute leukaemia. Frequently, in cases of grossly elevated white cell counts at presentation, the diagnosis is self-evident from the peripheral blood. However, a bone marrow aspirate, and often a biopsy, is still necessary for confirmation purposes and accurate classification.

Accurate classification has become increasingly important as therapeutic advances have been made in both the treatment and the management of the acute leukaemias. Phenotypic characterization of the leukaemic cells at presentation is essential to enable the selection of appropriate treatment and the monitoring of the progress of the disease during treatment. Because of this, a battery of techniques has developed which facilitate this process.

Rudolf Virchow (1821–1902)
The name leukaemia was coined by Virchow in 1847. He described the disease some 2 years earlier, the year before he lost his first university appointment in Berlin, apparently a victim of his 'uncompromisingly radical political attitudes'! His seminal observation was made at the autopsy table when he noted massive splenomegaly and a peculiar appearance of the blood in a recently deceased patient. The normal ratio of pigmented (red) cells and colourless (white) cells seemed to be reversed in the blood of the deceased. He described this condition as 'weisses blut' which translates as 'white blood' in English or 'leukaemia' in Greek.

Table 12.1 *The diagnosis and initial classification of acute leukaemia*

Full blood count (FBC)
Requested because of clinical symptoms such as bruising, organomegaly or
    bone pain
Occasionally a chance finding on medical screening
FBC usually shows anaemia, thrombocytopenia and variable WBC

Morphology
Peripheral blood film may show blast cells
Bone marrow smear shows more than 30% blast cells

Immunophenotyping
Flow cytometry or immunocytochemistry using panels of monoclonal
    antibodies
Classification into ALL, with T or B characteristics; AML M0–M7 subtypes
Biphenotypic if evidence of both lymphoid and myeloid markers
                    95% of cases are diagnosed by this point

Cytogenetics
For clonality and prognostic information

DNA analysis
Needed for rare cases
                    99.9% of cases are diagnosed by this point

---

John Bennett (1812–1875)

It is generally believed that John Bennett in Edinburgh simultaneously discovered leukaemia with Virchow. Bennett was described as 'a man of brilliance but short temper, certain of his own virtues, pugnacious, and unable to suffer fools'! Bennett also made his original observation at the autopsy table in a patient with a very similar case history. Bennett felt the blood had pus in it because microscopic examination revealed the presence of a huge number of cells usually associated with the presence of pus. He described the condition as 'pyaemia'. A major disagreement between Virchow and Bennett was conducted in the journals for several years. During the decades that followed Virchow, now reinstated to his position but still maintaining his enlightened social and political views, made some seminal observations about leukaemia. These were all made without the ability to stain and count blood cells and it is remarkable how close his guesses were to the truth as it is known today.

These technologies, including cytomorphology, electron micros-copy, cytochemistry, immunocytochemistry, cytogenetics, fluores-cent in-situ hybridization (FISH) and molecular genetics techniques, are utilized to define cellular characteristics or markers and the precise nature of the leukaemic proliferation or clone as shown in Table 12.1.

The morphological and cytochemical approach to classification

This approach to the classification of acute leukaemia relies on the examination of the morphology of the leukaemic cells using light microscopy. The information gleaned in this way is supplemented using a battery of cytochemical stains to detect subcellular com-ponents as shown in Table 12.2. Electron microscopy is also required in some cases. Using this approach, it is possible to differentiate lymphoblastic (ALL) and non-lymphoblastic (ANLL), and to subdivide each into a number of subtypes.

Classification of individual cases is far from straightforward, however. The disordered growth and differentiation which char-acterizes the leukaemic process increases the likelihood of aberrant expression of cell markers and can make recognition of the different subtypes difficult. Interpretation of the results obtained requires significant skill and, ultimately, relies upon the experience and judgement of a trained haematologist.

Table 12.2 *The substances stained by and applications of basic cytochemical stains*

Method	Substances stained	Main uses
Sudan black	Neutral fats, phospholipids and lipoproteins	Identification of granulocyte precursors
Peroxidase	Myeloperoxidase	Identification of neutrophil and eosinophil precursors
Periodic acid Schiff (PAS)	Glycogen	Block positive in M6 erythroblasts
Chloroacetate esterase	Esterase isoenzymes 1,2,7 and 8	Differentiation of granulocytic and monocytic maturation (M4 and M5)
Non-specific esterase	Esterase isoenzymes 3,4,5 and 6	
Acid phosphatase	Acid phosphatase	Useful in TALL and HCL
TdT	Terminal deoxynucleotidyl transferase (TdT)	Differentiation of ALL and ANLL*

* Rarely positive in ANLL.

In an attempt to improve the reproducibility and comparability of the classification process, a group of expert haematologists from France, America and Britain (FAB) collaborated to define a more objective set of criteria for the classification of the acute leukaemias. The FAB group recommended that the acute lymphoblastic leukaemias should be coded into three variants, which are designated L1–L3 according to the predominant morphology of the leukaemic lymphoblasts, and that the non-lymphoblastic leukaemias should similarly be coded into eight subtypes, which are designated M0–M7. The classification should only be made after the examination of both peripheral blood and bone marrow films, including the performance of a 500 cell differential count. In addition, a myeloperoxidase or Sudan black stain should be used to facilitate the recognition of myeloblasts. The FAB classification scheme is summarized in Table 12.3.

In extremely rare circumstances it is impossible to classify the acute leukaemia into either ALL or ANLL with any technology. This unusual entity, not included in the FAB scheme, is therefore termed acute undifferentiated leukaemia (AUL). In cases of AUL it is important to confirm that the disease is of haemopoietic origin and to exclude other non-haemopoietic malignancies that have spread to the bone marrow.

The immunological and genetic approach to classification

With advances in diagnostic technology, further classification schemes have emerged. For example, the application of immuno-cytochemistry techniques which employ monoclonal antibodies to recognize lineage and differentiation markers on leukaemic cells has enabled the subdivision of ALL into at least four separate entities: early pre-B ALL, pre-B ALL, B ALL and T ALL. The most important of these subdivisions is between T ALL and B ALL. Prognostic and therapeutic significance has been attached to these

The study of haematological morphology parallels developments in microscopy and chemistry. The simple microscope of Van Leeuwenhoek (c. 1700) revealed the red blood cells, whereas the colourless white blood cells were not reliably identified until about 1830 by Addison and Gulliver. A major breakthrough occurred with the work of Paul Ehrlich (1854–1915), who is regarded as one of the founding fathers of cytochemistry. It was his interest and enthusiasm, including the testing of thousands of new stains, which led to the reliable identification of the subtypes of white blood cells. The early stains developed detected lipids and carbohydrates and assessed the acidic or basic nature of the cell. Enzyme detection did not really progress until the 1940s with the development of the azo dyes which can be used to detect intracellular enzymes such as esterases, phosphatases and dehydrogenases. By the mid 1970s cytochemistry was the best diagnostic tool available for acute leukaemia. The next advance came with the use of monoclonal antibodies and immunocytochemistry, which resulted in improvements in diagnosis and reclassification of some types of leukaemia.

Table 12.3 *Summary of the FAB classification scheme for the acute leukaemias*

Acute lymphoblastic leukaemia

Designation	Alternative	Bone marrow appearances
L1		Homogeneous population of small lymphoblasts with scanty cytoplasm and scanty nucleoli. Nucleus occasionally cleft
L2		Heterogeneous population of large lymphoblasts with moderately abundant cytoplasm and one or more nucleoli. Nucleus commonly indented or cleft
L3	Burkitt's type	Homogeneous population of large lymphoblasts with prominent nucleoli and deeply basophilic, vacuolated cytoplasm

Acute non-lymphoblastic leukaemia

M0		Identified by ultrastructural myeloperoxidase activity
M1	AML without maturation	Monomorphic with one or more distinct nucleoli, occasional Auer rod and at least 3% myeloperoxidase positivity
M2	AML with maturation	50% or more myeloblasts and promyelocytes with single Auer rods common. Dysplastic myeloid differentiation may also be present
M3	APL	Dominant cell type is promyelocyte with heavy azurophilic granulation. Bundles of Auer rods confirm diagnosis. Micro-granular variant exists (M3v)
M4	AMMoL	As M2 but 20% promonocytes and monocytes
M5	AMoL	> 80% monoblasts is poorly differentiated (M5a); > 80% monoblasts, promonocytes and monocytes is well differentiated
M6	AEL	> 50% bizarre, dysplastic nucleated red cells with multinucleate forms and cytoplasmic bridging. Myeloblasts usually > 30%
M7	AMegL	Fibrosis, heterogeneous blast population with cytoplasmic blebs. Platelet peroxidase positive

subtypes but, unfortunately, little correlation exists between the immunological subtypes and the morphological subtypes of ALL according to the FAB scheme.

A summary of blast cell markers in ALL subtypes, using the technologies of morphology, cytochemistry, immunocytochemistry and recombinant DNA, is shown in Table 12.4.

The immunological classification of ANLL is not as clear-cut as that of ALL. The specificity of myeloid-associated markers is not as strong and the correlation with the widely accepted FAB subgroups of ANLL is poor. The exceptions to this generalization are M7, M6 and M0. These are now identified using immunocytochemistry. Anti-glycophorin A detects the erythroid component in M6 acute leukaemia. Anti-platelet glycoprotein antibodies (anti-CD41, anti-CD42 and anti-CD61) detect the megakaryoblastic component in M7 acute leukaemia. A combination of a stem cell-associated antibody (anti-CD34) with a myeloid-associated antibody (anti-CD33) detects the only evidence of myeloid differentiation in M0 acute leukaemia.

Table 12.4 *Blast cell markers of the acute lymphoblastic leukaemias*

	Early pre-B	Pre-B	B	T
Incidence	9%	70%	1%	20%
Morphology				
L1	90%	90%	10%	95%
L2	10%	10%	15%	5%
L3	0%	0%	75%	0%
Cytochemistry				
Acid phosphatase	−	−	−	+
5′-Nucleotidase	+	+	−	−
Nuclear TdT	+–|	++	+/−	++
Immunophenotype				
Cytoplasmic μ chains	−	+	−	−
Membrane immunoglobulin	−	−	+	−
CD2	−	−	−	++
CD10	+++	+	+/−	−
HLA-DR	+++	++	++	+/−
CD19, cytoplasmic CD22	+	+	+	−
CD7, cytoplasmic CD3	−	−	−	+++
Gene rearrangement				
Immunoglobulin heavy chain	+	+	+	−
Immunoglobulin light chain	+/−	+/−	+	−
T cell receptor	−/+	−/+	−/+	+

A major advantage with the immunocytochemistry techniques, when compared to the traditional morphology and cytochemistry, is that they can be automated in a flow cytometry analytical system using lasers and fluorescence detection. A summary of blast cell markers in ANLL subtypes using the technologies of morphology, cytochemistry and immunocytochemistry is shown in Table 12.5.

A major shortcoming of the markers described to date is that they are markers of normal haemopoietic differentiation and can therefore only be described as leukaemia-associated markers. Unfortunately, no leukaemia-specific antigenic marker is currently available for classification purposes.

/ Cytogenetics, the study of chromosomes, has been applied to the acute leukaemias for many years. Numerous non-random patterns of chromosomal alterations have been demonstrated in bone marrow cells from the majority of patients with acute leukaemia. Routinely prepared metaphase preparations have shown clonal karyotypic abnormalities in about 50% of patients with ANLL and 60% of patients with ALL. High-resolution chromosome banding techniques have shown clonal cytogenetic abnormalities in virtually all patients with either ANLL or ALL. Cytogenetic abnormalities of leukaemic cells can be characterized as changes involving chromosome number (ploidy) or chromosome structure,

Flow cytometry involves the detection of particles such as cells, bacteria or chromosomes as they move in a liquid stream through a laser-controlled 'sensing' zone. The particles of interest are often rare 'events' in a mixture of normal or contaminating particles. As each particle passes through the laser beam, it scatters some of the light in all directions. If the particle has been marked with a fluorescent dye, the laser will cause it to fluoresce. The pattern of scattered and fluorescent light produced reveals much about the particle. For example, forward-angle light scatter (FALS) gives an indication of cell size, while right-angle light scatter (RALS) gives an indication of cell granularity. Modern flow cytometers can make several separate measurements on each particle, at the rate of several thousands of particles per second. The results can be displayed using single histograms or more complex multiparametric diagrams. Some flow cytometers are even capable of sorting out of the main particles of special interest, which can then be used in further experiments.

Table 12.5 *Blast cell markers of the acute non-lymphoblastic leukaemias*

	M0	M1	M2	M3	M4	M5	M6	M7
Cytochemistry								
Myeloperoxidase	−	+	++	+++	+	+/−	−	−
Chloroacetate esterase	−	+/−	+	++	+	−	−	−
Non-specific esterase	−	−	−	−	+	++	−	−
Immunocytochemistry								
HLA-DR	+	+	+	−	−	+	+/−	+
CD34	++	++	−/+	−	−	−	−	+
CD33	+/−	+/−	+	+	+	+	−/+	−/+
CD13	+	+	+	++	++	++	+/−	−
CD14	−	−	−	−	−/+	+	−	−
CD11b	−	+/−	+/−	−/+	+	+	−	−
CD71	−	−	−	−	−	−	+	−
CD41, CD42 or CD61	−	−	−	−	−	−	−	+

Table 12.6 *Non-random structural chromosome abnormalities in the acute leukaemias*

Type of leukaemia	Chromosome abnormality	FAB type
ALL	t(9;22)(q34;q11)	L1, L2
Pre-B ALL	t(1;19)(q23;p13)	L1
	t(4;11)(q21;q23)	L1, L2
B ALL	t(8;14)(q24;q32)	L3
	t(2;8)(p12;q24)	L3
	t(8;22)(q24;q11)	L3
T ALL	t(11;14)(p13;q11)	L1, L2
	t(8;14)(q24;q11)	L1, L2
AML	t(8;21)(q22;q22)	M2
APL	t(15;17)(q22;q12)	M3
	t(15;17)(q22;q21)	M3
AMoL	del/t(11)(q23)	M5
AMMoL	inv16, 16q−, t(16;16)	M4
AEL	t(8;16)(p11;p13)	M6

for example translocation (t), inversion (inv) and deletion (del). The demonstration and typing of chromosomal abnormalities is becoming increasingly important as an aid to diagnosis and classification and as a prognostic indicator in the leukaemias.

A summary of some of the most important chromosomal abnormalities associated with acute leukaemia is shown in Table 12.6. A large number of other chromosomal abnormalities have been reported in association with acute leukaemia. However, these do not show the same strong correlation with a particular leukaemic subtype as those shown and so are less useful in the classification of the disease. Hyperdiploidy and hypodiploidy are very important numerical observations, particularly in early pre-B cell ALL.

Pathophysiology of the acute leukaemias

Acute leukaemia causes morbidity and mortality through three general mechanisms:

- Deficiency in normal blood cell number or function.
- Invasion of vital organs with impairment of organ function.
- Systemic disturbances shown by metabolic imbalance.

The treatment of leukaemia with cytotoxic chemotherapy is also associated with significant morbidity. In fact, it is often difficult to distinguish between the effects of treatment and the pathophysiology of the disease itself.

Infection

Infection is one of the most common causes of death and a significant cause of morbidity in acute leukaemia. The increased infection risk is caused by impaired host defence due to neutropenia or neutrophil dysfunction. Neutropenia may be caused by the 'crowding out' of normal neutrophil production by leukaemic tissue in the bone marrow or cytoreductive therapy. The usual hallmark of infection is fever. Unfortunately, the leukaemic process itself can cause fever, leading to complications in the recognition of infection. Differentiation between fever caused by infection and fever caused by the leukaemia process itself is often difficult. Typically, humoral and cell-mediated immunity are normal in acute leukaemia but, as the disease progresses, immune function deteriorates and the frequency and severity of infection increases.

The prevention of infection is a vital part of the treatment of acute leukaemia. Antibiotic regimes are implemented at the first sign of fever because of the association of infection with mortality. In some cases, severely neutropenic patients are treated with prophylactic antibiotics, regardless of signs of infection.

Haemorrhage

Haemorrhage is a common problem in acute leukaemia both at presentation and during treatment. Usually it is the direct result of thrombocytopenia but it may be secondary to qualitative defects of platelets or disseminated intravascular coagulation (DIC). The risk of severe haemorrhage is inversely related to the circulating platelet count: life-threatening haemorrhage is unlikely until the platelet count falls below 20×10^9/l. Occasionally, platelet dysfunction can result in bleeding problems at higher platelet counts. In either case, the most effective form of treatment is platelet transfusion. Some

In-situ hybridization is a technique by which specific portions of chromosomes can be marked by hybridization with a labelled nucleic acid probe. The label used can be a radioisotope, an enzyme or a fluorochrome. Fluorescent in-situ hybridization (FISH) is revolutionizing molecular cytogenetics. It is now possible to detect structural and numerical aberrations in disorders where conventional karyotyping is very difficult or impossible. The important feature of FISH is that the nucleic acid is retained *in situ* and not degraded during processing. FISH techniques can be applied to most biological tissues, including whole cells, tissue sections, chromosomes and bare nuclei. The probes used are usually between 10 and 25 kilobases in length. Longer probes give weaker signals, probably because they penetrate less efficiently into crosslinked tissue and smaller probes may be difficult to visualize. Chromosome 'paints' which label complete chromosomes are useful in the detection of numerical abnormalities.

treatment centres aim to prevent haemorrhage by a regime of prophylactic platelet transfusion.

Disseminated intravascular coagulation is particularly troublesome in M3 leukaemia due to the presence of thromboplastin-like substances in the abnormal granules of the leukaemic promyelocytes, but it may be seen in any form of acute leukaemia. As described in Chapter 18, Gram-negative septicaemia is associated with intractable DIC, which commonly results in death.

Anaemia

Normocytic, normochromic anaemia is extremely common in acute leukaemia and is responsible for the symptoms associated with fatigue and a sense of ill-health. The severity of the anaemia typically reflects the severity of the disease. The unregulated proliferation of leukaemic tissue results in the physical 'crowding out' of normal haemopoietic elements, leading to a reduction in erythropoiesis, thrombopoiesis and leukopoiesis. In some cases, ineffective erythropoiesis or, more rarely, haemolysis may exacerbate the anaemia. In most anaemic individuals, erythropoietin levels are raised in proportion to the degree of anaemia but the normal erythroid precursors show diminished responsiveness to this hormone. It is thought that leukaemic cells elaborate one or more inhibitors of normal haemopoiesis.

Infiltration of vital organs

The organs infiltrated at presentation and during the course of acute leukaemia vary according to the subtype involved, but may include liver, spleen, lymph nodes, meninges, brain, skin, eyes and testes. In contrast to the solid tumours, the frequency of organ infiltration by acute leukaemia far exceeds the frequency of symptomatic complications associated with such infiltration. Broadly, there are three types of complication associated with organ infiltration in acute leukaemia:

- **Hyperleucocytosis.** The extremely high white cell count sometimes seen at presentation in acute leukaemia is associated with 'sludging' in the microcirculation, and predisposes to the formation of microthrombi or acute haemorrhage. The organs most commonly involved are the brain, lungs and eyes. The increase in whole blood viscosity is usually partially offset by the presence of anaemia.
- **Leucostatic tumours.** Rarely, leukaemic blast cells may lodge in the vascular system of infiltrated organs and proliferate, forming macroscopic pseudotumours, which eventually erode the vessel wall resulting in haemorrhage. Leukostatic tumours are associated with hyperleukocytosis, particularly where expansion of

the leukaemic cell load occurs rapidly. The organs most commonly affected are the brain, liver and lungs.

- **Sanctuary site relapse.** Leukaemic infiltration of the testes and meninges is observed in all forms of acute leukaemia but is most common in ALL. These organs provide an effective sanctuary for resident leukaemic blasts because cytotoxic drugs penetrate them poorly. In the absence of specific additional prophylactic therapy to these organs, they may provide a source for the resurgence of leukaemic proliferation, leading to relapse. Meningeal and testicular relapse are most commonly seen in childhood ALL.

Important characteristics of the acute leukaemias

Acute lymphoblastic leukaemia

Acute lymphoblastic leukaemia is the most common malignant disease affecting children, accounting for approximately 30% of childhood cancers. The age distribution of the disease is skewed with 75% of cases occurring in children under the age of 15 years. Beyond childhood, the age distribution is uniform with a median between 30 and 40 years. Before the 1960s ALL was almost always fatal whereas now at least 50% of childhood cases are considered curable. Unfortunately, this is not the case with adult ALL, which is much more refractory to treatment.

A number of prognostic indicators have been identified which can be used to stratify individual cases into different risk groups and to tailor treatment accordingly. Broadly, those individuals who are judged to have a relatively poor prognosis by these criteria are treated more aggressively than those judged to have a good prognosis. The most widely accepted prognostic indicators are summarized in Table 12.7.

These prognostic indicators are most useful at presentation and have greater predictive power in children. The most important prognostic feature at presentation is the white cell count because this provides an indication of the size of the tumour load and the likelihood of successful remission induction. The next most important factor in terms of its predictive power is age at presentation. Infants have a poor prognosis because of the high tumour load relative to their body mass and a greater incidence of extramedullary involvement. Adults have a poorer prognosis than children because of differences in the biology of ALL in adults. Males have a slightly poorer prognosis than females because of the possibility of testicular relapse. Extramedullary involvement typically only occurs in the presence of a high tumour load and so is an indicator of a poor prognosis. The presence of a mediastinal mass on chest X-ray is indicative of the presence of a hypertrophic thymus and is associated with T ALL. The presence of anaemia at presentation indicates a slowly progressing tumour: there is no time for anaemia

Table 12.7   *Prognostic indicators in acute lymphoblastic leukaemia*

Prognostic indicator	Favourable	Unfavourable
White cell count	$< 10 \times 10^9/l$	$> 50 \times 10^9/l$
Age	3–7 years	< 1 year or > 10 years
Sex	Female	Male
Race	White	Black
Time to remission	< 14 days	> 28 days
Lymphadenopathy	Absent	Massive
Organomegaly	Absent	Massive
Mediastinal mass	Absent	Massive
CNS leukaemia	Absent	Massive
FAB type	L1	L3
Haemoglobin	$< 7\,g/dl$	$> 10\,g/dl$
Platelet count	$> 100 \times 10^9/l$	$< 30 \times 10^9/l$
Serum immunoglobulins	Normal	Decreased
Immunological markers	Early pre-B ALL	B or T ALL
Cytogenetic markers	Hyperdiploidy	Pseudodiploidy
	6q−	t(9;22), t(8;14), t(4;11), t(14q+)

The discovery of common ALL antigen (CALLA) by Dr M. Greaves in 1975 caused a great deal of excitement among leukaemologists because it appeared to be the first leukaemia-specific marker to be identified. He produced a polyclonal antibody that reacted with up to 80% of cases of childhood ALL by immunization of a rabbit with ALL blast cells. However, as the use of monoclonal antibodies to type ALL progressed, it became apparent that there was no specific antibody to detect leukaemic cells: all antibodies produced to date detect a normal cell at some stage of differentiation. The structure and function of CALLA has been established and it has been renamed CD10. It is a zinc metalloprotease of mol. wt 100 000 that hydrolyses peptide bonds, thereby reducing cellular responses to peptide hormones. Among the many biologically active peptides it cleaves are bradykinin, endothelin, angiotensin and oxytocin. CD10 is encoded by a gene on chromosome 3q21–q27. CD10 positivity is widely distributed in normal tissue: it is found in precursor T and B lymphocytes, granulocytes, brain, kidney and muscle, but its main diagnostic utility is as a marker of ALL.

to develop before the onset of symptoms in more aggressive tumours.

The majority of cases of ALL present with clinical symptoms of bone marrow failure and organ infiltration. Bone pain is common in childhood ALL. Superficial lymphadenopathy and moderate enlargement of the spleen and liver occur at some time in the course of the disease in most cases of ALL. Leukocytosis (predominantly leukaemic blast cells) and thrombocytopenia are common at presentation.

Early pre-B acute lymphoblastic leukaemia

More than 70% of cases of ALL in children and about 50% of cases in adults type as early pre-B ALL. This form of ALL is characterized by a lack of immunoglobulin markers on the cell surface or within the cytoplasm and, in about 90% of cases, by the presence on the cell surface of CD10, and is typically associated with a good prognosis. Because of its frequency, this form of ALL has been called 'common ALL' in earlier classification systems. Very occasionally, the phenotype of early pre-B cell ALL is observed with no expression of CD10. This may be referred to as 'null ALL'. Hyperdiploidy is most frequently documented in early pre-B cell ALL. Chromosomal translocations are more often associated with the other subtypes of ALL.

Pre-B acute lymphoblastic leukaemia

The leukaemic blast cells in pre-B ALL are characterized by the presence of cytoplasmic immunoglobulin heavy (μ) chains in the absence of light chains or surface immunoglobulin. Most cases are coded as FAB subtype L1 and 90% of cases are CD10 positive. Approximately 30% of cases exhibit the karyotype characterized by t(1;19)(q23;p13), which has been reported to convey a risk of early relapse during standard therapy.

B acute lymphoblastic leukaemia

B ALL is a relatively rare condition, representing less than 2% of cases of ALL. The leukaemic blasts in this subtype of ALL show signs of greater maturity than those in the other subtypes: CD10 expression is weak; immunoglobulins are expressed on the cell surface and molecular genetic analysis reveals a clonal rearrangement of both heavy and light chain immunoglobulin genes. The blast cells in the majority of cases of B ALL are FAB subtype L3. B ALL is associated with chromosomal translocations involving the c-*myc* oncogene and the immunoglobulin genes, i.e. t(8;14) (q24;q32), t(8;22)(q24;q11), t(2;8)(p12;q24). This form of ALL is associated with a uniformly poor prognosis.

T acute lymphoblastic leukaemia

T ALL accounts for between 10 and 15% of ALL in both children and adults. This subtype of ALL is rarely seen in children under the age of 1 year or in adults over the age of 50 years. T ALL occurs more frequently in males and is usually associated with a high white cell count and mediastinal mass at diagnosis. The incidence of central nervous system involvement is higher than in other types of ALL. T ALL is associated with a poor prognosis. The most sensitive marker of T ALL is the finding of a clonal rearrangement of the T cell receptor β (Tiβ) gene. Chromosomal translocations are relatively common in T ALL, with the genes encoding Tiα, Tiβ and Tiγ chains frequently involved. The genes that code for Tiβ and Tiγ chains are located on chromosome 7, while those for Tiα and Tiδ are located on chromosome 14.

Acute non-lymphoblastic leukaemia

Acute non-lymphoblastic leukaemia can occur at any age but is more common in adults, showing an increasing frequency with advancing age. ANLL accounts for 12% of cases of acute leukaemia in children under the age of 10 years and 28% between 10 and 15 years. In adults, ANLL accounts for 80–90% of cases of acute leukaemia. ANLL often occurs as a secondary event, particularly following a period of myelodysplasia or treatment for other neoplasms. ANLL diagnosed as a primary disorder is known as *de novo* ANLL.

The clinical features of ANLL are similar at all ages and are the consequence of the replacement of normal marrow elements by malignant blasts, often resulting in impaired haemopoiesis and organomegaly. The most common presenting symptoms are pallor and fatigue secondary to anaemia, bleeding problems secondary to thrombocytopenia, infection secondary to neutropenia and unexplained weight loss. Infiltration of the skin and gums occurs in approximately 10% of patients with ANLL and is particularly associated with M4 and M5 subtypes. Disseminated intravascular coagulation occurs more commonly in ANLL than ALL and is most closely associated with the M3 subtype. About 1 in 4 individuals with ANLL present with white cell counts in excess of $100 \times 10^9/l$, leading to problems associated with leukostasis, particularly within the pulmonary, CNS and genitourinary systems.

The recognition of prognostic indicators in ALL stimulated the search for similar indicators in ANLL but consistent findings have been difficult to obtain.

The cell of origin in ANLL most often shows myeloid or monocytic differentiation. Approximately 5–10% of cases have erythroid or megakaryocytic differentiation. Morphology and cytochemistry are usually sufficient to permit the recognition and classification of the majority of cases of ANLL. The presence of Auer rods, crystalline structures derived from primary granules by coalescence of primary granules, is a characteristic of myeloblasts in ANLL. Electron microscopy and immunocytochemistry are necessary to diagnose the remaining cases of ANLL. Cytogenetic abnormalities are common in ANLL and are frequently associated with a particular morphological subtype and clinical presentation.

Acute myeloblastic leukaemia (AML)

This subgroup includes the three FAB subtypes M0, M1 and M2 and is characterized by the presence of myeloblasts with increasing cytochemical and morphological evidence of myeloid differentiation. The most differentiated, M2, is associated with the cytogenetic abnormality t(8;21). This entity occurs mostly in children or young adults and is associated with anaemia, thrombocytopenia and splenomegaly at diagnosis. The myeloblasts usually contain Auer rods and the mature myeloid cells are dysplastic.

Acute promyelocytic leukaemia (APL)

Approximately 6% of patients with ANLL present with APL (FAB subtype M3) which is characterized by the predominance of promyelocytes in the bone marrow. The leukaemic promyelocytes are frequently abnormal in their granulation pattern and possess multiple Auer rods. APL is most common in young adults and is characterized by a low white cell count and thrombocytopenia at presentation, coupled with disseminated intravascular coagulation (DIC). The recognition and intensive treatment of the associated DIC in APL has improved its prognosis. The chromosomal translocations t(15;17)(q22;q21) or (q22;q11–12) are present in almost all cases of APL and have not been described in any other condition.

Acute myelomonoblastic leukaemia (AMMoL)

The AMMoL subtype (FAB subtype M4) is characterized morphologically by the presence of both myeloid and monocytic differentiation. The latter is best demonstrated by the use of non-specific esterase cytochemistry, in particular a naphthyl butyrate esterase, and positive reactions with the CD14 monocyte-associated surface marker. Abnormalities of chromosome 16 are associated with a variant of AMMol with abnormal eosinophil morphology (designated $M4_{Eo}$) which is associated with a good prognosis.

Acute monoblastic leukaemia (AMoL)

AMoL accounts for between 2 and 10% of cases of ANLL and is characterized by the presence of monoblasts that are either poorly differentiated (FAB subtype M5a) or well differentiated (FAB subtype M5b). Cytogenetic abnormalities in AMoL often involve translocations between chromosome 11 and chromosomes 9, 10 or 17.

Acute erythroleukaemia (AEL)

AEL (FAB subtype M6) most commonly affects those over the age of 50 years and is more common in men than in women. This subtype is regarded as ANLL with predominant erythroid differentiation and accounts for approximately 3% of cases of ANLL. The morphology of the erythroid cells is typically severely dysplastic with multinucleated erythroblasts and cytoplasmic bridging. AEL frequently represents an erythroleukaemic transformation of myelodysplasia. Aneuploidy has been reported in 63% of patients and abnormalities often involve either chromosome 5 or 7.

Acute megakaryoblastic leukaemia (AMegL)

AMegL (FAB subtype M7) represents between 3 and 12% of adult cases of ANLL and occurs as *de novo* leukaemia, secondary leukaemia following cytotoxic chemotherapy and as transformed myeloproliferative and myelodysplastic syndromes. Cytogenetic abnormalities are variable but have included abnormalities of chromosomes 8 and 21. A subset of AMegL occurs in infants

A typical tumour cell load at diagnosis for ANLL is about $5 \times 10^{11} - 5 \times 10^{12}$ cells: this compares to a total normal haemopoietic stem cell load of less than 1×10^9.

Cytotoxic drugs belong to one of seven categories:

- Alkylating agents such as cyclophosphamide, chlorambucil and busulfan which crosslink the side chains of proteins and nucleic acids.

- Antimetabolites such as methotrexate, 5-fluorouracil and cytosine arabinoside which inhibit intracellular enzyme activity.

- Anthracycline antibiotics such as daunorubicin, actinomycin D and adriamycin which inhibit DNA and RNA synthesis and generate oxygen free radicals.

- Steroid hormones such as prednisone which are lympholytic.

- Plant alkaloids such as vincristine and vinblastine which inhibit mitosis and etoposide which induces DNA strand breaks.

- Enzymes such as L-asparaginase which deprives ALL blasts of the amino acid L-aparagine.

- Miscellaneous agents such as bleomycin which causes DNA strand breaks and 2'-deoxycoformycin which inhibits adenosine deaminase.

and is characterized by extensive organomegaly and the chromosomal translocation t(1;22)(p13;q13).

Treatment and management of acute leukaemia

The treatment of acute leukaemia can be divided into three categories: cytotoxic drug therapy and radiotherapy to eradicate the leukaemic cells, bone marrow transplantation and general supportive therapy for bone marrow failure. There are significant differences between ALL and ANLL in terms of age of incidence, drug sensitivity, treatment approach and overall prognosis, which justify a different therapeutic strategy in each case. The use of haemopoietic growth factors is being assessed in clinical trials in conjunction with cytotoxic drug therapy and bone marrow transplantation.

Cytotoxic chemotherapy

The aim of cytotoxic drug therapy is to induce a remission (an absence of any clinical or conventional laboratory evidence of disease) and then to progressively eradicate the residual leukaemic cells by courses of consolidation, intensification and maintenance therapy. Several cytotoxic drugs are combined to increase the cytotoxic effect, improve remission rates and the length of remission, and to reduce the frequency of drug resistance. Drug combinations are given in cycles with treatment-free intervals to allow the recovery of normal haemopoietic tissue. Standard treatment regimes specific for ALL and ANLL have been devised from multicentre trials of cytotoxic drug combinations. These may be varied to take into account the prognostic factors of each case at diagnosis and classification.

Maintenance cytotoxic drug therapy has been found to be effective in treating ALL but not ANLL. A feature of treatment regimes for ANLL is prolonged and severe bone marrow failure due to the lack of selectivity of the myelotoxic drugs used. Intensive supportive care is necessary during this period of treatment. Treatment of relapse is more successful in ALL than ANLL.

Leukaemic cells in the CNS are beyond the reach of most cytotoxic drugs. Consequently prophylactic treatment consisting of intrathecal methotrexate and cranial irradiation is included in most treatment regimes for ALL to prevent CNS relapse of the leukaemia. Meningeal relapse occurs less commonly in ANLL overall, but is most closely associated with AMMoL and AMoL. Testicular leukaemia occasionally occurs in ALL, necessitating irradiation with reinduction cytotoxic drug therapy.

Supportive therapy

The availability of separate blood components (red cells, platelets and fresh frozen plasma) has radically improved the general supportive therapy of patients with acute leukaemia. Packed red cells are used to treat anaemia; platelets to treat the haemorrhagic complications associated with thrombocytopenia, which can be particularly severe during cytotoxic drug therapy; and fresh frozen plasma, usually combined with platelets, is used to treat the DIC which is often troublesome in APL. Patients with acute leukaemia are highly susceptible to infection. The prompt and effective treatment of established infection and attempts to prevent infection are vitally important components of leukaemia treatment. The infections are usually bacterial but viral, fungal and protozoal infections also occur with increased frequency. Measures taken to reduce the risk of infection include nursing in isolation facilities, antibiotic therapy to reduce gut and other commensal flora, and vigorous microbiological surveillance.

Bone marrow transplantation

Bone marrow transplantation (BMT) involves the elimination of host haemopoietic stem cells using large doses of cytotoxic drugs and total body irradiation and the subsequent infusion of replacement bone marrow cells. The transplanted marrow may be from an HLA-matched donor (**allogeneic transplant**) or from a sample of stored patient bone marrow 'harvested' during disease remission (**autologous transplant**). BMT is used in some centres to treat ANLL in first remission in patients under 45 years of age, and to treat ALL in successful second remission. It is also considered for other cases of acute leukaemia with particularly poor prognostic indicators.

The rigours of bone marrow transplantation are such that it is only offered to those under the age of 45 years who are physically in good condition. The conditioning process involves the administration of large doses of cyclophosphamide as a cytotoxic and immunosuppressive agent followed by either total body irradiation (TBI) or total lymphoid irradiation (TLI) to induce marrow ablation. The dose of radiation employed needs to be as high as possible but is limited by the damage it causes to the lungs, gastrointestinal tract and central nervous system. The conditioning process is associated with a range of severe toxic effects such as nausea, vomiting, diarrhoea, abdominal pain, haemorrhagic cystitis, lung and heart damage, hair loss, reddening of the skin, sterility, thyroid dysfunction and, in children, impairment of growth and intellectual ability. TLI is associated with lower pulmonary toxicity than TBI.

A major cause of failure in any form of organ transplantation is the possibility of rejection of the graft by the host immune system.

It is now standard practice to prescribe cytotoxic drugs in combinations with the intention of inducing an additive or a synergistic effect on the tumour cells. Combinations of drugs are selected according to the following principles:

- Each drug employed must be effective when used as a single agent.

- Drugs with different modes of action should be used.

- The major toxicity of each drug should differ from others in the combination.

- There should be no synergistic toxicity. Each drug must be used in its optimum dose and treatment schedule.

In practice, compromises are often required, but each combination should be as close to this ideal as possible. Widely used combinations include **CHOP** – **C**yclophosphamide, **H**ydroxydaunomycin, **O**ncovin and **P**rednisolone; **MAZE** – **M**-amsacrine, **AZ**acytidine and **E**toposide; and **DAT** – **D**aunorubicin, **A**ra-C and 6-**T**hioguanine.

One of the most important limitations to the successful use of cytotoxic chemotherapy is the development of multidrug resistance. MDR is common in relapsed leukaemias and secondary ANLL and is associated with a poor prognosis. The development of the MDR phenotype is associated with the expression of a 170 kDa transmembrane protein (P-glycoprotein), encoded by a gene located at 7q21–23 called *mdr*-1. A structurally related gene, *mdr*-2, is located nearby. P-glycoprotein acts as an energy-dependent efflux pump for a wide range of cytotoxic drugs, thereby reducing their toxic effects. The function of the *mdr*-2 gene product is unknown but it does not act as an efflux pump. Atypical patterns of MDR have also been described, associated with alterations in topoisomerase, glutathione-S-transferase or CTP synthetase activity.

Graft rejection can be minimized by only using HLA-matched tissue and by the use of immunosuppressive agents such as cyclosporin. However, because bone marrow transplantation involves the engraftment of immunocompetent tissue, an additional complication exists, i.e. the possibility of rejection of the host by the graft. This phenomenon is known as **graft versus host disease (GVHD)** and is an important cause of morbidity and mortality in bone marrow transplant recipients. The incidence of GVHD can be reduced by post-transplant immunosuppressive therapy or by pre-transplant purging of T lymphocytes from the donor marrow. Unfortunately, the reduction in the incidence of GVHD achieved using T lymphocyte-depleted bone marrow is offset by a concomitant increase in the rate of graft rejection. Acute GVHD is associated with T lymphocyte-mediated attack of skin, liver and lung tissue. There is some evidence that a minor degree of chronic GVHD may contribute to a reduction in the risk of leukaemic relapse following bone marrow transplantation by a '**graft versus leukaemia effect**'.

In the absence of a suitable donor, transplantation of autologous bone marrow harvested during disease remission may be used. This form of treatment is associated with a higher rate of engraftment and the absence of GVHD. However, a greater risk of leukaemic relapse and the absence of the graft versus leukaemia effect balance these advantages. Pre-transplant purging of the leukaemic cells from the marrow sample using monoclonal antibodies can reduce the risk of leukaemic relapse following autologous bone marrow transplantation.

Haemopoietic growth factors

A further development in the treatment of acute leukaemia, the use of recombinant human haemopoietic growth factors, is being assessed by clinical trials. Haemopoietic growth factors are administered in conjunction with cytotoxic drug therapy to improve the eradication of leukaemic cells and to accelerate the recovery of normal haemopoiesis. An important consideration in the trials is the potentially adverse effect of the growth factors in accelerating the proliferation of the leukaemic cells, although recent studies suggest that this is not a problem. The utility of haemopoietic growth factors is also being assessed in BMT where it is envisaged that they will accelerate the haemopoietic reconstitution process.

Suggested further reading

Alexander, F. (1998). Clustering of childhood acute leukaemia – The EUROCLUS project. *Radiation and Environmental Biophysics* **37(2)**, 71–74.

Bain, B.J. (1990). *Leukaemia Diagnosis: A Guide to the FAB Classification*. London: Gower Medical Publishing.

Macey, M. (1998). Flow cytometry in haematology. In *Progress in Haematology* (C.D.R. Dunn and C.J. Pallister, eds). London: Greenwich Medical Media.

Pinto, A., Zulian, G.B. and Archimbaud, E. (1998). Acute myelogenous leukaemia. *Critical Reviews in Oncology/Hematology* 27(2), 161–64.

Reid, M. (1998). Whither leukaemia classification? In *Progress in Haematology* (C.D.R. Dunn and C.J. Pallister, eds). London: Greenwich Medical Media.

http://www.leukaemia.demon.co.uk/

Self-assessment questions

1. Which FAB type acute leukaemia is associated with:
   (a) bundles of Auer rods;
   (b) poorly differentiated monoblasts;
   (c) vacuolated lymphoblasts with deeply basophilic cytoplasm?
2. Which acute leukaemia characteristically demonstrates:
   (a) acid phosphatase +, CD2+;
   (b) cytoplasmic μ chains +, membrane immunoglobulin –;
   (c) CD71 +;
   (d) t(15;17)(q22;q12).
3. Distinguish between the sources of bone marrow for allogeneic and autologous transplant.
4. Distinguish between the graft versus host (GVH) and graft versus leukaemia (GVL) effects.

Key Concepts and Facts

- Classification of acute leukaemic is essential to facilitate appropriate treatment and disease monitoring.

- In the FAB system, ALL is divided into three subtypes (L1–L3) and ANLL into eight subtypes (M0–M7) based on morphology and cytochemistry.

- Ancillary approaches to classification include the use of immunophenotyping and cytogenetic analysis. Concordance between classification systems is relatively poor.

- Acute leukaemia causes morbidity and mortality through three general mechanisms: deficiency in normal blood cell number or function, invasion of vital organs and metabolic imbalance.

- Treatment of acute leukaemia can be divided into three categories: cytotoxic drug therapy and radiotherapy to eradicate the leukaemic cells, bone marrow transplantation and general supportive therapy for bone marrow failure.

Chapter 13
Chronic leukaemias

Learning objectives

After studying this chapter you should confidently be able to:

List the different types of chronic leukaemia.

Identify characteristic features of the different forms of chronic leukaemia.

Outline the pathophysiology of the chronic leukaemias.

Outline the approaches to treatment of the chronic leukaemias.

The chronic leukaemias are malignant disorders that are characterized by the unbridled clonal proliferation of relatively well-differentiated blood cells. The chronic leukaemias can be divided on the basis of the lineage of the malignant clone into chronic myeloid leukaemias and chronic lymphoid leukaemias. Each of these groups is capable of further division as described below.

Chronic myeloid leukaemia

Chronic myeloid leukaemia (CML) is a clonal myeloproliferative disorder of the totipotential haemopoietic stem cell and is almost invariably characterized by the presence of a chromosomal marker, the **Philadelphia chromosome** t(9;22)(q34;q11), in the leukaemic cells. CML occurs with an annual incidence of about 1 per 100 000 of the population with no apparent geographic variation. There is a slight excess incidence of CML in males. There was a significant increase in the incidence of CML in survivors of the atomic explosions in Hiroshima and Nagasaki. No other universally accepted predisposing factors have been identified.

CML is characterized by an insidious onset of ill-health and is associated with a massive increase in the circulating granulocyte count and splenomegaly. CML affects all age groups but is seen most frequently in middle age. Until recently, the prognosis of patients with CML was poor with a median survival of 3 years. However, recent reports have indicated an improved prognosis due

In 1960, an abnormally small group G chromosome, the Philadelphia chromosome (Ph′), named after the city of its discovery, was identified in the bone marrow cells of patients with CML. About 90% of CML patients are Philadelphia positive using conventional cytogenetic techniques. With the introduction of Giemsa banding techniques in 1973, the Ph′ chromosome was shown to result from a reciprocal translocation between chromosomes 9 and 22, t(9;22)(q34;qll).

to earlier detection, improved anti-CML therapy and better supportive care.

Leukaemogenesis of CML

Much of the research into the causation of CML has centred on the role of the Philadelphia chromosome. The typical reciprocal translocation t(9;22)(q34;q11) involves the translocation of the c-*abl* oncogene from 9q34 to a point within the breakpoint cluster region of the *bcr* gene at 22q11, forming a chimeric *bcr-abl* gene.

The normal *abl* gene product (p145^{abl}) is a tyrosine kinase while the normal *bcr* gene product (p160^{bcr}) is a serine/threonine kinase. Both molecules are important intracellular signal transduction proteins and are expressed in virtually all types of normal cells.

The chimeric *bcr-abl* fusion gene produces a novel 8 kb *m*RNA transcript which encodes a chimeric protein of molecular weight 210 000 (p210$^{bcr-abl}$). This protein contains 1104 amino acids encoded by the translocated *abl* gene and either 927 or 902 amino acids encoded by the disrupted *bcr* gene. The chimeric p210$^{bcr-abl}$ has a much more powerful tyrosine kinase activity than p145^{abl} and has been shown to interact with its substrates in an altered manner. Although the way in which p210$^{bcr-abl}$ brings about malignant change is unknown, there is little doubt that it plays a pivotal role in CML, particularly in the chronic phase.

CML is typically a triphasic disease. It can be separated on the basis of various clinical and laboratory characteristics into a **chronic phase**, an **accelerated phase** and a terminal **blastic phase**. During the chronic phase of CML the t(9;22)(q34;q11) typically is the only chromosomal abnormality present. However, progression into the accelerated phase is accompanied by the acquisition of additional chromosomal abnormalities in about 80% of cases. The most common additional abnormalities are the acquisition of an extra Philadelphia chromosome (+Ph), trisomy 8 (+8) and i(17q).

Disease progression occurs as a consequence of activation of additional oncogenes within leukaemic stem cells, thereby favouring the establishment and expansion of new malignant clones which have the characteristics of acute leukaemia. A number of oncogenes have been shown to be altered in blastic phase cells, including the recessive tumour suppressor gene *p53* and *myc*. There is, as yet, no convincing evidence that these oncogenes are directly implicated in the induction of the blastic phase of CML.

Current evidence suggests that the genesis of CML is a multistep process:

- The first step involves the clonal proliferation of a genetically unstable, Philadelphia chromosome-negative totipotential stem cell. The abnormal clone that results has a proliferative advantage over normal haemopoietic stem cells. The cause and nature of the stimulus for this clonal proliferation is unknown.

Recent work has implicated the novel chimeric protein p210$^{bcr-abl}$ in the pathogenesis of CML. The human *bcr-abl* gene has been successfully expressed in murine bone marrow cells. When these transfected cells were reinfused into lethally irradiated mice, the majority developed chronic phase CML and a further group developed acute leukaemia. Furthermore, experiments using human CML cells in *in vitro* culture have shown that blocking the expression of the chimeric p210$^{bcr-abl}$ protein by antisense oligonucleotides abolishes the leukaemic phenotype. These observations suggest that cure of CML requires complete elimination or suppression of the Ph' positive clone. Novel treatment strategies such as the use of antisense oligonucleotides or synthetic peptides directed against p210$^{bcr-abl}$ *m*RNA or its protein product are currently under evaluation.

- Chronic phase CML is triggered by the acquisition of a Philadelphia chromosome and the expression of $p210^{bcr-abl}$ in a single member of the expanded totipotential stem cell clone.
- Progression of the disease to the accelerated and blastic phases is prompted by the subsequent accumulation of proto-oncogene mutations. The processes involved in the evolution of the malignant clone towards the blastic phase are poorly understood at present.

Recognition and classification of CML

Recognition of CML requires the examination of appropriately stained blood and bone marrow smears and cytogenetic studies. Frequently, in cases of grossly elevated white cell counts at presentation, the diagnosis is self-evident from the peripheral blood. However, a bone marrow aspirate is still required to provide material for cytogenetic evaluation and to assess the degree of fibrosis. About 90% of cases of CML have clear cytogenetic evidence for the presence of the Philadelphia chromosome. The application of molecular genetic techniques to cases of atypical CML in which the Philadelphia chromosome cannot be identified by conventional means has revealed evidence for the rearrangement of the *bcr* and *abl* genes in at least 35% of cases. The division of CML into typical and atypical forms is clinically relevant because atypical CML has a relatively poor prognosis.

Pathophysiology of CML

Chronic phase CML

The three defining features of typical chronic phase CML are a raised granulocyte count, the presence of the Philadelphia chromosome and splenomegaly. The total WBC at presentation often exceeds $100 \times 10^9/l$ and may be as high as $1000 \times 10^9/l$. All stages of granulocyte differentiation are present in the peripheral blood but a rise in the level of circulating myelocytes and mature neutrophils is especially prominent. The proportion of myeloblasts and promyelocytes is low during the chronic phase. The absolute basophil, eosinophil and monocyte count may all be increased. The leukaemic cells have an increased rate of cytoplasmic maturation relative to nuclear maturation, which is manifest as heavy granulation of promyelocytes. A variety of functional abnormalities may be present including defects of chemotaxis and phagocytosis and deficiency of granule contents such as lactoferrin, myeloperoxidase and alkaline phosphatase. This last observation is exploited in the differentiation of early CML from other causes of leukocytosis where the level of alkaline phosphatase is normal or increased.

Other commonly observed peripheral blood cell abnormalities

include normocytic, normochromic anaemia and thrombocytosis. Broadly, the severity of both abnormalities increases with increasing total WBC count. Paradoxically, bleeding secondary to an acquired defect of platelet function is a common complication of CML. The circulating levels of CFU-GEMM, CFU-GM, BFU-E and CFU-Meg are greatly increased in CML. These cells all carry the Philadelphia chromosome and thus reflect expansion of the leukaemic clone. The serum vitamin B_{12} level is typically massively increased, reflecting synthesis of transcobalamins I and III by the leukaemic granulocytes. Hyperuricaemia is also common and reflects the increased white cell turnover.

Bone marrow examination reveals extreme hypercellularity with loss of fat spaces, extension of haemopoietically active marrow into the long bones and extramedullary haemopoiesis, resulting in splenomegaly. An increase in marrow reticulin fibres is common at presentation, progressing in most cases to outright fibrosis.

The typical physical features of chronic phase CML include pallor, lethargy and fatigue which are secondary to the anaemia; abdominal distension or discomfort secondary to splenomegaly; sternal tenderness or more generalized bone pain secondary to expansion of haemopoietically active marrow; and purpura or bleeding secondary to platelet dysfunction.

Accelerated phase CML

There are no universally agreed objective criteria for defining the point at which CML enters the accelerated phase. Broadly speaking, most workers accept that the transition to accelerated phase is accompanied by increasing refractoriness to treatment, which may be reflected in one or more of the changes listed in Table 13.1. The median duration of the chronic phase from presentation is 3 years. Transition to the accelerated phase is usually a gradual process, with minimal physical symptoms. Once the accelerated phase is clearly established, however, progression to the blastic phase is inexorable and usually occurs within a few months.

Blastic phase CML

In most cases, establishment of the accelerated phase of CML is followed by a sustained downward spiral in which the disease becomes progressively refractory to treatment, the blast cell count rises inexorably and physical symptoms steadily worsen. Progression of chronic phase to blastic phase CML has been likened to the evolution of a chronic leukaemia into an acute leukaemia. The accumulation of blast cells that results is accompanied by the development of progressive anaemia, neutropenia and thrombocytopenia. Most cases of blastic phase CML show features of M1 or M2 ANLL, but monoblastic, erythroblastic, megakaryoblastic and lymphoblastic transformation also occur. The treatment for blastic

The earliest known cases of leukaemia involved a 28-year-old slater called John Mentieth and a 50-year-old cook called Marie Straide. Mentieth was admitted to the Edinburgh Royal Infirmary on 27 February 1845 and Straide was admitted 2 days later to the Charite Hospital in Berlin. Both succumbed shortly after admission and were examined *post mortem* by Drs Bennet and Virchow respectively. With the benefit of hindsight, it seems likely that both were suffering from CML. Both complained of progressive lethargy and a painful, swollen abdomen, probably reflecting anaemia and massive splenomegaly. Straide also had a severe cough and Mentieth had numerous solid tumours scattered about his body, a classical feature of end-stage untreated CML.

Table 13.1 *Objective criteria for the recognition of transition to accelerated phase CML*

Laboratory features
>15% blasts in bone marrow or peripheral blood
>30% blasts + promyelocytes in peripheral blood
>20% basophils in peripheral blood
$< 100 \times 10^9/l$ platelets (not treatment-related)
Acquisition of additional cytogenetic abnormalities
Increasing collagen fibrosis of bone marrow

Clinical features
Increasing splenomegaly which is refractory to treatment
Increasing chemotherapy requirement

The earliest agent that could clearly be shown to be effective in the treatment of leukaemia and lymphoma was a 1% aqueous solution of AsO_3, known as **Fowler's solution**. This highly toxic substance had been in use for almost a hundred years as a general tonic and cure-all. Its first use in a case of leukaemia was in 1865 when a German physician called Lissauer administered it to a woman with CML. The temporary remission that resulted prompted others to repeat the experiment with similar success. Unfortunately, the remissions were short-lived and arsenic fell into disuse when, at the turn of the century, radiotherapy became available.

phase CML is the same as that for the acute leukaemia that it most closely resembles but is usually much less successful. The most common causes of death in blastic phase CML are infection secondary to neutropenia and haemorrhage secondary to thrombocytopenia.

Atypical CML

The absence of the Philadelphia chromosome in an individual with an otherwise CML-like picture is the defining feature of atypical CML. The 6% of cases of CML which show no evidence of $p210^{bcr-abl}$ expression have a much poorer prognosis with a median duration of survival from presentation of about 18 months.

Juvenile CML

Typical CML is rare in children but, where present, is clinically indistinguishable from the adult disease. A distinct form of CML occurs in infants with a peak incidence between 1 and 5 years of age. Juvenile myelomonocytic leukaemia (JMML), as this form is known, is characterized by a CML-like blood picture with a prominent monocytic component, thrombocytopenia and a raised foetal haemoglobin concentration, which may exceed 50% of the total. Typical clinical features at presentation include anaemia, hepatosplenomegaly, respiratory tract infection and eczematous rash. JMML is associated with a uniformly poor prognosis: most affected infants die within 18 months of presentation.

Treatment and management of CML

The mainstays of conventional cytotoxic chemotherapy of CML are busulphan and hydroxyurea. Rapid and prolonged haematological remission with resolution of physical symptoms can be achieved in at least 80% of cases of CML using either of these drugs. However, disease progression is not significantly altered by such treatment: the median duration of the chronic phase of CML is much the same in treated and untreated individuals. In addition, cytogenetic studies have revealed the persistence of the Philadelphia chromosome-containing clone, even during apparently complete remission. For these reasons, conventional cytotoxic chemotherapy of CML must be considered to be palliative rather than curative.

Recombinant human α-interferon can induce haematological remission in up to 70% of newly diagnosed cases of CML. This drug selectively suppresses the leukaemic clone and improved survival and durable cytogenetic remission is obtainable in about 20% of cases. The toxicity of α-interferon is relatively mild, consisting of flu-like symptoms.

The only form of treatment for CML which currently offers the prospect of a cure is bone marrow transplantation. Allogeneic transplantation offers significantly improved disease-free survival times, particularly when transplantation is performed early in the chronic phase. The use of T lymphocyte-depleted bone marrow reduces the incidence of graft versus host disease but is associated with an increased incidence of graft failure and relapse because of the reduction in the graft versus leukaemia effect. When an HLA-matched donor is unavailable, autologous marrow transplantation may be attempted using bone marrow harvested following successful treatment with α-interferon.

Chronic lymphoid leukaemias

Chronic lymphoid leukaemia can be subdivided into three main subtypes: chronic lymphocytic leukaemia (CLL), prolymphocytic leukaemia (PLL) and hairy cell leukaemia (HCL). Each of these subtypes can be further subdivided on the basis of immunological phenotype. The distinction between the chronic lymphoid leukaemias and other lymphoproliferative disorders such as lymphoma frequently is unclear, particularly when the latter presents or relapses in a 'leukaemic phase' caused by overspill of the lymphoma cells from the tissues into the circulation. The non-leukaemic lymphoproliferative disorders are described in Chapter 15.

Recognition and classification of chronic lymphoid leukaemias

Chronic lymphoid leukaemias are classified using a combination of morphology and immunophenotyping. The primary distinction to be made in each case is between T and B lineage disease. Further subdivision into differentiation or maturation stage can then be performed to provide the classification scheme shown in Table 13.2. CLL, PLL and HCL are predominantly B lymphoid diseases: T lymphoid variants account for about 5% and 25% of cases respectively. THCL has been reported only twice. Immunophenotyping can be performed on lymphoid cells derived from peripheral blood, bone marrow, lymph node biopsy or tissue biopsy or from other body fluids such as a pleural effusion.

Identification of a chronic lymphoid leukaemia by immunophenotyping of peripheral blood cells requires the demonstration and typing of the malignant lymphoid clone against a background of normal, polyclonal lymphocytes. Recognition of a B lymphoid clone is relatively simple in such circumstances because the proportion of circulating B lymphocytes is normally low. One reliable way to identify a B lymphoid clone is to demonstrate immunoglobulin light chain restriction. In contrast, recognition of a malignant T lymphoid clone must take place against a dominant background of normal, mature T lymphocytes and is often inconclusive. Definitive demonstration of a clonal T lymphoid disorder relies upon the

It was Virchow who first proposed that there was more than one form of leukaemia. He suggested that one form was characterized by massive splenomegaly and marked expansion of the numbers of one type of colourless cells in the blood while the other was characterized by swelling of the lymph nodes and an increase in the other main type of colourless blood cells (remember that Romanowsky staining was not yet available and the distinctions between the types of leukocyte were far from clear). Virchow coined the terms splenic leukaemia and lymphatic leukaemia to describe these two types. Several years later, in 1879, it was suggested that the predominant cells in the splenic form of leukaemia emanated from the bone marrow and so the term myeloid leukaemia was coined and gradually came to replace the term splenic leukaemia.

Table 13.2 *Immunophenotype classification of chronic B lymphocytic leukaemias*

Marker	BCLL	TCLL	PLL	TPLL	HCL
CD2	−	+	−	+	−
CD3	−	+	−	+	−
CD5	+	+	+/−	+	−
CD7	−	+	−	+	−
CD10	−	−	−	−	−
CD11c	−	−	−	−	+
CD19	+	−	+	−	+
CD20	+	−	+	−	+
CD22	+/−	−	+	−	+
CD25	−	−	+/−	−/+	+
CD38	−	−	−	−	−
FMC7	−/+	−	−	−	+ +
SIgM	−	−	+	−	+

demonstration of a clonal rearrangement of the T lymphocyte receptor.

Chronic lymphocytic leukaemia

Chronic lymphocytic leukaemia (CLL) is by far the most common of the chronic lymphoid leukaemias, comprising about 70% of cases. CLL most commonly affects the elderly inhabitants of developed countries. This may be partly due to the increased life expectancy in such countries but there also appears to be a genetic component because the disease is rare in expatriate as well as indigenous Japanese. CLL is twice as common in men as in women. There have been rare reports of a familial tendency towards the development of CLL.

Leukaemogenesis of CLL

Research into the molecular and cytogenetic changes that accompany the development of CLL has been hampered by the low mitotic rate of the leukaemic cells. Even following stimulation with mitogenic factors, metaphase preparations can be obtained in little more than half of cases. Because of these technical difficulties, there is far less agreement about the frequency, nature and significance of non-random chromosomal abnormalities in CLL than for CML or the acute leukaemias. The most widely accepted non-random chromosomal abnormalities in CLL are +12, 14q+ and 13q− which are seen in about 33%, 25% and 10% of cases respectively.

Recognition and classification of CLL

Recognition of classical CLL is based on the presence of an absolute lymphocytosis and typical morphology. Lymphocyte counts at presentation range widely but most commonly lie between 20 and 50×10^9/l. The leukaemic cells in BCLL characteristically are small, round, mature cells, with a thin rim of featureless sky blue cytoplasm. The microscopic hallmark of CLL is the presence of a large number of 'smear' cells on the blood film. This artefact is caused by damage to exceptionally fragile BCLL cells during spreading of the blood film and is not associated with other chronic lymphoid disorders.

The bone marrow is always involved in CLL: an infiltrate that occupies 30–50% of the available space is common. As the disease progresses, the leukaemic clone progressively squeezes out normal haemopoiesis, resulting in anaemia and thrombocytopenia. Erythroid hyperplasia in the bone marrow is strongly indicative of the presence of autoimmune haemolysis, a common complication of CLL. Sensitive techniques such as immunophenotyping, flow cytometry and dual labelling of cells have enabled the reliable recognition of CLL, even in the absence of an absolute lymphocytosis.

CD5 expression is considered to be essential for a diagnosis of CLL. CD5 is a pan T cell marker that is involved in T lymphocyte activation. This marker has also been demonstrated on foetal splenic lymphocytes and on a small subset of adult lymph node germinal centre lymphocytes. These CD5+ B lymphocytes are postulated to be involved in the regulation of autoimmunity, which accords well with the observed excess of autoimmune disease in CLL. The clonal nature of BCLL is easily confirmed by the demonstration of immunoglobulin light chain restriction (the leukaemic cells express either κ or λ light chains, but never both) or the presence of a clonal immunoglobulin gene rearrangement.

Pathophysiology of CLL

CLL is an insidious and slowly progressive disease. Typical presenting features include general malaise and fatigue secondary to anaemia, mild hepatosplenomegaly and painless, symmetrical lymphadenopathy. Splenomegaly in CLL is minimal; massive enlargement of the spleen is associated with HCL or PLL. In contrast to the acute leukaemias and lymphomas, symptoms such as unexplained fever, severe weight loss and night sweats are uncommon in CLL. However, susceptibility to bacterial or fungal infection increases as the disease advances due to progressive immunodeficiency, neutropenia and hypogammaglobulinaemia. As many as 25% of cases of CLL are free of physical symptoms at diagnosis.

The most common cause of anaemia in CLL is bone marrow failure but autoimmune haemolytic anaemia (AIHA), haematinic deficiency and pure red cell aplasia are all potential complications. AIHA occurs in about one-third of cases but, if recognized early and treated successfully, does not confer a poor prognosis. Several triggers of pure red cell aplasia have been documented including parvovirus infection, T lymphocyte suppression of erythropoiesis and the development of auto-antibodies directed against erythropoietin.

Treatment and management of CLL

A wide selection of treatment options exists for CLL, ranging from minimal supportive care to aggressive cytotoxic chemotherapy and radiotherapy. Age and clinical stage largely determine which option is selected in an individual case. For example, an 85-year-old man presenting with minimal disease requires supportive therapy and haematological monitoring to provide early warning of disease progression. In contrast, a much younger patient with advanced disease requires aggressive treatment.

The mainstay of treatment is a combination of chlorambucil or cyclophosphamide and prednisolone, which achieves a good response in about 50% of early disease cases, but complete remission in less than 30% of individuals with advanced disease. Because the aim of treatment is palliative rather than curative, secondary symptoms such as anaemia, thrombocytopenia and infections must be treated promptly and effectively. Splenic irradiation or splenectomy may be indicated for troublesome splenomegaly, refractory AIHA or autoimmune thrombocytopenia. Alternative approaches, which are still the subject of clinical trials, include drugs such as fludarabine, $2'$-deoxycoformycin and 2-chlorodeoxy-adenosine and immunotherapy using a monoclonal antibody such as CD52 which lyses CLL cells.

Prolymphocytic leukaemia

Prolymphocytic leukaemia (PLL) is a relatively uncommon condition which afflicts the elderly of developed countries and affects men more commonly than women. It accounts for less than 10% of the chronic lymphoid leukaemias. The T lymphoid variant of PLL accounts for about 25% of cases.

Leukaemogenesis of PLL

PLL was, for many years, thought to be an unusual variant of CLL. However, with the advent of immunophenotyping, it became clear that PLL is a separate disease.

The incidence of clonal chromosomal rearrangements in PLL is very high, with rearrangements of 14q being particularly common. In BPLL the most common breakpoint is at 14q32, the site of the immunoglobulin heavy chain gene locus, whereas in TPLL the breakpoint usually is located at 14q11, the locus of the T lymphocyte receptor α chain gene.

Recognition and classification of PLL

Recognition of PLL is relatively straightforward and is based on the presence of a markedly raised white cell count, which is composed of more than 55% of prolymphocytes. The white cell count at presentation typically is greater than $100 \times 10^9/l$ and may reach as high as $1000 \times 10^9/l$. TPLL usually is associated with higher white counts than BPLL. Most cases are thrombocytopenic and anaemic secondary to marrow infiltration at presentation. The peripheral blood picture seen in BPLL is characteristic: examination of the bone marrow is seldom required for diagnostic purposes. The prolymphocytes of BPLL are relatively large cells with abundant pale blue cytoplasm which is free of granules, and a central nucleus with a prominent, single nucleolus. PLL is characterized at presentation by moderate splenomegaly in the absence of lymphadenopathy and typically follows a more aggressive course than CLL.

Treatment and management of PLL

PLL is a more aggressive disease than CLL and is moderately refractory to treatment. Effective treatment for PLL is hampered by the advanced age of those affected. In most cases, the first step of treatment is to reduce the circulating white cell count by leukopheresis or splenic irradiation. The latter option causes a significant reduction in the splenomegaly, appears to lengthen the duration of subsequent remission and is generally well tolerated by elderly patients. Splenectomy may further improve the duration of remission but, in contrast to HCL, does not impede disease progression. Disease debulking is insufficient to induce remission in PLL: supplementary cytotoxic chemotherapy, most commonly using CHOP (cyclophosphamide, hydroxydaunomycin (adriamycin), oncovin (vincristine) and prednisolone), is usually required. This aggressive treatment schedule necessitates energetic supportive care in these elderly patients. Most individuals will have some, generally short-lived, response to treatment but complete remissions are rare. Several other treatments have been tried in PLL with limited success, including α-interferon, immunotherapy, 2′-deoxycoformycin, 2-chlorodeoxyadenosine and fludarabine.

Hairy cell leukaemia

Hairy cell leukaemia (HCL) is an uncommon B lymphoid disorder, accounting for no more than 10% of cases of chronic lymphoid leukaemia. It has a similar age distribution to CLL and shows a male:female ratio of about 6:1.

> The name hairy cell leukaemia was coined by Schrek and Donnelly in 1966, but the disease was first described by Bouroncle in 1958 and was then called leukaemic reticuloendotheliosis. The lineage and normal counterpart of the hairy cell was the subject of heated scientific debate for many years. However, advances in immunophenotyping and genotyping have finally confirmed the cell as being of B lymphoid origin.

Leukaemogenesis of HCL

All of the technical problems associated with cytogenetic analysis of CLL apply equally well to HCL, but the pancytopenia which accompanies this condition and the difficulty of obtaining an adequate bone marrow sample impose extra difficulties. The most common abnormalities are rearrangement of chromosome 14q, with the breakpoint occurring at 14q32, and defects of chromosome 12.

Recognition and classification of HCL

HCL typically presents with pancytopenia (neutropenia and monocytopenia being especially prominent), variable normochromic, normocytic anaemia and thrombocytopenia. Identification of the diagnostic hairy cells is mandatory for a diagnosis of HCL. However, these are usually evident on careful examination of a well-stained blood film. Hairy cells are almost twice as large as normal lymphocytes and have an eccentric nucleus which rarely contains nucleoli. The abundant, pale blue cytoplasm, which may contain azurophilic cytoplasmic inclusions that superficially resemble Auer rods, is characteristically demarcated by long 'hair-like' projections. Electron microscopy reveals the presence of cylindrical structures which contain rows of ribosomes known as ribosome-lamellar complexes in about 50% of cases. These complexes are not unique to HCL; they can, on occasion, be demonstrated in other B lymphoid disorders. Attempts to aspirate bone marrow often result in a dry tap because of increased marrow fibrosis. Hairy cells express a characteristic pattern of cell surface antigens which confirms their mature, functional B lymphocytic origin (Table 13.2).

Pathophysiology of HCL

Most cases of HCL present with fatigue and general malaise secondary to anaemia, severe infections secondary to leukopenia or bleeding problems secondary to thrombocytopenia. Mycobacterial and other uncommon opportunistic infections are a particular feature. Infection and autoimmune disease are the leading causes of death in HCL. Some degree of splenomegaly is present in virtually all cases and is accompanied by minimal hepatomegaly in about 50% of cases. Lymphadenopathy is rare except in the terminal phase of the disease.

Treatment and management of HCL

Most individuals with HCL are symptomatic at presentation and require immediate treatment. The most common first-line treatment for HCL is splenectomy, which has been shown to relieve the

Supplementary evidence for a diagnosis of HCL can be obtained by staining a peripheral blood film for the enzyme acid phosphatase. The addition of tartaric acid to the reaction mixture inhibits all of the common isoenzymes of acid phosphatase, except isoenzyme 5, which is found in hairy cells. Tartrate resistant acid phosphatase (TRAP) activity is located in the Golgi area and in the nuclear membrane of hairy cells, and is characteristic. Although TRAP positivity has rarely been demonstrated in other T and B lymphoid disorders, its presence is highly suggestive of HCL, particularly when accompanied by the other signs of this disease.

pancytopenia and induce remission in most cases. The 40% of cases with progressive disease post-splenectomy require second-line chemotherapy to induce and maintain remission. Promising results have been obtained with recombinant human α-interferon, 2′-deoxycoformycin and 2-chlorodeoxyadenosine.

Suggested further reading

Goldman, J. (1997). ABC of clinical haematology – Chronic myeloid leukaemia. *British Medical Journal* **7081**, 657–660.

Hamblin, T.J. and Oscier, D.G. (1997). Chronic lymphocytic leukaemia: the nature of the leukaemic cell. *Blood Reviews* **11**(3), 119–128.

Macey, M. (1998). Flow cytometry in haematology. In *Progress in Haematology* (C.D.R. Dunn and C.J. Pallister, eds). London: Greenwich Medical Media.

http://www.leukaemia.demon.co.uk/

http://walden.mvp.net/~lackritz/

Self-assessment questions

1. Which chronic leukaemia is associated with:
   (a) t(9;22)(q34;q11);
   (b) AIHA;
   (c) ribosome-lamellar complexes?
2. Which chronic leukaemia characteristically demonstrates:
   (a) CD5 +, CD19 +;
   (b) CD5 +, SIgM +;
   (c) CD5 −, FMC7 +;
   (d) moderate splenomegaly in the absence of lymphadenopathy and a moderately aggressive course?

Key Concepts and Facts

- Chronic leukaemias are characterized by unbridled clonal proliferation of relatively well-differentiated blood cells.

- The chronic leukaemias can be divided into myeloid and lymphoid leukaemias. Each of these groups is capable of further division.

- CML is a clonal disorder of the totipotential haemopoietic stem cell and is characterized by the presence of the Philadelphia chromosome $t(9;22)(q34;q11)$.

- CML is a triphasic disease: chronic, accelerated and blastic phases are recognized.

- The only form of treatment for CML that offers the prospect of cure is bone marrow transplantation.

- A distinct form of CML, juvenile myelomonocytic leukaemia (JMML), occurs in infants and is associated with a uniformly poor prognosis.

- Chronic lymphoid leukaemias are classified using a combination of morphology and immunophenotyping.

- CLL, PLL and HCL are predominantly B lymphoid diseases, although less common T lymphoid variants exist.

- CLL is an insidious and slowly progressive disease.

- PLL is a more aggressive disease than CLL and is moderately refractory to treatment.

- Hairy cell leukaemia (HCL) is an uncommon B lymphoid disorder that is characterized by 'hairy cells' which express a characteristic pattern of cell surface antigens.

Chapter 14
The myelodysplastic syndromes

Learning objectives

After studying this chapter you should confidently be able to:

List the different subtypes of myelodysplastic syndrome.

Describe in detail the FAB classification system for the myelodysplastic syndromes.

Identify characteristic features of the different forms of myelodysplastic syndrome.

Outline current knowledge about the aetiology of the myelodysplastic syndromes.

Outline the pathophysiology of the myelodysplastic syndromes.

Outline the approaches to treatment of the myelodysplastic syndromes.

The myelodysplastic syndromes (MDSs) are a heterogeneous group of neoplastic disorders which are characterized by varying degrees of pancytopenia and dysplasia in the presence of a normocellular or hypercellular bone marrow. The MDSs vary from a mild, refractory anaemia to a condition that closely resembles ANLL. Some cases evolve into acute leukaemia. The FAB classification recognizes five subtypes of MDS: **refractory anaemia (RA), refractory anaemia with ring sideroblasts (RARS), refractory anaemia with excess of blasts (RAEB), refractory anaemia with excess of blasts in transformation (RAEB-t) and chronic myelomonocytic leukaemia (CMML).**

The myelodysplastic syndromes are predominantly diseases of the elderly, although MDS secondary to monosomy 7 is seen in children, and rare congenital chromosome fragility states such as Fanconi's anaemia are associated with MDS. The median age at presentation of MDS is 65 years. Fewer than 10% of cases are younger than 50 years of age at presentation. Overall, the incidence of MDSs is about 1 per 100 000 persons, with males being affected slightly more often than females.

Recognition and classification of the MDSs

The presentation of the MDSs is highly variable, but about 90% of cases are anaemic and up to 50% are pancytopenic. In addition, a wide range of dysplastic and dysfunctional states may be present, as shown in Tables 14.1 and 14.2. None of these features are, in themselves, diagnostic of MDS. Rather, it is the pattern of

Table 14.1 *Commonly observed dysplastic features in MDS*

Red cells	Granulocytes	Platelets
Ovalomacrocytes	Hypogranularity	Micromegakaryocytes
Dimorphic population	Abnormal granulation	Megakaryocyte fragments in peripheral
Megaloblastic change	Pseudo Pelger–Huët	blood
Gross poikilocytosis	Nuclear appendages	Platelet dysfunction
Multinuclearity	Gross hypersegmentation	Agranular platelets
Nuclear budding	Decreased myeloperoxidase activity	Giant platelet granules
Ring sideroblasts	Abnormal esterase activity	
Raised HbF concentration	Neutrophil dysfunction	
Presence of HbH	Abnormally localized immature	
Reticulocytopenia	myeloid precursors in marrow	
Howell Jolly bodies	Monocytosis	
Pappenheimer bodies	Abnormal monocytes	
Basophilic stippling		
Decreased pyruvate kinase activity		

Table 14.2 *Frequency of the more commonly observed dysplastic features in MDS*

Affected cell line	Observed abnormality	Frequency (%)
Peripheral blood		
Red cells	Ovalomacrocytosis	100
	Hypochromia	20
	Erythroblastosis	25
White cells	Promyelocytes in peripheral blood	25
	Neutrophil hyposegmentation	15
Platelets	Large, dysplastic forms	75
Bone marrow		
Red cells	Erythroid hyperplasia	70
	Erythroid hypoplasia	10
	Megaloblastic change	85
	Dyserythropoiesis	80
	Excess sideroblasts	20
White cells	Abnormal monocyte maturation	80
	Granulocyte maturation bulge	85
Platelets	Megakaryocytosis	50
	Megakaryocytopenia	30
	Dysthrombopoiesis	85

refractory cytopenia with dysplastic features affecting all three cell lines in an elderly person which suggest the diagnosis. However, before a diagnosis of MDS can be made, it is important to exclude all other potential causes of cytopenia or dysplasia.

When the original FAB classification scheme for acute leukaemia was proposed in 1976, a group of conditions called the dysmyelo-poietic syndromes were defined, but were not included in the scheme. At this stage two types of dysmyelopoietic syndrome were recognized: refractory anaemia with excess of blasts (RAEB) and chronic myelomonocytic leukaemia (CMML). In the years that followed, it rapidly became apparent that the range of morphological appearances in the MDS was very wide and that there was some correlation between morphological subtypes and the risk of transformation to ANLL. In 1982, a more detailed FAB classification scheme for the MDS was proposed which took account of these findings. Classification according to the FAB scheme requires careful examination of both peripheral blood and bone marrow films, as shown in Figure 14.1. The current FAB classification scheme is shown in Table 14.3. The FAB subtypes carry prognostic significance, as shown in Table 14.4.

Refractory anaemia

Up to 35% of MDS cases are classified as RA. The typical picture includes a macrocytic or, less commonly, normocytic anaemia and reticulocytopenia which does not respond to haematinic therapy. Basophilic stippling is commonly present. In some cases, dysplastic features are restricted to the red cells but, typically, features such as neutropenia with hypogranular and hypolobulated neutrophils and thrombocytopenia with large, agranular platelets also are present. Up to 90% of cases of RA at presentation are pancytopenic. Bone marrow examination typically reveals hypercellularity with dysplastic, normoblastic or megaloblastic erythropoiesis. Ring sideroblasts are seen but do not exceed 15% of the erythroblasts present. The blast cell count always is less than 5% of the total nucleated cells.

Refractory anaemia with ring sideroblasts

RARS constitutes about 20% of cases of MDS. It is characterized at presentation by the presence of anaemia and a dual red cell population: a major population of normochromic macrocytes and a minor population of hypochromic microcytes. Typically, the serum iron, ferritin concentration and transferrin saturation are all raised and Pappenheimer bodies and basophilic stippling are present. Neutropenia, thrombocytopenia and trilineage dysplasia are much less common than in RA. The bone marrow is typically

The term **basophilic stippling** describes red cell inclusions which are composed of ribonucleoprotein and mitochondrial remnants. They are seen on Romanowsky-stained blood films as diffuse or punctate cytoplasmic granules. These inclusions are not specific for MDS. They are also seen in toxic states such as lead poisoning.

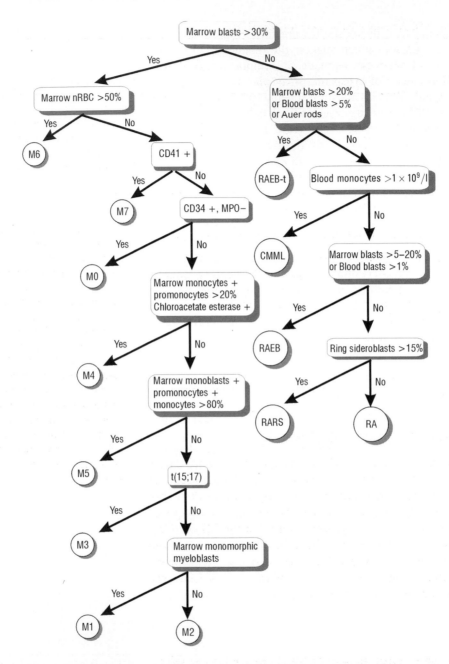

Figure 14.1 *Standardized assessment to differentiate MDS from ANLL*

hypercellular with prominent normoblastic or megaloblastic erythroid hyperplasia and dysplasia. The defining feature for a diagnosis of RARS is that ring sideroblasts should comprise at least 15% of the erythroblasts present and that blast cells should comprise less than 5% of the total of nucleated cells in the bone marrow.

Table 14.3   *The FAB classification scheme for the MDSs*

Disorder	Blasts (%)		Blood monocytes ($\times 10^9/l$)	Ring sideroblasts (%)	Other features
	Blood	*Marrow*			
RA	<1	<5	<1.0	<15	Anaemia
RARS	<1	<5	<1.0	<15	Anaemia, refractory cytopenia
RAEB	<5	5–20	<1.0	<15	Anaemia, refractory cytopenia
RAEB-t	<5	20–30	<1.0	<15	Auer rods in blast cells
CMML	<5	<20	>1.0	<15	Increased blood granulocyte and marrow promonocyte counts

Table 14.4   *Rates of progression to acute leukaemia and median survival for FAB subtypes of MDS*

FAB subtype	Rate of transformation (%)	Median survival (months)
RA	15	32
RARS	10	76
RAEB	30	10
RAEB-t	48	5
CMML	20	18

Refractory anaemia with excess of blasts

RAEB constitutes up to 25% of MDSs and is a much more aggressive disease than RA or RARS. It is characterized at presentation by symptomatic anaemia, neutropenia and thrombocytopenia. Trilineage dysplasia is more common and tends to be more severe than in the relatively benign forms of the MDSs. Blast cells are typically present in the peripheral blood but do not exceed 5% of the total of nucleated cells. Bone marrow examination reveals a variable number of ring sideroblasts and a blast cell count of between 5 and 20% of the total nucleated cell count.

Refractory anaemia with excess of blasts in transformation

A case of RAEB is said to be in transformation to acute leukaemia (RAEB-t) when any of three markers is present:

- A peripheral blood blast cell count that exceeds 5% of the total of nucleated cells.
- Auer rods in the blast cells in the peripheral blood.
- A bone marrow blast cell population that exceeds 20% of the total of nucleated cells.

A **sideroblast** is a nucleated red cell that contains stainable iron granules. These granules are iron-laden mitochondria. A **ring sideroblast** occurs when the poisoned mitochondria encircle the nucleus, forming a necklace-like appearance. Ring sideroblasts are not specific to MDS. They are seen in a wide range of haematological conditions but usually are relatively few in number. A mature red cell with stainable iron granules (Pappenheimer bodies) is known as a **siderocyte**.

If blast cells exceed 30% of the total nucleated cells in the bone marrow, transformation to acute leukaemia is complete. Typically, such cases are profoundly neutropenic and thrombocytopenic and trilineage dysplasia is almost universal. Some degree of hepato-splenomegaly is commonly present.

Although both RAEB and ANLL are associated with peripheral blood cytopenia despite the presence of a hypercellular bone marrow, the mechanisms involved are quite different. In acute leukaemia, the pancytopenia is directly related to the dominance of leukaemic blast cells in the marrow whereas in RAEB it is the result of ineffective haemopoiesis, i.e. a large proportion of the cells produced are morphologically and functionally defective and are doomed to die in the bone marrow. Furthermore, trilineage dysplasia is invariably present in RAEB while it is infrequent in *de novo* ANLL.

Chronic myelomonocytic leukaemia

CMML is characterized at presentation by hepatosplenomegaly, a peripheral blood monocyte count that exceeds $1 \times 10^9/l$ and monocytic dysplasia. Anaemia and thrombocytopenia are much less common than in other types of the MDS. Where present, the anaemia is usually normocytic and normochromic but macrocytes, microcytes and siderocytes may all be present. Dysplastic features commonly are present but trilineage dysplasia is not as common as in other types of the MDSs. Typically, the bone marrow is hypercellular with dysplastic promonocytes being especially prominent. The blast and ring sideroblast counts vary but seldom exceed 20% of the total.

Aetiology of the MDS

The mechanisms that underlie the genesis and progression of the MDSs remain obscure. It is clear that these disorders are clonal and originate at the level of the pluripotent stem cell. However, the state of knowledge about the nature of the primary stem cell mutation and the molecular mechanisms involved remains relatively rudimentary.

Epidemiological evidence

The heterogeneity of the MDSs and the lack of an agreed classification system until 1982 has hampered epidemiological study of these conditions. Petroleum industry workers and those exposed to benzene or its derivatives show a slight excess of MDS. Isolated reports exist of RAEB in individuals exposed to thorium dioxide (Thorotrast), an early radioactive X-ray contrast medium. At *post-mortem*, these cases showed histological evidence of resid-ual Thorotrast in the spleen, lymph nodes and bone marrow. It is plausible that chronic exposure of such sensitive sites to ionizing radiation may have contributed to the induction of MDS in these cases.

Treatment of primary malignancies with alkylating agents such as melphalan, chlorambucil, cyclophosphamide and busulphan is associated with the induction of secondary ANLL. In almost 70% of cases, secondary ANLL is preceded by a myelodysplastic phase. Secondary MDS is even more refractory to treatment than *de novo*, or primary, MDS and is associated with a shorter time-course. The majority of cases present as RAEB or RAEB-t, have a greater incidence of cytogenetic abnormalities and at least 60% progress to ANLL. The median delay between the therapeutic exposure and presentation is about 4 years but may be as long as 12 years. The risk of secondary MDS or ANLL following exposure to alkylating agents is substantial. For example, about 10% of cases of Hodgkin's disease treated with alkylating agents develop this complication within 9 years of the start of therapy.

Cytogenetic and molecular evidence

Chromosomal abnormalities are present in up to 50% of cases of *de novo* MDS and in virtually all cases of secondary MDS. The variety of abnormalities observed is extensive but the most common abnormalities are 5q−, +8 and −7. None of these chromosomal abnormalities is specific for the MDSs and there is no absolute relationship with a particular subtype. However, a number of non-random associations can be discerned:

- 5q− is seen in all MDS subtypes but is strongly associated with RA, accounting for about 70% of cytogenetic abnormalities in this subtype. This chromosomal abnormality is associated with a clinical subtype of RA, the **5q− syndrome**, which is seen most commonly in elderly women and is characterized by a refractory macrocytic anaemia, thrombocytosis, splenomegaly and a low rate of progression to acute leukaemia. The median survival time for the 5q− syndrome is greater than 5 years.

- −7 and 7q− are also seen in all MDS subtypes but are most strongly associated with secondary and paediatric MDS. Monosomy 7 is associated with a very poor prognosis – the median survival time from presentation is less than 1 year.

- 11q− accounts for 20% of chromosomal abnormalities in RARS. This abnormality is associated with raised iron stores and high ring sideroblast counts. The molecular basis for this association is unknown but the presence of the gene that encodes the H-subunit of ferritin at 11q13 may be significant.

Despite the variety of cytogenetic abnormalities observed in the MDSs, their presence does not, in most cases, provide a useful additional indicator of prognosis. Generally, however, multiple

> The q arm of chromosome 5 contains the genes that encode the growth factors IL-3, IL-4, IL-5, IL-9, IL-12B and IL-13, GM-CSF and the M-CSF receptor. It seems likely that the loss of these factors would contribute to dysplastic growth. Similarly, the q arm of chromosome 7 contains the genes which encode EPO and the epidermal growth factor receptor (EGFR).

cytogenetic abnormalities are associated with a poorer prognosis than single abnormalities. This is consistent with a multi-step hypothesis for the development of the MDSs, in which progressive genetic instability and the acquisition of cytogenetic abnormalities are relatively late events. Three patterns of evolution of the MDSs have been described:

- A stable group with no increase in bone marrow blasts and a normal karyotype.
- Rapid blast transformation with the acquisition of new cytogenetic changes after an initial, stable phase.
- Gradually increasing blasts count in the absence of new cytogenetic changes.

Pathophysiology of the MDS

Erythrodysplasia

Ferrokinetic studies have demonstrated major defects in erythropoiesis in all of the MDS groups, with ineffective erythropoiesis often being evident prior to the development of anaemia and obvious erythrodysplasia. The MDS can be divided into three groups based on plasma iron turnover, marrow iron turnover, red cell iron utilization and red cell survival. The lowest erythroid output and the poorest red cell survival times are seen in RAEB and RAEB-t. At the other extreme, cases of RARS are marked by profound erythrokinetic abnormalities with greatly increased plasma and marrow iron turnover secondary to ineffective erythropoiesis but longer red cell survival times. One of the major contributors to premature red cell death in RARS is mitochondrial iron accumulation, which leads to an increase in the generation of free radicals with concomitant damage to mitochondrial function. The other forms of MDS form a heterogeneous intermediate group.

Other frequently observed changes in the red cells in the MDSs include a variety of secondary metabolic abnormalities such as pyruvate kinase deficiency and increased concentration of foetal haemoglobin. Isolated reports exist of an acquired form of HbH disease secondary to defective α globin gene transcription. Changes in red cell antigen expression are occasionally seen, most commonly involving increased i antigen expression and complement sensitivity.

Leucodysplasia

Neutropenia and dysplasia of the granulocytic cells in the presence of a normocellular or hypercellular bone marrow is a common finding in MDS. This contrasts with CML and hypoplastic anaemia where dysplastic features are minimal or absent and marrow cellularity is reflected in the peripheral blood. A proportion of Philadelphia chromosome negative CML cases in which a *bcr-abl* rearrangement cannot be identified show prominent leukodysplastic features and probably should be reclassified as MDS. Enzyme and functional defects parallel the morphological abnormalities of granulocytes and monocytes.

Lymphocyte morphology typically is normal in the MDSs, despite the demonstrable involvement of lymphoid cells in some cases. However, a fall in CD4+ T lymphocytes and NK cells and a lack of Epstein–Barr virus receptors on B lymphocytes are all common. Occasionally, lymphoproliferative disorders such as myeloma, B and T cell lymphomas and hypogammaglobulinaemia have been described in coexistence with the MDS.

Thrombodysplasia

Thrombodysplasia is manifest as the presence of morphologically bizarre megakaryocytes and peripheral blood platelets. Abnormalities of platelet function such as defective adhesion and aggregation responses are common. Acquired platelet glycoprotein defects such as those seen in Bernard–Soulier syndrome have been described in juvenile MDS.

Treatment and management of the MDSs

The age of the individual and the severity of the condition determine the treatment offered for the MDS. Broadly speaking, the aim of treatment in young patients is curative while in elderly patients with aggressive disease it is palliative. A number of factors have been suggested to have prognostic value in the MDSs, as shown in Table 14.5.

Those cases identified as having a good prognosis are usually offered supportive treatment such as blood and platelet transfusions to correct the anaemia and thrombocytopenia and antimicrobial chemotherapy to combat infections. As described above, a proportion of these cases progress to acute leukaemia but it is currently impossible to predict with certainty which will follow this course. Poor prognosis cases are typically offered some form of treatment but there is currently little agreement about which approach affords the best prospect of cure or prolongation of life. The most common causes of death in the MDSs are infectious and haemorrhagic complications secondary to peripheral cytopenia or leukaemic transformation.

Suggested further reading

Aul, C., Gattermann, N. and Schneider, W. (1995). Epidemiologic

Table 14.5 *Presenting features which have been suggested to signify poor prognosis in the MDSs*

Excess of bone marrow blasts
Abnormal localized immature myeloid precursors
Pancytopenia
Abnormal chromosome 7
Complex or multiple cytogenetic abnormalities
Increased age at presentation

and etiologic aspects of myelodysplastic syndromes. *Leukemia and Lymphoma* **16**(3–4), 247–262.

Gallagher, A., Darley, R.L. and Padua, R.A. (1997). The molecular basis of myelodysplastic syndromes. *Haematologica* **82**(2), 191–204.

Kouides, P.A. and Bennett, J.M. (1996). Morphology and classification of the myelodysplastic syndromes and their pathologic variants. *Seminars in Hematology* **33**(2), 95–110.

Lowenthal, R.M. and Marsden, K.A. (1997). Myelodysplastic syndromes. *International Journal of Hematology* **65**(4), 319–338.

Sanz, M.A. and Sempere, A. (1996). Immunophenotyping of AML and MDS and detection of residual disease. *Bailliere's Clinical Haematology* **9**(1), 35–55.

Self-assessment questions

1. List the five different subtypes of myelodysplastic syndrome.
2. Which FAB subtype of MDS is associated with:
   (a) >5% blasts in the peripheral blood;
   (b) a blood monocyte count of $>1.0 \times 10^9$/l;
   (c) 10% blasts in the marrow, <15% ring sideroblasts?
3. Which of the following is associated with a poor prognosis in MDS:
   (a) abnormalities of chromosome 7;
   (b) >15% ring sideroblasts in the marrow;
   (c) complex or multiple cytogenetic abnormalities;
   (d) hypogranulated neutrophils;
   (e) abnormal localized immature myeloid precursors?
4. Which FAB subtypes are the most likely and the least likely to transform into ANLL?

Key Concepts and Facts

- The MDS are a heterogeneous group of neoplastic disorders, characterized by pancytopenia and dysplasia in the presence of a normo- or hypercellular bone marrow.

- The MDSs vary from a mild, refractory anaemia to a condition that closely resembles ANLL.

- Five subtypes of MDS exist: refractory anaemia (RA); refractory anaemia with ring sideroblasts (RARS); refractory anaemia with excess of blasts (RAEB); refractory anaemia with excess of blasts in transformation (RAEB-t); and chronic myelomonocytic leukaemia (CMML).

- Chromosomal abnormalities are present in 50% of *de novo* MDS and virtually all cases of secondary MDS. The most common abnormalities are 5q−, +8 and −7.

- Some cases of MDS evolve into ANLL. Evolution is most common for RAEB-t and least common in RA and RARS.

Chapter 15
Non-leukaemic malignant disorders

Learning objectives

After studying this chapter you should confidently be able to:

List several examples of non-leukaemic myeloproliferative and lymphoproliferative disorders.

Demonstrate knowledge of the distinguishing features of the different forms of polycythaemia.

Outline the pathophysiology of the polycythaemias, primary thrombocythaemia and myelofibrosis.

Demonstrate knowledge of the pathophysiology of multiple myeloma and related plasma cell disorders.

Demonstrate knowledge of the pathophysiology of the lymphomas.

Outline the REAL classification of the lymphoproliferative disorders.

The non-leukaemic malignant disorders are an extremely diverse group of disorders which can be divided according to the origin of the malignant clone into myeloproliferative and lymphoproliferative types. The malignant myeloproliferative disorders include **primary proliferative polycythaemia (PPP)**, which is one of many different types of polycythaemia, **primary thrombocythaemia** and **myelofibrosis**. The malignant lymphoproliferative disorders include **multiple myeloma (MM)** and related plasma cell disorders, **Hodgkin's disease (HD)** and the various **non-Hodgkin's lymphomas (NHL)**.

The non-leukaemic myeloproliferative disorders

Primary proliferative polycythaemia

Primary proliferative polycythaemia is a malignant disorder of haemopoietic stem cells which is characterized by absolute erythrocytosis and, commonly, a moderately increased granulocyte count and platelet count. It is predominantly a disease of middle age: the median age at diagnosis is 55 years. Males are affected slightly more commonly than females.

Recognition and classification of the polycythaemias

The defining criterion of polycythaemia is a rise in the venous packed cell volume (PCV) to more than 0.53 in males or more than 0.51 in females, reflecting an increase, real or apparent, in the circulating red cell count. Normally, the red cell count is under tight hormonal control and is maintained within remarkably narrow limits. Alterations in the venous PCV can be caused by a reduction in plasma volume or by a true increase in red cell numbers. An absolute increase in the rate of erythropoiesis can be caused by malignant transformation, which frees the haemopoietic stem cells from hormonal control, or via hypoxic or physiologically inappropriate stimulation of erythropoietin release. Thus, the polycythaemias are a large and diverse group of disorders, only one member of which, PPP, is a malignant disorder. However, an understanding of the aetiology and classification of all types of polycythaemia is essential because recognition of PPP is based largely upon exclusion of the other types. The classification of the polycythaemias is illustrated schematically in Figure 15.1.

Apparent polycythaemia

Apparent polycythaemia occurs where an increased venous PCV is explained by a reduction in the plasma volume (PV). Alternative names for this condition include relative polycythaemia, pseudo-polycythaemia, stress polycythaemia, spurious polycythaemia and Gaisböck's syndrome. Red cell mass and plasma volume are under separate physiological control and so may vary independently of each other. Plasma volume may fall as a result of dehydration secondary to diuretic therapy, severe diarrhoea and vomiting, burns or alcohol ingestion. Prolonged stress, hypertension and smoking have a similar effect. Other clinical and laboratory signs that can be used to differentiate between apparent polycythaemia and the other forms are summarized in Table 15.1.

Secondary polycythaemias

The secondary polycythaemias are the result of increased stimulation of erythropoiesis, either in response to hypoxia or to another physiologically inappropriate stimulus. Leukocytes and platelets are not involved. Physiologically appropriate release of erythropoietin occurs in response to tissue hypoxia which results from persistently low atmospheric oxygen tension, inadequate uptake of atmospheric oxygen due to cardiovascular or respiratory disease, or defective transport of absorbed oxygen from the lungs. A variety

---

The references ranges for venous haematocrit (PCV) are as follows:

Cord blood	0.44–0.62
Child (10 years)	0.37–0.44
Adult male	0.40–0.54
Adult female	0.36–0.47

The venous haematocrit overestimates the whole body haematocrit (WBPCV) because of normal changes in the ratio of plasma:cells in arterial and venous blood. As a general guide, the WBPCV is about 91% of the venous PCV, but this value varies considerably, for example, in pregnancy, splenomegaly and congestive cardiac failure.

Animal species that are indigenous to high altitudes such as the llama and vicuña do not normally have high red cell counts. They have adapted to the low oxygen tension of their environment by synthesizing a form of haemoglobin with an extraordinarily high oxygen affinity. This helps to maximize the extraction of atmospheric oxygen in the lungs, but the mechanisms involved in maintaining optimal oxygen delivery to the tissues in these animals are much less clear.

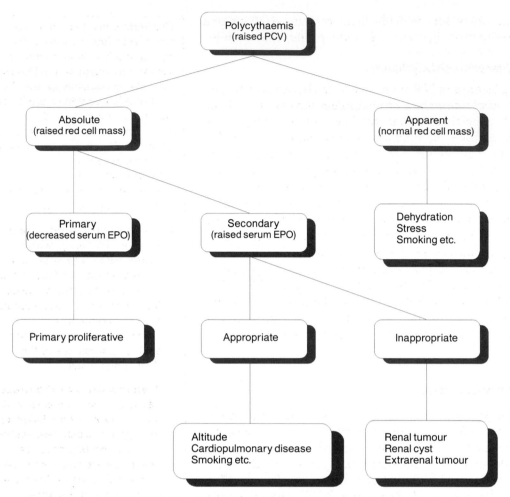

Figure 15.1 *Recognition and classification of the polycythaemias*

Table 15.1 *Differential diagnosis of the polycythaemias*

Laboratory/clinical variable	PPP	Apparent polycythaemia	Secondary polycythaemia
Packed cell volume	↑	↑	↑
Red cell mass	↑	N	↑
Serum erythropoietin	↓	N	↑
White cell count	↑	N	N
Platelet count	↑	N	N
Bone marrow	Hyperplastic	N	Erythroid hyperplasia
Spleen	Enlarged	N	N
Arterial pO_2	N	N	↓ or N
Serum ferritin	↓	N	N
Serum vitamin B_{12}	↑	N	N
Leukocyte alkaline phosphatase	↑	N	N
Serum lysozyme	↑	N	N

N = normal; ↑ = raised; ↓ = decreased.

of disorders are associated with the inappropriate synthesis and release of erythropoietin, e.g. polycystic kidneys and renal tumours.

Primary proliferative polycythaemia

The presenting features of PPP are related to the hypervolaemia and hyperviscosity that accompanies the absolute increase in red cell mass. Typical complaints include ruddiness of the complexion, headaches, blurred vision, dizziness, mental impairment and a feeling of congestion in the head. Splenomegaly secondary to vascular engorgement, extramedullary haemopoiesis and fibrosis is common. Hyperviscosity causes an increased incidence of arterial and venous thrombosis. Paradoxically, platelet dysfunction with a tendency to bruise and bleed excessively following trauma is also common in all of the non-leukaemic myeloproliferative disorders. The laboratory characteristics of PPP are shown in Table 15.1.

Up to 25% of cases of PPP transform to chronic myelofibrosis and of these up to one-third eventually progress to ANLL. The duration of PPP prior to transformation in these cases has varied from less than 2 years to more than 20 years. Treatment with alkylating agents is associated with a higher rate of progression to ANLL.

Primary thrombocythaemia

Primary thrombocythaemia is a malignant clonal disorder that is characterized by megakaryocytic hyperplasia and a markedly increased circulating platelet count. Alternative names for this disorder include **essential thrombocythaemia, idiopathic thrombocythaemia** and **primary haemorrhagic thrombocythaemia**. The median age at diagnosis is 60 years: primary thrombocythaemia is rare in children and young adults. Men and women appear to be affected with equal frequency.

Primary thrombocythaemia characteristically presents with a platelet count greater than $1000 \times 10^9/l$ but platelet counts as high as $10\,000 \times 10^9/l$ are not rare. Examination of a blood film reveals the presence of platelet clumping and bizarre morphological abnormalities of the platelets with marked variation in size, shape and granulation. Megakaryocyte fragments may be present in the peripheral blood. Typically, a moderate neutrophilia is present, but the white cell count seldom exceeds $35 \times 10^9/l$. The red cell count and haemoglobin concentration are normal in most cases but some degree of iron deficiency may be present, secondary to chronic blood loss. Examination of the bone marrow reveals hypercellularity with pronounced megakaryocytic hyperplasia, granulocytic hyperplasia and, sometimes, erythroid hyperplasia. The major clinical problems of primary thrombocythaemia are thromboembolic complications secondary to the extremely high platelet count and haemorrhagic complications secondary to platelet dysfunction. Paradoxically, both

---

The normal heart is a muscular pump with four chambers. The right and left atria receive blood from the systemic and pulmonary circulations respectively and the right and left ventricles discharge blood into the aorta and pulmonary artery respectively. The left and right sides of the heart are separated by a septum.

Congenital cardiac malformations that are associated with erythrocytosis include:

- **Ventricular septal defect** (hole in the heart), where malformation of the septum permits shunting of blood from the left to the right ventricle. VSD is frequently accompanied by other congenital cardiovascular abnormalities such as persistence of the ductus arteriosus.

- **Transposition of the great vessels**, where the aorta and pulmonary artery are linked to the opposite ventricles, leading to dyspnoea (shortness of breath) and a grey complexion (cyanosis) due to suboptimal oxygenation of the arterial blood.

Thrombotic complications in PPP are manifest as an increased incidence of:

- **Transient ischaemic attacks** (TIA) which are secondary to emboli in the cerebral circulation and present as a sudden neurological deficit. TIAs normally resolve completely within 24 h.

- **Intermittent claudication** which is secondary to atherosclerosis of the arteries of the lower limbs and presents as painful cramping of the legs and feet following exercise.

Myelofibrosis is also known as **agnogenic myeloid metaplasia**.

thromboembolic and haemorrhagic complications may be present in the same individual. Significant splenomegaly is present in up to 80% of cases. Some degree of hepatomegaly is also common.

Up to 25% of cases of primary thrombocythaemia transform to myelofibrosis or, rarely, PPP or ANLL. By far the most common cause of death in this disorder is thromboembolic complications. The median duration of survival with primary thrombocythaemia is about 10 years.

Myelofibrosis

Myelofibrosis is predominantly a disease of the middle-aged and elderly. It is characterized by progressive collagen fibrosis of the bone marrow spaces, megakaryocytic hyperplasia and massive splenomegaly secondary to extramedullary haemopoiesis. Myelofibrosis affects men and women equally.

The onset of myelofibrosis is insidious. Typical complaints at presentation include lethargy and exercise intolerance secondary to anaemia; weight loss and night sweats secondary to metabolic derangement; bruising secondary to platelet dysfunction; and splenomegaly secondary to extramedullary haemopoiesis. Marked splenomegaly is present at diagnosis in at least 50% of cases.

Examination of the blood reveals leukoerythroblastic anaemia with prominent polychromasia, anisocytosis and 'teardrop' poikilocytosis. The white cell count and platelet count are variable but are frequently raised. Platelet morphology is frequently grossly atypical, suggesting overlap with primary thrombocythaemia. Attempts to aspirate bone marrow frequently fail because of the fibrotic overgrowth of the marrow space. Trephine biopsy typically reveals large areas of fibrosis with patchy areas of hypercellularity which contain prominent clusters of dysplastic megakaryocytes. The median survival from diagnosis in myelofibrosis is about 3 years. About 10% of cases progress to ANLL.

The non-leukaemic lymphoproliferative disorders

The non-leukaemic lymphoproliferative disorders are malignant clonal disorders of the lymphopoietic system.

Multiple myeloma and related plasma cell disorders

Multiple myeloma (MM) is a B lymphoid malignancy and is characterized by the proliferation of a malignant clone of plasma cells which synthesize and secrete excessive amounts of monoclonal immunoglobulin. MM is a disease of the elderly, with the median age at diagnosis being about 62 years. The disease is more common in blacks than in whites and shows a slight excess incidence in men.

In many respects, MM behaves as a solid tumour with a particular predilection for bone marrow. All of the many sequelae of MM are attributable to two causes:

- The uncontrolled growth of a plasma cell tumour which secretes a substance which suppresses B lymphocyte function and promotes osteolysis.

- The inexorable and pointless synthesis and secretion of large quantities of monoclonal immunoglobulin by the malignant plasma cells.

Thus, the most common presenting features in MM are bone pain and hypercalcaemia secondary to osteolysis; anaemia and uraemia secondary to renal impairment caused by deposition of immunoglobulin in the tubules; and respiratory tract infection secondary to defective humoral immunity.

Diagnosis of myeloma requires the demonstration of a monoclonal immunoglobulin or immunoglobulin light or heavy chain in serum and, where proteinuria is present, in the urine. Determination of the immunoglobulin subclass and light chain class of the monoclonal protein provides important prognostic information. IgG mycloma is associated with a slower tumour growth rate than the other types of myeloma. However, the rate of synthesis of monoclonal immunoglobulin is highest in this form, so the total serum immunoglobulin concentration is also highest in IgG myeloma. IgA myeloma is associated with hyperviscosity because of the tendency of this form of immunoglobulin to polymerize. IgD myeloma is a particularly malignant form which is associated with a younger age group and is most common in men. The median survival time for this form of myeloma is about a year. IgE myeloma is extremely rare and is associated with the presentation of **plasma cell leukaemia** (PCL). This rare disease presents as an acute leukaemia with a circulating plasma cell count greater than 2×10^9/l, anaemia, thrombocytopenia, hepatosplenomegaly, osteolysis and renal failure. The white cell count at presentation frequently exceeds 80×10^9/l of which more than half are atypical plasma cells. **Bence–Jones (BJ) myeloma** occurs when immunoglobulin light chains are synthesized in the absence of heavy chains. This form of myeloma is associated with the most rapid tumour growth. The prognosis is particularly grim for λ chain BJ myeloma.

The presence of a monoclonal immunoglobulin does not necessarily equate with myeloma; almost 1% of individuals over the age of 25 years and at least 3% over the age of 70 years express such a band. Some of these cases probably represent very early myelomas but a significant proportion are completely stable and show no evidence of malignant progression, even after many years. These individuals are said to have a **monoclonal gammopathy of undetermined significance (MGUS)**.

Multiple myeloma was first described in 1844 by Solly, almost a year before the first descriptions of leukaemia by Virchow and Bennett. Solly called the condition *mollities ossium*.

Plasma cell leukaemia is a rare condition which is characterized by a peripheral blood plasma cell count in excess (often greatly) of 2×10^9/l, anaemia, thrombocytopenia and many of the clinical features of multiple myeloma. The disease typically occurs *de novo* but is also seen as a terminal event of pre-existing multiple myeloma. The prognosis for PCL is poor.

Rouleaux describes a condition where the red cells coalesce into long chains which characteristically resemble 'stacks of coins'. Rouleaux formation is triggered by an increase in the concentration of plasma proteins such as immunoglobulins.

Haematological examination typically reveals rouleaux formation secondary to the increased immunoglobulin concentration, normocytic, normochromic anaemia secondary to depression of erythropoiesis, variable thrombocytopenia and leukopenia. In a minority of cases, a leukoerythroblastic blood picture with atypical plasma cells in the peripheral blood is strongly suggestive of the diagnosis. The plasma viscosity is raised, occasionally markedly so. Examination of the bone marrow reveals an increased number of atypical plasma cells. Immunofluorescent staining of the myeloma plasma cells confirms that they are all synthesizing a single form of immunoglobulin heavy chain and light chain.

Waldenström's macroglobulinaemia

Waldenström's macroglobulinaemia (WM) is an uncommon B lymphoid malignant disorder which is characterized by hyperviscosity secondary to the excessive secretion of a monoclonal IgM immunoglobulin by the malignant clone. The malignant cells of WM are rather more immature than those in MM. WM is a disease of the elderly, with a peak incidence occurring in the seventh decade of life.

WM is an indolent disease which typically presents with variable combinations of weight loss, hepatosplenomegaly, lymphadenopathy and a bruising or bleeding tendency, following a long history of vague malaise, weakness and weight loss. Because of the large size and chemical properties of IgM the most common cause of morbidity is hyperviscosity.

Haematological examination reveals marked rouleaux and normocytic, normochromic anaemia. The total white cell count may be normal or depressed but relative lymphocytosis is common. The platelet count is normal at presentation in 50% of cases. However, neutropenia and thrombocytopenia often become more troublesome as the disease advances. Attempts to aspirate bone marrow frequently fail due to hypercellularity and the extremely high viscosity of the marrow blood. The malignant cells are pleomorphic: some resemble lymphocytes whereas others clearly resemble plasma cells; most, however, have an intermediate appearance and are described as being lymphoplasmacytoid.

Hodgkin's disease

Hodgkin's disease (HD) is a malignant lymphoma and so differs from the leukaemias, myelodysplastic syndromes and non-leukaemic myeloproliferative disorders so far described in a number of important respects:

Lymphadenopathy means swollen lymph glands and may be indicative of infection, inflammation or malignancy.

- HD arises in lymph nodes, not in bone marrow.
- Disease progression in HD occurs by dissemination of the malignant cells via the lymphatic circulation; involvement of

blood and bone marrow occurs only as a late event in advanced disease.

- The putative malignant cell in HD is known as the **Reed–Sternberg cell**. The origin of this cell and its normal equivalent remain to be established.

- HD is curable in at least 70% of cases.

- HD is suspected of having an infectious aetiology, at least in the younger age group.

HD has an overall annual incidence of about 2.5 per 100 000 in the UK and has a bimodal age distribution in the developed countries of the world with peaks of incidence in the third decade of life and over the age of 55 years. A different age distribution is common in developing countries, where the highest incidence of

Hodgkin's disease was first described by Thomas Hodgkin of Guy's Hospital, London in 1832. His report was based on seven cases with massive lymphadenopathy and splenomegaly. Most of his colleagues thought that these were cases of tuberculosis but Hodgkin, with remarkable prescience, thought they were clinically distinct. The name Hodgkin's disease was not coined by Hodgkin himself: he was a modest and unassuming man. The eponymous title was coined 33 years later by Samuel Wilks, also of Guy's, when he published a more detailed account of several cases of this condition.

Table 15.2 *The revised European-American lymphoma (REAL) classification system*

Hodgkin's disease
  Classical types
    Nodular sclerosis
    Mixed cellularity
    Lymphocyte depletion
    Nodular lymphocyte predominance

B cell neoplasms
  Precursor B cell neoplasms
    Precursor B lymphoblastic leukaemia/lymphoma
  Peripheral B cell neoplasms
    B CLL/prolymphocytic leukaemia/small lymphocytic lymphoma
    Immunocytoma/lymphoplasmacytic lymphoma
    Mantle cell lymphoma
    Follicle centre cell lymphoma, follicular
    Marginal zone B cell lymphoma
    Hairy cell leukaemia
    Plasmacytoma/plasma cell myeloma
    Diffuse large B cell lymphoma
    Burkitt's lymphoma

T cell neoplasms
  Precursor T cell neoplasms
    Precursor T lymphoblastic leukaemia/lymphoma
  Peripheral T cell and NK cell neoplasms
    T CLL/prolymphocytic leukaemia
    Large granular lymphocytic leukaemia (LGL)
    Mycosis fungoides/Sézary syndrome
    Peripheral T cell lymphomas, unspecified
    Angioimmunoblastic T cell lymphoma (AILD)
    Angiocentric lymphoma (nasal NK/T cell lymphoma)
    Intestinal T cell lymphoma
    Adult T cell lymphoma/leukaemia (ATLL)
    Anaplastic large cell lymphoma (ALCL)

Table 15.3 *Major clinical and laboratory features of the leukaemia/lymphomas*

Disorder	Morphology	Genetics	Immunology	Clinical
B cell neoplasms				
Precursor B lymphoblastic leukaemia/lymphoma	Lymphoblasts	No consistent abnormality	TdT+, CD10+/−, CD19, 79a+, Cyt μ −/+	More common in children. Aggressive disease but frequently curable
B CLL/prolymphocytic leukaemia/small lymphocytic lymphoma	Predominantly small lymphocytes	Trisomy 12 or 13q abnormalities	SIgM±, CD5+, CD10−, CD19,20,79a+, CD22 +/−, CD23+	Usually leukaemic. Affects adults. Indolent course
Immunocytoma/lympho-plasmacytic lymphoma	Plasmacytoid lymphocytes, plasma cells, lymphocytes	No specific abnormality	SIgM+, Cyt Ig+, CD5,10−, CD19,20,22,79a+	Adults. Indolent course
Mantle cell lymphoma	Small irregularly shaped centrocyte-like cells	t(11;14), *bcl-1* rearrangement	SIg (λ > κ)+, CD5+, CD10−/+, CD19,20,22,79a+, CD23−, cyclin D1+	Adults. Moderately aggressive course (median survival 3–4 years)
Follicle centre cell lymphoma, follicular	Mixture of germinal centre blasts and cleaved cells	t(14;18) and *bcl-2* rearrangement in majority	SIg+, CD5−, CD10+/−, CD19,20,22,79a+	Adults. Indolent course (median survival 7–9 years)
Marginal zone B cell lymphoma	Small centrocyte-like cells, 'monocytoid' B cells, lymphocytes, plasma cells	Trisomy 3	SIg+, CD5,10−, CD23−, CD19,20,22,79a+	Indolent course, often localized. May transform to large cell lymphoma
Hairy cell leukaemia	Small lymphoid cells with bean-shaped nuclei and pale cytoplasm	No specific abnormality	SIg+, CD5,10,23−, CD11c,25+, CD19,20,22,79a+, CD103+	Adults. Often with splenomegaly and pancytopenia. Indolent course
Plasmacytoma/plasma cell myeloma	Plasma cells	t(11;14) in a few cases	SIg−, Cyt Ig+, EMA−/+, CD19,20,22, CD79a+/−	Adults. Lytic bone lesions, less common soft tissue tumour. Relapse after plateau phase
Diffuse large B cell lymphoma	Monomorphic large cells, prominent nucleoli and basophilic cytoplasm	t(14;18) in 30%, *bcl-6* rearranged in 40%	SIgM+/−, Cyt Ig−/+, CD5,10−/+, CD19,20,22,79a+	Children or adults. Aggressive course but may be curable
Burkitt's lymphoma	Medium-sized cells, basophilic cytoplasm. 'Starry sky' appearance. High mitotic rate	t(2;8), t(8;14) or t(8;22); *myc* rearrangement	SIgM+, CD5,23−, CD10+, CD19,20,22,79a+, Ki67 >85% of cells	More common in children. Aggressive but curable in children

T cell neoplasms

	Morphology	Cytogenetics/Genetics	Immunophenotype	Clinical features
Precursor T lymphoblastic leukaemia/lymphoma	Lymphoblasts, identical cytologically to B lymphoblasts	*scl/tal-1* rearrangements in 25%	TdT+, CD1a+/−, CD3+/−, CD7+, CD4 and/or 8+	Frequently involves mediastinum. Adolescents and young adults. Highly aggressive but potentially curable
T CLL/prolymphocytic leukaemia	Small lymphoid cells with some nuclear irregularity	Inv 14(q11;q32) in some cases	CD2,3,5,7+, CD4+, CD8−/+	Adults. Often leukaemic. More aggressive than B CLL
Large granular lymphocytic leukaemia (LGL)	Small/medium lymphoid cells with eccentric round or oval nuclei. Azurophilic cytoplasmic granules	No specific abnormality	CD2+, CD3,8+/−, CD16+, CD56,57−/+	Adults. Usually leukaemic. Neutropenia ±anaemia. Indolent course
Mycosis fungoides/Sézary syndrome	Small/medium cells with cerebriform nuclei. Epidermal infiltration	No specific abnormality	CD2,3,4,5+, CD7,8,25	Adults. Principally localized to skin but may involve blood and lymph nodes
Peripheral T cell lymphomas, unspecified	Atypical lymphocytes of varying size. Variable reactive background elements, e.g. macrophages, vessels etc.	No specific abnormality	CD3+/−, variable expression of other T cell markers	Adults. Aggressive course but potentially curable
Angioimmunoblastic T cell lymphoma (AILD)	Architecture effaced, arborizing high endothelial venules, no secondary follicles. Mixed infiltrate of lymphocytes, blasts and atypical clear cells	No specific abnormality	T cell phenotype. Large follicular dendritic cell clusters around proliferating venules	Systemic disease with lymphadenopathy, fever, weights loss and skin rash. Polyclonal hypergammaglobulinaemia. Aggressive course
Angiocentric lymphoma (nasal NK/T cell lymphoma)	Polymorphic lymphocytes infiltrating vessel walls. Necrosis of normal and neoplastic tissue	No specific abnormality. EBV genome present	CD2,56+, CD3−/+, CD5,7+/−, CD4 or 8+/−	Children and adults. Commoner in Asia. Extranodal sites involved, e.g. nose, palate, skin. Variable course
Intestinal T cell lymphoma	Neoplastic cells range from small lymphocytes to large bizarre cells	No specific abnormality	CD3,7+, CD8+/−, CD103+	Adults. Aggressive course, often with intestinal perforation
Adult T cell lymphoma/leukaemia (ATLL)	Pleomorphic infiltrate of small and large lymphoid cells	Integrated HTLV-I genome present	CD2,3,4,5,25+, CD7−	Adults. Commonest in Japan and Caribbean. Hypercalcaemia, osteolysis common. May be aggressive or indolent.
Anaplastic large cell lymphoma (ALCL)	Bizarre large cells, sometimes RS-like or multinucleate. Abundant cytoplasm. Cohesive cells, intrasinus spread	t(2;5) causing fusion of *alk* and nucleophosmin genes, especially in younger patients	T or null phenotype, CD30+, EMA+/−	Children and adolescents. Systemic form aggressive but potentially curable. Rare primary cutaneous disease in adults, indolent but incurable

HD occurs in children and a second, smaller, peak occurs in the elderly. HD is a rare condition in young adults in developing countries. There is a slight excess incidence of HD in males.

The most common presenting feature in HD is the presence of painless, asymmetrical lymphadenopathy, which may be accompanied by severe, generalized itching in the absence of a skin rash. In contrast to the non-Hodgkin's lymphomas, which are frequently disseminated at presentation, most cases of HD are restricted to a single anatomical site at presentation. The presence of pyrexia and drenching night sweats are usually associated with more advanced disease. Examination of the peripheral blood seldom affords any useful information in HD. The presence of anaemia, lymphocytopenia or leukoerythroblastosis all suggest the presence of advanced disease with bone marrow involvement, but this is uncommon at presentation.

Histological examination of an affected lymph node biopsy reveals the loss of normal architecture and the presence of a diffuse infiltrate of lymphocytes, histiocytes, eosinophils, plasma cells and neutrophils which are of normal appearance. Scattered among this infiltrate are variable numbers of Reed–Sternberg (RS) cells, the hallmark of HD. RS cells are typically large, with two or more large, oval nuclei, each of which contains a huge nucleolus that is separated from the thickened nuclear membrane by a clear zone. Although it is widely agreed that RS cells are the malignant cells in HD and that there is strong evidence for a lymphoid origin, the normal counterpart of this cell remains to be identified.

The natural history of untreated HD appears to involve the creeping advance of tumour from a single point of origin in a lymph node, first to contiguous nodes by direct contact, then to adjacent and more distant lymph nodes via the lymphatic circulatory system and, finally, to the spleen where further dissemination to the liver and bone marrow occurs via the blood circulatory system. With modern treatment, more than 80% of cases of early HD and 50% of cases of advanced HD survive for more than 10 years after presentation.

Non-Hodgkin's lymphomas

The term non-Hodgkin's lymphoma (NHL) encompasses a large number of disparate malignant clonal disorders of lymphoid tissue. Separation of NHL into smaller, more closely related groups has proved to be very difficult. As a group, NHL is the most common of the haemopoietic malignant disorders with an overall incidence of about 1 per 10 000. The incidence of NHL increases with increasing age and the median age at presentation is about 60 years. Men are affected more commonly than women.

About 80% of NHL are of B lymphoid origin while almost all of the rest are of T lymphoid origin (rare examples of true histiocytic lymphomas have been described). In general, lymphomas with a follicular pattern of growth are less aggressive than those with a diffuse pattern of growth and small lymphocytic lymphomas are less aggressive than large cell lymphomas. However, in common with the acute leukaemias, some forms of high grade lymphoma are more amenable to treatment than the more indolent or chronic types. In contrast to HD, most NHLs are disseminated to a greater or lesser extent at presentation.

Historically the classification of the NHLs has been both confused and confusing. Several classification systems have been proposed over the years, each with their inherent strengths and weaknesses, but none gained universal acceptance. In 1994, an international group of haematologists and histopathologists published the 'revised European-American lymphoma (REAL) classification system', which has since gained near universal acceptance. The REAL classification system is summarized in Table 15.2.

The REAL classification system recognizes the close relationship between the lymphoid leukaemias and the lymphomas. The major clinical and laboratory features of these disorders are summarized in Table 15.3.

Suggested further reading

Degos, L., Hermann, F., Linch, D.C. and Loewenberg, R. (1998). *A Textbook of Malignant Haematology*. London: Martin Dunitz.

Malpas, J.S., Bergsagel, D.E., Kyle, R.A. and Anderson, K.C. (1997). *Myeloma Biology and Management*, 2nd edn. Oxford: Oxford University Press.

van Heerde, P. Meijer, C.C.L.M., Noorduyn, L.A. and van der Valk, P. (1996). *Malignant Lymphomas*. London: Manson Publishing.

Self-assessment questions

1. List three non-leukaemic myeloproliferative and three lymphoproliferative disorders.
2. What tests would you need to perform to distinguish between a case of primary proliferative polycythaemia and a secondary polycythaemia due to chronic obstructive airways disease? Outline the results you would expect to see in each case.
3. Why is cardiopulmonary disease associated with an erythrocytosis?
4. Why is multiple myeloma associated with an increased plasma viscosity?
5. Why is Waldenström's macroglobulinaemia associated with hyperviscosity syndrome?
6. Outline the main presenting features of a case of Hodgkin's disease.
7. Name the malignant cell in Hodgkin's disease.

Key Concepts and Facts

- Primary proliferative polycythaemia (PPP) is a malignant disorder of haemopoietic stem cells.

- Apparent polycythaemia is explained by a reduction in the plasma volume.

- Secondary polycythaemias result from increased stimulation of erythropoiesis in response to hypoxia or a physiologically inappropriate stimulus.

- Up to 25% of cases of PPP transform to chronic myelofibrosis and about 8% progress to ANLL.

- Primary thrombocythaemia is a malignant clonal disorder that is characterized by megakaryocytic hyperplasia and a markedly increased circulating platelet count.

- Myelofibrosis is a malignant disorder that is characterized by progressive fibrosis of marrow spaces with megakaryocytic hyperplasia and extramedullary haemopoiesis.

- Multiple myeloma (MM) is a B lymphoid malignancy characterized by proliferation of plasma cells which secrete monoclonal immunoglobulin.

- Hodgkin's disease (HD) is a malignant lymphoma and arises in the lymph nodes.

- The putative malignant cell in HD is known as the Reed–Sternberg cell.

- The non-Hodgkin's lymphomas (NHL) are a disparate group of malignant disorders of lymphoid tissue.

- The lymphoproliferative disorders can be classified using the REAL system which recognizes the close relationship between the lymphoid leukaemias and the lymphomas.

Chapter 16
Hypoplastic anaemias

Learning objectives

After studying this chapter you should confidently be able to:

Define the scope and nature of the hypoplastic anaemias.

Outline the classification of the hypoplastic anaemias.

Compare and contrast the pathophysiology of selected inherited and acquired hypoplastic anaemias.

Outline the available treatment strategies for the hypoplastic anaemias.

The term hypoplastic anaemia encompasses all forms of peripheral blood cytopenia that are caused by a failure of haemopoiesis. Disorders such as the myelodysplastic syndromes which are characterized by bone marrow hypercellularity and ineffective haemopoiesis, or hypersplenism where cytopenia is secondary to peripheral blood cell destruction are specifically excluded by this definition. Hypoplastic anaemia is a rare condition with an overall incidence in Western Europe of about 1 per 200 000. Hypoplastic anaemia is a very rare condition in childhood, increases to a plateau of frequency between the ages of 20 and 65 years and thereafter becomes increasingly common with advancing age. The incidence of hypoplastic anaemia is greater in underdeveloped countries where it primarily affects children.

Classification of the hypoplastic anaemias

There is no universally agreed classification scheme for the hypoplastic anaemias. In this book they are classified according to three criteria:

- Whether they are inherited or acquired disorders.
- Whether the hypoplasia affects all haemopoietic cell lines or is restricted to a single cell type.
- Aetiology.

Table 16.1 *Classification of the hypoplastic anaemias**

Pancytopenia	Single cell line affected
Inherited	
Fanconi's anaemia	Diamond–Blackfan syndrome
Dyskeratosis congenita	Congenital dyserythropoietic anaemias
	Congenital neutropenias
	Congenital amegakaryocytic thrombocytopenia
Acquired	
Primary (idiopathic)	Chronic acquired pure red cell aplasia
Secondary to chemical or physical agents	Parvovirus infection
Dose-dependent	Acquired amegakaryocytic thrombocytopenia
Idiosyncratic	Acquired neutropenia
Infection	
Metabolic abnormalities	
T lymphocyte mediated	

* Only selected examples are described in this chapter.

The classification of the hypoplastic anaemias is summarized in Table 16.1.

The inherited hypoplastic anaemias

Fanconi's anaemia

Almost one-third of childhood cases of hypoplastic anaemia are inherited and most of these can be classified as Fanconi's anaemia. A range of congenital abnormalities is present including patchy brown skin pigmentation, stunting of growth, microcephaly, renal and skeletal malformations and, classically, absence or under-development of both thumbs. Typically, the onset of anaemia is delayed until childhood or early adolescence. Fanconi's anaemia is inherited as an autosomal recessive disorder but the nature of the genetic defect is unknown. The incidence of the gene that causes Fanconi's anaemia has been estimated to be as high as 1 in 400 of the population.

The most common presenting features for Fanconi's anaemia are bleeding secondary to thrombocytopenia and a request for investigation of short stature. Typically, thrombocytopenia develops first as an isolated abnormality, followed some months or even years later by the development of anaemia. Neutropenia is usually a relatively late manifestation of the disease. Bone marrow examination reveals hypocellularity with a reduction in the number of CFU-GEMM, CFU-GM and BFU-E and extensive fatty replacement of haemopoietic tissue. Dysplastic features are usually minimal and

Microcephaly is a medical term that means an abnormally small head in relation to the rest of the body.

reflect the stress imposed on the dwindling haemopoietic tissue in trying to maintain circulating blood cell counts.

More than 10% of Fanconi's anaemia cases progress to acute leukaemia or develop a tumour of the gastrointestinal tract or skin. Allogeneic marrow transplantation is a successful form of treatment for hypoplastic anaemia but does not correct the other congenital abnormalities or the tendency to develop non-haemopoietic malignancy. In the absence of a suitable bone marrow donor, administration of high dose anabolic steroids produces a temporary recovery in peripheral blood cell counts but at the cost of development of male secondary sexual characteristics in both boys and girls, liver damage and bouts of uncontrolled hyperactivity and aggression.

Dyskeratosis congenita

Dyskeratosis congenita is an inherited disorder which is associated with abnormal growth of skin, nails and hair. It usually is inherited as an X-linked recessive disorder although isolated reports of autosomal recessive inheritance exist. Typically, congenital abnormalities such as alopecia, abnormal sweating, telangiectasia and mental retardation are joined by the development of progressive hypoplastic anaemia in early adulthood. The nature of the genetic abnormality is unknown.

Diamond–Blackfan syndrome

Diamond–Blackfan syndrome typically presents in the first 2 years of life as a severe anaemia and reticulocytopenia in the presence of normal white cell and platelet counts. Bone marrow examination reveals either a complete absence of erythropoietic precursors or a maturation arrest in erythropoiesis. Diamond–Blackfan may be confused with Fanconi's anaemia, although cytogenetic abnormalities are absent. The pattern of inheritance in most cases is autosomal recessive, although the nature of the genetic defect is unknown.

The treatment of choice for Diamond–Blackfan syndrome is allogeneic marrow transplantation but, if this option is not available, most cases respond well to high dose corticosteroids or cyclosporin. The success of corticosteroid therapy in inducing prompt and sustainable remission of the anaemia suggests an immune-mediated pathogenesis.

The congenital dyserythropoietic anaemias

The congenital dyserythropoietic anaemias (CDAs) are a group of rare inherited disorders of unknown cause which are characterized by a variable degree of anaemia, reticulocytopenia, markedly

Standard cytogenetic preparations of bone marrow from cases of Fanconi's anaemia typically show some increase in the number of chromosomal breakages and complex rearrangements present. However, pretreatment of the bone marrow samples with cyclophosphamide or mitomycin C increases the incidence of these abnormalities markedly. Using this technique, Fanconi's homozygotes are readily and reliably detectable. The cells of Fanconi's heterozygotes may also show an increase in the number of chromosomal aberrations but cannot be separated from normal cells with absolute certainty.

Alopecia is a medical term meaning hair loss. A *telangiectasia* is a vascular lesion formed by dilatation of a group of small blood vessels.

In Ham's acidified serum test, the patient's red cells are incubated for 1 h at 37°C with a selection of ABO compatible acidified sera and the samples are examined for the presence of haemolysis. A 'positive' result (i.e. haemolysis) is obtained in cases of paroxysmal nocturnal haemoglobinuria (PNH) and HEMPAS.

ineffective erythropoiesis and erythroblast multinuclearity. Three types of CDA are recognized:

- **Type I CDA** is the mildest form and is associated with mild to moderate macrocytic anaemia, megaloblastoid bone marrow appearances and an autosomal recessive mode of inheritance. The hallmark of this form of CDA is the presence in the bone marrow of up to 3% binucleated erythroblasts with intranuclear chromatin bridges.

- **Type II CDA** is the most common and most severe form and is characterized by a mild to severe normocytic anaemia, the presence of up to 50% multinucleated erythroblasts in the bone marrow, enhanced expression of Ii antigens on red cells and an autosomal recessive mode of inheritance. Mature peripheral blood red cells in this disorder are highly susceptible to lysis in acidified serum. CDA type II is also known by the descriptive title **hereditary erythroblast multinuclearity with positive acidified serum test** (HEMPAS).

- **Type III CDA** is the rarest form and is associated with a mild macrocytic anaemia, the presence of highly multinucleate erythroblasts in the bone marrow and an autosomal dominant mode of inheritance. The abnormal erythroblasts may contain up to 12 nuclei and are sometimes known as **gigantoblasts**.

Inherited neutropenias

Cyclic neutropenia

Cyclic neutropenia is a rare congenital disorder which is characterized by recurrent neutropenia with oral ulceration, pharyngitis with lymphadenopathy and, in severe cases, pneumonia. The neutrophil count in affected individuals follows a regular cyclic pattern with bouts of neutropenia occurring at about 3 weekly intervals and lasting for about 4 days. A sharp fall in the numbers of CFU-GM present in the bone marrow and an arrest of granulopoietic activity occurs about 1 week before the neutropenic phase. These changes remit spontaneously after a few days and the neutrophil count climbs back into the lower reaches of normality for about 2–3 weeks before the cycle repeats itself.

Cyclic neutropenia is usually a congenital abnormality although occasional reports exist of the development of this condition in later life. In most cases, the mode of inheritance is uncertain but a minority show clear evidence of autosomal dominant inheritance. Typically, cyclic neutropenia is relatively benign, requiring only antimicrobial therapy to treat the minor infections that occur during the neutropenic phase of the cycle.

Kostmann's infantile genetic agranulocytosis

Infantile agranulocytosis is a rare, autosomal recessive trait characterized by profound neutropenia despite the presence of normal numbers of CFU-GM in the bone marrow which are capable of terminal differentiation in culture and a severe susceptibility to infection. Most affected infants die from overwhelming infection within the first year of life. Attempts to treat this condition with recombinant human G-CSF have given promising results.

Familial benign neutropenia

Familial benign neutropenia is a rare condition which is inherited in an autosomal dominant fashion and is characterized by chronic mild neutropenia with a compensatory increase in the cell count of the other leukocytes and a relatively mild clinical course. Bone marrow examination typically reveals mild granulocytic hypoplasia but normal erythropoietic and thrombopoietic activity.

Reticular dysgenesis

Reticular dysgenesis is a rare condition of unknown aetiology which is characterized by a selective and complete absence of leukopoiesis. Affected infants lack any identifiable granulocyte, monocyte or lymphocyte precursors in the bone marrow and lymphoid organs, and so are extremely immunosuppressed. Erythropoiesis and thrombopoiesis appear to be normal in this condition.

Congenital amegakaryocytic thrombocytopenia

Amegakaryocytic thrombocytopenia is a rare condition which is inherited as an autosomal recessive disorder and is characterized by a severe thrombocytopenia secondary to deficiency of megakaryocyte production, platelet dysfunction and, usually, absence of the bones of the lower arms. The condition is also known as the **thrombocytopenia with absent radii (TAR) syndrome.** Haemorrhage is a major cause of mortality in the first year of life. The nature of the underlying defect in this disorder is unknown.

The acquired hypoplastic anaemias

In about half the cases of hypoplastic anaemia, careful investigation reveals a likely cause for the depression in haemopoiesis, such as a history of exposure to ionizing radiation or to drugs or chemicals that are known to be myelotoxic. It follows that, in the remainder of cases, no clearly identifiable culprit can be found. Such cases are referred to as **idiopathic hypoplastic anaemias.**

Hypoplastic anaemia secondary to chemical or physical agents

A wide range of chemical and physical agents have been implicated in the causation of hypoplastic anaemia. Broadly speaking, these agents can be divided into two types:

- Those agents that always induce hypoplastic anaemia in all of those exposed and in whom the degree of hypoplasia induced is proportional to the degree of exposure.
- Those agents that are innocuous to most people but which induce hypoplasia in a minority of susceptible individuals. This is the larger group and includes a huge number of widely used drugs.

Ionizing radiation

Exposure to ionizing radiation such as X-rays, γ-rays, α particles and β particles inflicts serious damage to cellular DNA, involving the introduction of strand breaks, base deletions and the promotion of inappropriate base-pairing. The degree of damage inflicted is typically proportional to the dose of radiation received, although actively cycling cells are much more radiosensitive than those in G_0. Because of this, the most radiosensitive tissues are the haemopoietic stem cells, gut mucosal cells and testicular germ cells. A dose of 7 Gy or more of penetrating ionizing radiation such as X-rays completely ablates the bone marrow and other rapidly dividing tissue and, in the absence of bone marrow transplantation, is uniformly fatal. With lesser doses, the effect of the radiation is dose-related. Exposure to a single, short-lived dose of ionizing radiation may inflict serious damage to the bone marrow and mucosae leading to severe gastrointestinal disturbances, haemorrhage secondary to thrombocytopenia and infectious complications secondary to neutropenia, commonly resulting in death. However, given supportive care to maintain life, such individuals may recover following repopulation of the bone marrow by haemopoietic stem cells that were in G_0 at the time of exposure.

Chronic or repeated exposure to ionizing radiation is associated with the development of profound hypoplastic anaemia because, as resting haemopoietic stem cells are spurred into the cell cycle to replace damaged stem cells, they too are subject to the damaging effects of the radiation. This relentlessly destructive cycle eventually leads to severe depletion of the haemopoietic stem cell pool.

Cytotoxic chemotherapy

Cytotoxic drugs are extremely toxic substances that are used deliberately to kill malignant cells. However, they are not selective for malignant cells, and both normal and malignant cells are poisoned by such agents. The degree of hypoplasia that results is dose-related. Long experience with the therapeutic use of cytotoxic drugs has enabled the selection of dose regimens that induce temporary bone marrow hypoplasia so that recovery of normal haemopoietic tissue occurs quickly after withdrawal of the drug. Occasionally, prolonged use of alkylating agents such as busulphan

The biological damage inflicted by ionizing radiation is largely determined by the dosage, which is defined in terms of the amount of energy transferred to the irradiated tissue. Dosage is expressed in gray (Gy) where 1 gray is equivalent to the absorption of 1 joule of energy per kilogram of irradiated tissue. The older unit of dosage was the rad (1 Gy = 100 rad).

can lead to prolonged hypoplasia from which recovery is slow or incomplete.

Benzene

Chronic exposure to benzene is associated with the induction of hypoplastic anaemia and acute non-lymphoblastic leukaemia. Benzene is widely used as an organic solvent and a cleaning agent and is added to petrol as an antiknocking agent. It is unclear whether exposure to low levels of benzene is myelotoxic. Most recorded cases have been exposed to high concentrations of benzene over many years, usually at their place of work. In many cases, withdrawal of benzene exposure permits regeneration of the bone marrow without further intervention but the risk of leukaemogenesis may still be present in such cases.

Idiosyncratic responses

Many widely used drugs have been reported to induce hypoplastic anaemia in a tiny percentage of those taking them. The best known example is the antibacterial agent chloramphenicol which has been used with safety for decades. At the doses that are in everyday use, chloramphenicol therapy is not associated with clinically significant myelotoxicity. However, about 1 in 20 000 of the population are exquisitely sensitive to this drug: even the tiny amount present in eye drops is sufficient to cause profound and refractory hypoplastic anaemia which commonly results in death. The genetic basis for this idiosyncratic response is unknown and there is no way to predict which individuals are at risk. In the last few decades, chloramphenicol has been implicated in almost a quarter of cases of acquired hypoplastic anaemia in the UK. Recent years have seen a marked decline in the use of chloramphenicol.

Infection

Most infections are, to some degree, myelosuppressive. Chronic haemolytic states such as sickle cell disease and hereditary spherocytosis are occasionally complicated by a sudden arrest of erythropoietic activity. These so-called hypoplastic crises are thought to result from the myelosuppressive effects of infection on an already severely stressed bone marrow. The most common infective trigger is parvovirus B19, which specifically infects erythroid precursors. In the absence of chronic haemolysis, parvovirus B19 causes a flu-like illness which is variously known as **fifth disease**, **erythema infectiosum** or, more colourfully, **slapped-cheek disease**.

The recent upsurge in interest about green issues has had many effects, including the appearance of new, environmentally friendly products. One such product, lead-free petrol, was made available following the publication of several studies which showed that exposure to the small quantities of lead in exhaust emissions posed a potential threat to health, particularly for those who live in the inner cities. Most motorists now use lead-free petrol in their cars, secure in the knowledge that they are helping to rid the environment of toxic pollutants such as lead. However, what is seldom publicized is that, deprived of tetraethyl lead as an antiknocking agent, the oil companies simply increased the quantity of the known leukaemogen, benzene, in their new 'environmentally friendly' lead free petrol!

Pathophysiology and treatment of hypoplastic anaemia

The pathogenesis of hypoplastic anaemia is highly diverse: some cases appear to result from a functional defect of pluripotential haemopoietic stem cells; others from a defect of the haemopoietic inductive microenvironment; while others appear to be mediated by immune mechanisms.

The presenting features of hypoplastic anaemia are non-specific and predictable: pallor, lassitude and exercise intolerance secondary to anaemia; frequent and recurrent bacterial and fungal infections secondary to neutropenia; and a tendency to bruise easily secondary to thrombocytopenia. Lymphadenopathy and splenomegaly are typically absent. The diagnosis of hypoplastic anaemia can only be made when all other possible causes of the pancytopenia have been excluded by careful clinical and laboratory investigation.

Examination of the peripheral blood reveals pancytopenia. The concentration of foetal haemoglobin is commonly raised and may be as high as 20% of the total. Ferrokinetic studies reveal a delayed uptake and utilization of iron from the plasma and confirm the absence of extramedullary haemopoiesis. Bone marrow aspirates show patchy hypocellularity and replacement of haemopoietic tissue by fatty deposits. Attempts to culture bone marrow *in vitro* reveal a deficit of haemopoietic progenitor cells such as CFU-GM, CFU-E and BFU-E, and a diminished response to haemopoietic growth factors.

In the absence of treatment, the prognosis for hypoplastic anaemia is poor. The two main prognostic indicators in hypoplastic anaemia are age and disease severity at presentation. About 25% of those cases with severe disease at presentation will die within 4 months without treatment. Of the remainder, a further 25% will die within 4–12 months, and a further 35% will succumb at some later time, usually sooner rather than later. Only around 15% will remit spontaneously, and even then the remission is more likely to be partial rather than total. The median survival time in the absence of treatment for those with severe disease is 6 months: only about 20% of such cases survive much beyond a year. The treatment of choice for those with severe disease is bone marrow transplantation. Lasting restoration of haemopoiesis following bone marrow transplantation is achieved in more than 80% of cases. The success rate is somewhat lower in cases that have been given blood transfusions prior to transplantation.

If a suitable donor is not available, or if the patient is too old to withstand the rigours of the transplantation process, the treatment of choice is immunosuppressive therapy. Cyclophosphamide and antithymocyte globulin produce stable remission rates in more than 50% of those treated.

Supportive therapy during the pancytopenic period is extremely important. Antibiotics are required to treat established infection or, where the neutrophil count is very low, may be used prophylactically. Measures for the avoidance of infection are also important. Menstrual blood losses can be prevented or minimized by the administration of oral contraceptives. Transfusion therapy should be avoided if at all possible, especially in those cases that are eligible for a bone marrow transplant.

Suggested further reading

Brown, K.E. and Young, N.S. (1996). Parvoviruses and bone marrow failure. *Stem Cells* **14**(2), 151–163.

Kaufman, D.W., Levy, M. and Shapiro, S. (1991). *The Drug Etiology of Agranulocytosis and Aplastic Anemia*. New York: Oxford University Press.

Nakao, S. (1997). Immune mechanism of aplastic anemia. *International Journal of Hematology* **66**(2), 127–134.

Young, N.S. and Maciejewski, J. (1997). Mechanisms of disease – The pathophysiology of acquired aplastic anemia. *New England Journal of Medicine* **336**(19), 1365–1372.

Self-assessment questions

1. Hypersplenism is accompanied by peripheral cytopenia. Why is this condition not considered to be hypoplastic anaemia?
2. Which of the following conditions is an inherited hypoplastic anaemia?
   (a) Fanconi's anaemia
   (b) DiGeorge's syndrome
   (c) CDA type II
   (d) refractory anemia
3. What is the most common infective trigger of acquired hypoplastic anaemia?

Key Concepts and Facts

- Hypoplastic anaemias are caused by a failure of haemopoiesis.

- Hypoplastic anaemia is very rare in childhood, but becomes increasingly common with advancing age.

- Fanconi's anaemia accounts for almost one-third of childhood cases of hypoplastic anaemia.

- More than 10% of Fanconi's anaemia cases progress to acute leukaemia.

- Diamond–Blackfan syndrome is a red cell hypoplastic state.

- The CDAs are a group of rare inherited anaemias of unknown cause. Three distinct forms are recognized.

- Cyclic neutropenia is a rare congenital disorder which is characterized by recurrent neutropenia.

- About half of all acquired hypoplastic anaemias are idiopathic.

- Acquired hypoplastic anaemia is associated with exposure to ionizing radiation, cytotoxic drugs, benzene and related products and infection.

- Some hypoplastic anaemias result from an idiosyncratic response to a normally innocuous agent.

- The most common infective trigger of hypoplastic anaemia is parvovirus B19.

- The prognosis for untreated hypoplastic anaemia is poor.

- The treatment of choice for severe hypoplastic anaemia is bone marrow transplantation.

Chapter 17
Overview of haemostasis

Learning objectives

After studying this chapter you should confidently be able to:

Name the four main systems involved in the prevention and arrest of blood loss.

Differentiate between primary and secondary haemostasis.

Outline blood vessel structure and the contribution of the vascular system to haemostasis.

Outline platelet structure and the contribution of platelets to haemostasis.

Describe the classical and modern theories of blood coagulation.

Highlight the pivotal role of vitamin K-dependent factors in haemostasis.

Outline blood coagulation.

Outline the fibrinolytic system and the inhibitory mechanisms that limit fibrinolysis.

Highlight the mutual interdependence of the various systems involved in haemostasis.

Key dates

1686 First separation of blood clot fibres from cells and serum.

1731 Observation that clots stem blood loss.

1803 Recognition of sex-linking in haemophilia.

1819 First observation of the procoagulant effect of tissues (tissue factor).

1845 Recognition that fibrin is formed from plasma fibrinogen.

1905 Morawitz theory of blood coagulation.

1926 Description of von Willebrand's disease.

1935 Development of one-stage prothrombin time by Quick.

1935 Description of the antihaemorrhagic properties of vitamin K.

1944 Recognition that Christmas disease is distinct from haemophilia.

1947 Description of serum inhibitor to tissue thromboplastin.

1964 Waterfall hypothesis of coagulation proposed.

1971 Use of ristocetin to diagnose vWD.

1977 Purification of tissue factor.

Post-1981 Development of monoclonal antibody and molecular techniques leading to improved understanding of haemostasis.

1987 Pathways of blood coagulation revised to take account of central roles of tissue factor and TFPI.

One of the most important survival mechanisms in higher animals is the ability to minimize blood loss following injury. Set against this requirement is the necessity to maintain blood in a fluid state in the absence of injury. Thus, in health, a dynamic equilibrium exists between mechanisms that tend to promote clot formation and those that tend to oppose clot formation. When these mechanisms are in balance, blood is maintained in the fluid state and confined to the circulatory system. Events that disturb the balance between these opposing forces promote either haemorrhage or clot formation. This chapter presents an overview of the processes involved in maintaining the haemostatic balance.

The vascular system

Blood vessel walls are composed of three distinct, concentric layers as shown in Figure 17.1:

- The **intima** forms the inner layer and consists of a thin monolayer of flat vascular endothelial cells. Vascular endothelial cells are non-thrombogenic and contain **Weibel–Palade bodies**. The vascular endothelium is mounted upon an internal elastic membrane which is largely composed of collagen fibres.

- The **media** forms the central layer and is the most variable component of the blood vessel wall. In elastic arteries, such as the aorta, the media is composed of elastic fibres arranged in concentric, circumferential layers to absorb the huge changes in pressure as the heart beats. In muscular arteries, the media is composed of smooth muscle cells that permit rhythmic contraction and relaxation of the artery, which helps to maintain blood pressure. In arterioles and veins, the media is thin and of much less functional importance.

- The **adventitia** forms the exterior coat and is composed of collagen with a scattering of smooth muscle cells. The border between the media and the adventitia may be marked by a collection of elastic fibres which form the **external elastic lamina**.

Contribution of the vascular system to haemostasis

Constriction of the injured blood vessel to limit early blood loss is an early means of minimizing blood loss. Vasoconstriction is mediated by substances such as adrenaline, ADP, kinins and thromboxanes. Many of these vasoactive substances are derived from blood platelets.

The metabolic activities of vascular endothelial cells play an

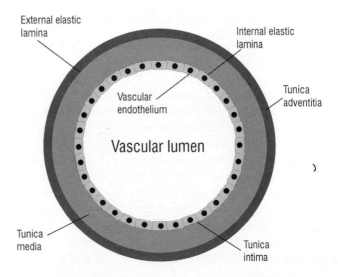

Figure 17.1 *The structure of a muscular artery*

important role in haemostasis. These cells are the major source of **von Willebrand factor (vWF), thrombomodulin** and **tissue factor pathway inhibitor (TFPI)**. The contribution of these substances to haemostasis is discussed later in this chapter. vWF is also synthesized by megakaryocytes. Endothelial cell prostaglandin metabolism produces **prostacyclin (PGI$_2$)** which is a very potent inhibitor of platelet aggregation and also acts as a vasodilator.

When the integrity of the vascular endothelial layer is breached, the subendothelial layers provide a surface for platelet activation and aggregation as well as activation of the coagulation system. More importantly, the adventitial cells express **tissue factor** which is now thought to be the primary activator of blood coagulation.

Blood platelets

Platelets are formed from the cytoplasm of bone marrow megakaryocytes and are the smallest of the blood cells. The normal platelet count lies between 150 and 400×10^9/l. They are disc-shaped, anucleate cells with a relatively complex internal structure reflecting the specific haemostatic functions of the platelet. The ultrastructure of the blood platelet is depicted in Figure 17.2.

Of particular importance are the two major types of intracellular granule, the α **granules** and the **dense granules**. The α granules contain the platelet glycoprotein **thrombospondin** as well as **fibrinogen, fibronectin, platelet factor 4 (PF4), vWF, β-thromboglobulin (β-TG), platelet-derived growth factor (PDGF)** and coagulation factors V and VIII. The dense granules, so called because of their appearance on electron microscopy, contain ADP, ATP and **serotonin (5-hydroxy-tryptamine or 5-HT)**. The contents of both the α and dense granules may be released, via a system of surface-connecting

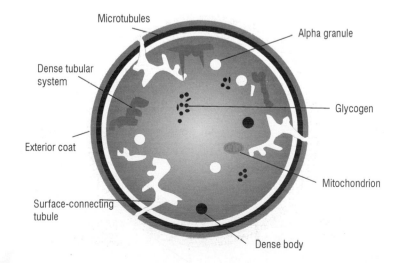

Figure 17.2 *Schematic of normal platelet ultrastructure*

Table 17.1 *Platelet granule constituents and their most important biological functions*

Location	Compound	Function
α Granule	Platelet factor 4	Neutralizes heparin effect
	β-thromboglobulin	Promotes fibroblast chemotaxis
	Platelet derived growth factor	Mitogen for fibroblasts; chemotaxin for neutrophils, fibroblasts and smooth muscle cells
	von Willebrand factor	Adhesion molecule; carrier for VIII
	Thrombospondin	Promotes platelet–platelet interaction
	Fibronectin	Adhesion of platelets and fibroblasts
Dense granules	ADP	Aggregation of platelets
	ATP	Source of ADP
	Serotonin	Vasoconstriction
	Calcium	Coagulation; platelet function

tubules, during platelet function. These granular contents have a variety of important biological activities as shown in Table 17.1.

Both platelets and vascular endothelial cells contain biochemical pathways for the metabolism of **arachidonic acid** (Figure 17.3). This polyunsaturated fatty acid is mainly present bound to membrane phospholipids but can be released by the enzyme phospholipase A_2 in activated platelets. The newly liberated arachidonic acid is converted to **thromboxane A_2 (TXA$_2$)** by the actions of the enzymes **cyclo-oxygenase** and **thromboxane synthetase**. TXA$_2$ is a

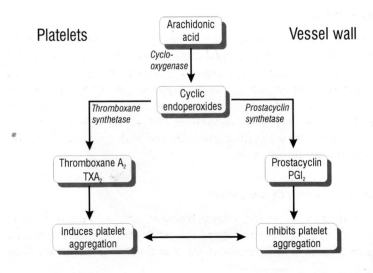

Figure 17.3 *Arachidonic acid metabolism in vascular endothelium and platelets*

powerful inducer of platelet aggregation but has a very short half-life (around 30 s). Arachidonic acid metabolism within vascular endothelium results in the generation of PGI_2, which is a potent inhibitor of platelet aggregation.

Platelet function

During primary haemostasis, there are four phases of platelet function:

- Adhesion to a surface.
- Shape change.
- Release of granule contents.
- Aggregation.

Adhesion

Blood platelets are activated by contact with a variety of physiological and non-physiological substances, including subendothelial tissue, foreign or charged surfaces, ADP, thrombin, TXA_2 and bacterial endotoxin. *In vivo*, damage to the vessel wall causes exposure of subendothelial fibres and results in the rapid adherence of circulating platelets to the surface of the wound. Normally, sufficient platelets would be present to completely cover the damaged area. The importance of platelet adhesion *in vivo* is illustrated by the relatively easy bruising and enhanced capillary fragility seen in patients with thrombocytopenia.

Platelet adhesion is mediated by interactions between specific platelet membrane receptors (designated GPIb and GPIIb/IIIa) and von Willebrand factor (vWF). Deficiency of vWF results in mucous membrane bleeding and easy bruising.

Shape change

Platelet adhesion is usually accompanied by a transformation in platelet shape from the normal discoid form to one of irregular outline with numerous cytoplasmic projections, the echinocytic configuration. In the early stages of platelet activation the shape changes are reversible, but with increased and continued stimulation the change becomes irreversible and is associated with centralization of the cytoplasmic granules and with degranulation and release of granule contents.

Release of granule contents

Platelet degranulation (the release reaction) occurs as a result of the fusion of the cytoplasmic granules with the surface-connected tubular system. The contents of the α and dense granules are thus

The most commonly prescribed antiplatelet drug is aspirin (acetylsalicylic acid) which acts by acetylating the enzyme cyclo-oxygenase, thereby inhibiting TXA production. Low-dose aspirin therapy is used as an effective prophylactic measure in cases of established thromboembolic disease.

Spiculated blood cells are called echinocytes because of their supposed resemblance to the spiny sea urchin *Echinus esculenta*.

made available at the platelet surface where they trigger further localized platelet adhesion and aggregation.

Aggregation

Platelet activation prompts the binding of plasma fibrinogen to specific platelet receptors (GPIIb/IIIa) and the formation of inter-platelet 'bridges'. A variety of compounds are capable of inducing platelet aggregation, including adrenaline, ADP, collagen, thrombin, arachidonic acid and TXA_2. *In vivo*, the ADP released from activated platelets and damaged red cells at sites of injury stimulates the activation of adjacent platelets, which undergo the release reaction and subsequently join the growing aggregate. This self-propagating activation rapidly results in the formation of a **primary haemostatic plug**, which physically blocks the breach in the vessel wall, thereby staunching blood loss.

The primary haemostatic plug is fragile and if it is not reinforced it quickly breaks down and bleeding recommences. The consolidation of the primary haemostatic plug is brought about by the enzymatic conversion of fibrinogen to fibrin and the subsequent stabilization of the resultant fibrin molecules by blood coagulation factor XIII. The activation and regulation of the blood coagulation system is discussed in greater detail below, although it should be remembered that the platelets themselves are capable of providing many of the components of this system at the local level.

The blood coagulation system

The blood coagulation system is composed of a series of functionally specific plasma proteins (coagulation factors) which interact in a highly ordered and predetermined sequence with the sole object of converting the soluble protein fibrinogen to an insoluble network of fibrin which consolidates and stabilizes the primary haemostatic plug. The coagulation factors are, by convention, referred to by an internationally agreed system of Roman numerals. These numbers are related to the order of discovery of the individual coagulation factors, not the order in which they take part in the coagulation process. Each coagulation factor also has one or more synonyms as shown in Table 17.2. The coagulation factors are synthesized primarily in the liver, although von Willebrand factor is produced by endothelial cells and megakaryocytes. Platelets also contain coagulation factors V, XIII, vWF and fibrinogen.

There are two types of coagulation factor:

- **Zymogens,** which are inactive plasma proteins (proenzymes) and which, after cleavage by a specific enzyme, are transformed into active enzymes. Coagulation factors that fall into this category include factors II, X, XI, XII and XIII. Most of the coagulation enzymes are **serine proteases**, i.e. the active site of the proteolytic

Although the presence of factor VIII in plasma was first demonstrated in 1911, its detailed biochemical and structural characteristics have only recently been elucidated. Factor VIII circulates in plasma complexed to von Willebrand factor. Without vWF as a protective carrier, factor VIII is rapidly broken down. Before this structure was clearly recognized, there was considerable confusion over nomenclature and understanding of the separate roles of these factors in haemostasis. The currently recommended nomenclature is as follows:

Factor VIII protein	FVIII
Factor VIII procoagulant activity	FVIIIAct
Factor VIII antigen	FVIIIAg
von Willebrand factor	vWF
von Willebrand factor antigen	vWFAg

The term **ristocetin cofactor** is also used to describe the attribute of vWF required for platelet aggregation by the antibiotic ristocetin. However, the use of specific terminology to indicate functional activities of vWF is not recommended.

Table 17.2 *Nomenclature of the coagulation factors*

Coagulation factor	Most commonly used synonym
I (not normally used)	Fibrinogen
II	Prothrombin
III (not used)	Tissue factor (thromboplastin)
IV (not used)	Calcium ions
V	Labile factor
VII	Stable factor
VIII	Antihaemophilic factor
IX	Christmas factor
X	Stuart–Prower factor
XI	Plasma thromboplastin antecedant (not normally used)
XII	Hageman factor
XIII	Fibrin stabilizing factor
None assigned	Prekallikrein
None assigned	High molecular weight kininogen

enzyme contains a serine residue. Factor XIII is a transglutaminase.

- **Accelerators,** which are not converted to an active enzyme during the coagulation process but act as accelerators or catalysts for other enzymatic reactions. Factors V and VIII fall into this category.

Two coagulation factors, fibrinogen and factor VII, cannot strictly be classified as either zymogens or accelerators. Fibrinogen is converted to fibrin, which has no enzymatic properties, and factor VII normally circulates as an active enzyme, although its activity is potentiated by tissue factor. By convention, activated coagulation factors are denoted by a subscript suffix a, e.g. XII_a is the activated form of factor XII.

The role of vitamin K in blood coagulation

Coagulation factors II, VII, IX and X as well as proteins C and S are dependent on vitamin K for their normal function. These factors are synthesized in an inactive form that cannot bind calcium ions. This ability is conferred by a post-translational modification which involves γ-carboxylation of glutamic acid residues. Vitamin K *in vivo* continuously cycles between three forms: vitamin K quinone, vitamin K hydroquinone and vitamin K epoxide. The γ-carboxylation reaction is coupled to the conversion of vitamin K hydroquinone to the epoxide form. Thus, in vitamin K deficiency, γ-carboxylation fails and non-carboxylated forms of factors II, VII, IX and X and proteins C and S are released into the circulation. Although they are immunologically identical to

During the winter of 1921–22, herds of Canadian cattle fed on stored sweet clover suffered an epidemic of a haemorrhagic disease secondary to prothrombin deficiency. During a subsequent outbreak in the USA, Wisconsin chemist Karl Link identified the agent responsible as bis-hydroxycoumarin (dicoumarol). This substance, under the name of warfarin, is widely used as a rat poison and oral anticoagulant for the treatment of thromboembolic disease. Warfarin acts by inhibiting the vitamin K-dependent carboxylation of factors II, VII, IX and X and proteins C and S, without which they are inactive.

the normal proteins, these proteins induced by vitamin **K** absence or antagonism (PIVKAs) cannot bind calcium ions, and thus cannot bind to phospholipid surfaces. Because of this, they are activated much more slowly than their normal counterparts, giving rise to the anticoagulant effect seen, for example, following oral anticoagulant therapy. PIVKAs can, however, be activated *in vitro* with the venom of certain snakes such as *Echis carinatus* and this property can form the basis for their laboratory measurement.

Mechanisms of blood coagulation

The classical blood coagulation cascade

Classical blood coagulation theory has divided the coagulation process into the **intrinsic pathway** and the **extrinsic pathway**, as shown in Figure 17.4.

The intrinsic pathway

Intrinsic blood coagulation is initiated by contact of the flowing blood with a foreign surface. A variety of foreign surfaces, both physiological (e.g. collagen, basement membranes and lipopolysaccharide) and non-physiological (e.g. glass and kaolin), are capable of activating blood coagulation via this pathway. Surface activation

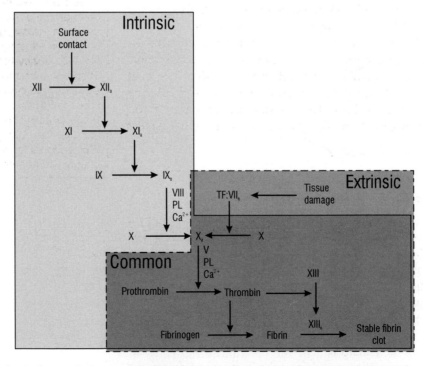

Figure 17.4   *The classical coagulation cascade illustrating the division into intrinsic, extrinsic and common pathways. This theory ascribes the major physiological role to surface contact activation via the intrinsic pathway. PL, phospholipid surface*

plays a key role in initiating many of the component pathways of the haemostatic system.

Exposure of a negatively charged surface to blood causes activation of factor XII, which then converts factor XI to XI_a. The factor XI for this reaction is also bound to the activating surface. Factor XI_a activates factor IX in a process requiring two proteolytic cleavages. Factor IX_a forms a complex with factors VIII and X, calcium ions and platelet membrane phospholipid, which results in the activation of factor X. This complex is sometimes referred to as the **tenase complex**. The resultant factor X_a forms a complex with factor V, prothrombin, calcium ions and phospholipid in a manner analogous to the formation of the factor X-activating complex. This complex is sometimes known as the **prothrombinase complex**. In these reactions, factors V and VIII act as accelerators. The activity of factors V and VIII is greatly increased by trace amounts of thrombin but higher thrombin concentrations degrade these factors. Thus, the concentration of thrombin acts as a regulator of the rate of coagulation via the intrinsic pathway.

The prothrombinase complex converts phospholipid-bound prothrombin to the active enzyme, **thrombin**. The primary function of thrombin is the conversion of fibrinogen to fibrin. This is achieved by the cleavage and release of two small peptides from the $A\alpha$ and $B\beta$ chains of fibrinogen, called fibrinopeptides A and B. This process reduces the overall negative charge of the molecule and allows the spontaneous polymerization of the resultant fibrin monomers. At this stage, however, the fibrin clot is held together by hydrophobic and electrostatic bonds alone and is relatively unstable. The final stage of blood coagulation is the stabilization of the fibrin clot by thrombin-activated factor XIII. This enzyme acts as a transglutaminase by catalysing the formation of crosslinks between adjacent fibrin molecules.

In 1955 a railway worker named John Hageman required surgery for a peptic ulcer but laboratory tests showed that his blood clotting time was prolonged. Further investigation revealed that he was deficient in a hitherto unknown plasma protein which was involved in contact activation of coagulation. This protein was named **Hageman factor**. Ten years later, several members of the Fletcher family were shown to have similarly prolonged clotting times and to be deficient in another plasma protein involved in contact activation. This factor was subsequently called **Fletcher factor**. A further 10 years passed before a Mr Fitzgerald, being treated for gunshot wounds, was shown to have a defect of contact activation and to be deficient in a plasma protein which became known as **Fitzgerald factor**. All three cases, separated by 20 years, have one important facet in common: gross prolongation of laboratory clotting times but an absence of any bleeding tendency. This apparent anomaly cannot be explained by classical blood coagulation theory. Hageman factor is now known as factor XII, Fletcher factor as prekallikrein and Fitzgerald factor as high molecular weight kininogen.

The extrinsic pathway

In the presence of calcium ions, tissue factor (TF) forms a complex with both factor VII (TF:VII) and factor VII_a (TF:VII_a). The formation of these complexes results in the rapid activation of complexed VII and the enormous potentiation of the action of VII_a, i.e. the activation of factors IX and X. Following factor X activation, coagulation proceeds as described above.

The classical concept of blood coagulation has been exceptionally important as a means of understanding the results of laboratory screening tests of coagulation. However, it is now clear that separate coagulation pathways do not exist *in vivo* and that tissue factor is the major physiological activator of blood coagulation. This has led to a revision in our concepts of coagulation *in vivo*.

Figure 17.5 *A simplified schematic of the current concept of coagulation. The inhibitory action of TFPI is shown in grey*

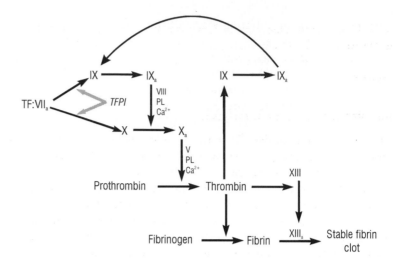

Current concept of the coagulation cascade

The observation that severe deficiency of factor XII, high molecular weight kininogen or kallikrein is not accompanied by the expected severe bleeding disorder, and the unexpected presence of a severe bleeding tendency in haemophilia cast doubt on the validity of the classical concept of blood coagulation. The discovery of a specific inhibitor of the TF : VII$_a$ complex (tissue factor pathway inhibitor, TFPI) triggered a revision of our concepts of the coagulation cascade. The biochemical details remain the same; it is just the order of events that is now believed to be different. The revised scheme of blood coagulation is shown in Figure 17.5.

In the current model, coagulation is initiated when factor VII or VII$_a$ in flowing blood comes into contact with tissue factor, which is expressed by subendothelial cells exposed at sites of vascular damage. The resultant TF : VII$_a$ complex activates a small amount of factors X and IX before the intervention of TFPI which blocks further factor X$_a$ generation through this route. The small amount of IX$_a$ present is soon exhausted. Further X$_a$ generation can only be achieved by the action of factor XI$_a$. Factor XI, now placed at the end of the coagulation cascade, is activated by the trace amounts of thrombin generated earlier.

Contact activation via factor XII, prekallikrein and HMW kininogen plays no role in this model of the coagulation cascade. The importance of these factors lies in orchestrating other inflammatory responses such as complement, kinin and fibrinolytic activation.

In this way, TFPI-mediated feedback inhibition of the TF : VII$_a$ complex explains the clinical importance of both 'intrinsic' and 'extrinsic' coagulation factors. Furthermore, it appears that the tissue factor–factor VII pathway is responsible for the rapid generation of thrombin sufficient to cause localized platelet aggregation and activation of the critical cofactors factor V and factor

Tissue factor pathway inhibitor (TFPI) is also referred to in older literature as extrinsic pathway inhibitor (EPI) and lipoprotein-associated coagulation inhibitor (LACI).

VIII. Continuing haemostasis, however, certainly requires ongoing generation of factor X_a through the actions of factors VIII and IX, thereby explaining the clinical importance of these coagulation factors.

Inhibitors of blood coagulation

The blood coagulation system is a multifactorial biological pathway consisting of zymogens and accelerators. Because of the natural amplification of the enzyme products of the coagulation cascade there is always a danger that the process may run out of control. A variety of inhibitory mechanisms exist which act to limit coagulation to the site of injury. The major inhibitors of the blood coagulation pathway are **antithrombin III, heparin cofactor II**, activated **protein C** and **tissue factor pathway inhibitor**.

Antithrombin III

Antithrombin III (ATIII) is a single-chain glycoprotein of molecular weight 61 000 which is synthesized in the liver and endothelium. ATIII is the main physiological inhibitor of activated coagulation serine proteases. It acts by forming a complex with thrombin and other serine proteases in which both components are inactivated. Complex formation is greatly accelerated (about 2000-fold) by the presence of the anticoagulant heparin. Because of this, ATIII is sometimes known as **heparin cofactor I**.

Heparin cofactor II

Heparin cofactor II is a single-chain glycoprotein of molecular weight 65 000 which is synthesized in the liver. It complexes with thrombin in a $1:1$ stoichiometric ratio, thereby inactivating the protease. In contrast to ATIII, heparin cofactor II is specific for thrombin, having no inhibitory activity against the other serine proteases. The activity of heparin cofactor II is amplified 1000-fold by the presence of heparin.

The protein C pathway

Protein C is a vitamin K-dependent protein that plays a dual role in haemostasis by inhibiting blood coagulation and stimulating fibrinolysis. Protein C is activated by thrombin in the presence of a cofactor called thrombomodulin. Activated protein C inhibits the coagulation cascade by inactivating factor VIII_a and factor V_a, thereby reducing the rate of thrombin generation.

Thrombomodulin has a molecular weight of 68 000 and is present in tight association with vascular endothelium. It forms complexes with thrombin in a $1:1$ stoichiometric ratio. Complexed thrombin activates protein C several thousand times faster than free

Protein C derives its name from the chromatographic separation of the vitamin K-dependent factors from plasma. Using this method, four peaks are obtained, and these are labelled A, B, C and D. Protein C is the major constituent of the third peak. Protein S is named after the city of its discovery, Seattle.

thrombin, but does not clot fibrinogen, activate factors V and VIII or aggregate platelets. Thrombomodulin-bound thrombin can still be inhibited by antithrombin III.

Protein S is a single-chain glycoprotein of molecular weight 69 000 which is synthesized in the liver and endothelium. It is a vitamin K-dependent protein but is not a serine protease. Activated protein C complexes with protein S and calcium ions on platelets and at the endothelial surface. The inhibitory activity of complexed protein C is greatly amplified.

Tissue factor pathway inhibitor

Tissue factor pathway inhibitor is synthesized by endothelial cells and circulates in plasma bound to low density lipoproteins. It is also present in platelets and bound to heparan sulphate at the endothelial surface. TFPI inhibits coagulation by binding to factor X_a and the $TF:VII_a$ complex, thereby inhibiting their proteolytic activity.

The fibrinolytic system

The major function of the fibrinolytic system is the degradation and dissolution of formed fibrin within the circulation. This is achieved by the rapid and localized formation of a powerful proteolytic enzyme called plasmin. As shown in Figure 17.6, the fibrinolytic system has four main components:

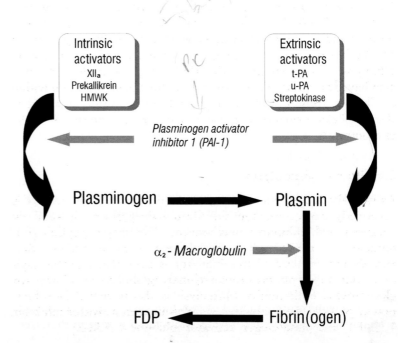

Figure 17.6 *The fibrinolytic system. Inhibitory pathways are shown in italics. HMWK, high molecular weight kininogen. FDP, fibrin(ogen) degradation products.*

- Plasminogen activators
- Plasminogen
- Plasmin
- Fibrinolytic inhibitors

Plasminogen activators

Plasminogen activation may occur via an intrinsic pathway, possibly mediated by components of contact activation, or via an extrinsic mechanism involving activators released from the blood vessel wall. Plasminogen activators are present in many different human and animal tissues and secretions. This form is known as **tissue-type plasminogen activator (t-PA)**. The other major activator is found predominantly in urine and is known as **urokinase-type plasminogen activator (u-PA)**.

Tissue plasminogen activator has a molecular weight of 70 000 and is synthesized and stored by vascular endothelial cells, ready for release into the bloodstream when required. It functions as a serine protease in the conversion of plasminogen to plasmin, a process greatly accelerated by the presence of fibrin.

Urokinase (u-PA) is a trypsin-like protease synthesized in the kidney and is found mainly in urine. It converts plasminogen directly to plasmin in a reaction that does not require the presence of fibrin.

Plasminogen and plasmin

Plasminogen is a single-chain glycoprotein with a molecular weight of about 92 000. The molecule contains five homologous triple-loop structures known as **kringles** which mediate binding to fibrin and fibrinogen. Both plasminogen and plasmin have a very strong affinity for fibrinogen and fibrin. This means that a fibrin clot will also have plasminogen activator and plasminogen bound up within it. Thus, activation of plasminogen to form plasmin is localized to the site of clot formation and digestion occurs from the inside of the clot outwards.

Inhibitors of fibrinolysis

As with the coagulation system, uninhibited proteolytic activity is potentially dangerous, and the fibrinolytic pathway is similarly equipped with inhibitory mechanisms. The major physiological inhibitor of plasmin is α_2-**antiplasmin**; enzyme activity that exceeds the capacity of this inhibitor is neutralized by the high molecular weight plasma protein α_2-**macroglobulin** or **histidine-rich glycoprotein**. Inhibition of fibrinolysis is also mediated by inhibition of plasminogen activators via **plasminogen activator inhibitor 1 (PAI-1)** and **plasminogen activator inhibitor 2 (PAI-2)**.

> In addition to the physiological activators of fibrinolysis, a number of exogenous activators exist. For example, **streptokinase** is derived from β-haemolytic streptococci and has been used as a therapeutic agent for the treatment of established thrombi for many years. However, streptokinase therapy is difficult to control and is complicated by the antigenicity of bacterial products. It is likely to be superseded by genetically engineered tissue plasminogen activator, although currently this is extremely expensive.

Suggested further reading

Amiral, J. (1997). Molecular markers in thrombosis and hemostasis. *Clinical and Applied Thrombosis–Hemostasis* **3**(2), 87–102.

Bloom, A.L., Forbes, C.D., Thomas, D.P. and Tuddenham, E.G.D. (1994). *Haemostasis and Thrombosis*. Edinburgh: Churchill Livingstone.

Broze, G.J. (1995). Tissue factor pathway inhibitor and the revised theory of coagulation. *Annual Review of Medicine* **46**, 103–112.

Roddie, P.H. and Ludlam, C.A. (1997). Recombinant coagulation factors. *Blood Reviews* **11**(4), 169–177.

Self-assessment questions

1. Name the four main systems involved in haemostasis.
2. Differentiate between the structure and content of the adventitial, medial and intimal layers in blood vessels.
3. Name three substances synthesized by vascular endothelial cells.
4. Which of the following substances are stored in platelet α granules:
   (a) ADP;
   (b) thrombospondin;
   (c) fibrinogen;
   (d) serotonin;
   (e) platelet factor 4 (PF4);
   (f) von Willebrand factor;
   (g) β-thromboglobulin (β-TG);
   (h) coagulation factors V and VIII?
5. Name the specific platelet membrane receptors for vWF that mediate platelet adhesion.
6. Which of the following coagulation factors are vitamin K-dependent:
   (a) V;
   (b) VII;
   (c) VIII;
   (d) II;
   (e) fibrinogen?
7. Which coagulation factor acts as a transglutaminase?
8. Name three components of the protein C inhibitory pathway.
9. What property of plasminogen helps to localize fibrinolysis to the site of clot formation?

Key Concepts and Facts

- In health, a dynamic equilibrium exists between mechanisms that promote clot formation and those that oppose clot formation.

- Blood vessel walls are composed of three distinct, concentric layers: the **intima**, the **media** and the **adventitia**.

- Substances such as adrenaline, ADP, kinins and thromboxanes mediate vasoconstriction.

- Vascular endothelial cells are the major source of **von Wille-brand factor (vWF)**, **thrombomodulin** and **tissue factor pathway inhibitor (TFPI)**.

- Vascular endothelial cells produce **prostacyclin (PGI$_2$)**, a vasodilator and potent inhibitor of platelet aggregation.

- Adventitial cells express **tissue factor**, the primary activator of blood coagulation.

- There are four phases of platelet haemostatic function: adhesion to a surface, shape change, release of granule contents and aggregation.

- Platelet activation rapidly results in the formation of a **primary haemostatic plug**.

- The blood coagulation system is composed of a series of functionally specific plasma proteins that interact in a pre-determined sequence to produce fibrin which consolidates and stabilizes the primary haemostatic plug.

- The coagulation factors are synthesized primarily in the liver, although von Willebrand factor is produced by endothelial cells and megakaryocytes.

- Coagulation factors II, VII, IX and X as well as proteins C and S are dependent on vitamin K for their normal function.

- In vitamin K deficiency, inactive forms of these factors, known as PIVKAs, are produced.

- In the intrinsic pathway, coagulation is triggered by contact with collagen or negatively charged surfaces and proceeds via stepwise activation to the formation of a stable fibrin clot.

- The extrinsic pathway requires the presence of tissue factor to bypass the early stages of the intrinsic pathway.

- The classical concept of coagulation has been superseded, although it remains conceptually important for the interpretation of laboratory tests.

- In the current model, coagulation is initiated by contact between factor VII or VIIa and tissue factor which is expressed by subendothelial cells exposed at sites of vascular damage.

- Contact activation via factor XII, prekallikrein and HMW kininogen plays no role in the current model of the coagulation cascade. These factors orchestrate complement, kinin and fibrinolytic activation.

- In this way, TFPI-mediated feedback inhibition of the TF:VII$_a$ complex explains the clinical importance of both 'intrinsic' and 'extrinsic' coagulation factors. Furthermore, it appears that the tissue factor–factor VII pathway is responsible for the rapid generation of thrombin sufficient to cause localized platelet aggregation and activation of the critical cofactors factor V and factor VIII. Continuing haemostasis, however, certainly requires ongoing generation of factor X$_a$ through the actions of factors VIII and IX, thereby explaining the clinical importance of these coagulation factors.

- The major inhibitors of the blood coagulation pathway are **antithrombin III**, **heparin cofactor II**, activated **protein C** and **tissue factor pathway inhibitor**.

- The major function of the fibrinolytic system is the degradation and dissolution of formed fibrin within the circulation.

Chapter 18
Disorders of haemostasis

Learning objectives

After studying this chapter you should confidently be able to:

List selected examples of inherited and acquired haemorrhagic disorders.

List selected examples of inherited and acquired thrombotic disorders.

List several examples of disorders of primary and secondary haemostasis.

Outline the pathophysiology of disorders of primary and secondary haemostasis.

Compare and contrast the pathophysiology of Bernard–Soulier syndrome, von Willebrand's disease and haemophilia.

Outline the molecular basis of haemophilia and the approach to screening for carrier detection.

Discuss the pathophysiology of selected inherited thrombotic disorders.

Discuss the pathogenesis and pathophysiology of disseminated intravascular coagulation.

Outline the prophylaxis and treatment of thrombosis.

Optimal haemostasis requires the interaction of numerous components of the blood vessel wall, platelets, coagulation system and the fibrinolytic system. Defects affecting any of these mechanisms can cause either a haemorrhagic or a thrombotic disorder which may be hereditary or acquired.

Inherited haemorrhagic disorders

Haemostasis requires a dynamic equilibrium between clot-promoting and clot-preventing activities. A haemorrhagic diathesis results from any alteration in the haemostatic balance which either impairs clot-promoting activities or potentiates clot-inhibiting activities. A variety of such defects exist including:

- Structural defects of the vascular system, resulting in easy disruption.
- Quantitative (thrombocytopenia) or qualitative (thrombocytopathy) defects of platelets, resulting in impaired platelet plug formation.
- Deficiency or dysfunction of coagulation factors (coagulopathy), resulting in impaired clot formation.
- Deficiency or dysfunction of fibrinolytic inhibitors, resulting in hyperfibrinolysis.

Inherited structural defects of the vascular system

Hereditary haemorrhagic telangiectasia

Hereditary haemorrhagic telangiectasia (HHT) is inherited as an autosomal dominant condition and is characterized by malformed, thin-walled capillaries, known as **telangiectases**, which are highly susceptible to rupture. Telangiectases are most obvious on the tongue, lips and nose but they occur throughout the body. Clinically, HHT presents as recurrent nosebleeds (epistaxes) and gastrointestinal blood loss. Enlargement and coalescence of telangiectases leads to bleeding in the lungs or brain, which may be life-threatening. No treatment is available for HHT other than correction of the recurrent anaemia and cautery of troublesome bleeding points.

> HHT is also known as Osler–Rendu–Weber syndrome.

Ehlers–Danlos syndrome

Ehlers–Danlos syndrome is the name given to a group of collagen disorders characterized by extreme elasticity and fragility of the skin, hypermobility of the joints and a haemorrhagic tendency. In the most serious variant type III collagen, the form that predominates in blood vessels, is deficient leading to a pattern of acute and severe internal bleeding which may be life-threatening. There is no treatment for this condition.

Inherited defects of platelets

A deficiency of platelet activity may be caused by severe thrombocytopenia or defective platelet function. The thrombocytopenias are described in Chapter 16 and later in this chapter.

Inherited thrombocytopathies

The clinical manifestations of congenital platelet disorders all follow a similar pattern: easy bruising, petechial rash, mucous membrane bleeding (epistaxis, gastrointestinal bleeding, menorrhagia) or excessive bleeding following minor trauma. The severity of these symptoms varies from a severe, life-long haemorrhagic diathesis to a much milder condition.

Bernard–Soulier disease

Bernard–Soulier disease (BSD) is a rare, autosomal recessive trait which is characterized by the presence of giant platelets, variable thrombocytopenia, impairment of vWF-mediated platelet adhesion, prolonged bleeding time and a bleeding tendency of variable severity. Bernard–Soulier platelets are deficient in certain platelet membrane glycoproteins (GPIb, GPIX and GPV) that are required for optimal platelet activation and function and have a shortened lifespan. There is no specific curative treatment for BSD. Supportive therapy includes red cell transfusions to combat anaemia, hormonal control of ovulation to minimize heavy menstruation and platelet transfusions when required.

Pseudo von Willebrand's disease

Pseudo von Willebrand's disease is inherited as an autosomal dominant condition and is characterized by mild thrombocytopenia, moderately reduced plasma vWF concentration and a prolonged bleeding time. Pseudo vWD is caused by an abnormality of platelet membrane glycoproteins that bind to plasma vWF. Careful laboratory testing is required to distinguish between pseudo von Willebrand's disease, true von Willebrand's disease and Bernard–Soulier disease.

Glanzmann's thrombasthenia

Glanzmann's thrombasthenia is inherited as an autosomal recessive trait and is characterized by a normal platelet count and morphology, impairment or absence of clot retraction and near absence of platelet aggregation. The disorder is caused by a profound deficiency or defect of the platelet membrane glycoprotein complex (GPIIb : GPIIIa) that mediates platelet aggregation responses by functioning as a surface receptor for fibrinogen and vWF. Although Glanzmann's thrombasthenia is a very uncommon disorder, it is one of the most frequently encountered inherited qualitative platelet defects.

Storage pool disease

Storage pool disease is a relatively mild autosomal dominant platelet disorder and is caused by a deficiency of platelet dense granules (δ-SPD) or α granules (α-SPD) or, rarely, both. This causes a deficiency of the important substances stored in these granules and consequent impairment of functional responses.

Petechiae are pinpoint haemorrhages which represent blood which has leaked from intact capillaries because of increased vascular permeability or failure of platelet function. Petechiae typically occur in clusters.
Purpura describes the appearance of confluent patches of petechiae.
Ecchymoses are commonly known as bruises and represent larger amounts of extravasated blood under the skin.
A **haematoma** is a large ecchymosis that involves subcutaneous tissue or muscle, producing localized swelling and deformity.
Haemarthrosis describes haemorrhage into a joint.

The first case of Bernard–Soulier disease was reported in 1948 by two French physicians, Jean Bernard and Jean-Pierre Soulier, in a 5-month-old child with recurrent haemorrhagic problems.

α-SPD is also known as **grey platelet syndrome** because, when stained with Romanowsky dyes and viewed by light microscopy, the absence of α granulation in the platelets results in a uniform grey appearance.

Inherited coagulopathies

The inherited coagulopathies are rare, with an overall incidence of about 0.02%, but disorders such as haemophilia are both scientifically and clinically important. Much of our current knowledge of the physiology of coagulation has been derived by studying the pathophysiology of cases of isolated coagulation factor deficiency. The two most commonly encountered inherited coagulopathies are associated with an abnormality or deficiency of the FVIII:vWF complex. Plasma FVIII and vWF normally circulate as a non-covalently bound complex. Formation of this complex is essential for the survival of FVIII in plasma. Von Willebrand's disease (vWD) is caused by a deficiency or defect of vWF, while haemophilia is caused by a deficiency or defect of FVIII.

Von Willebrand's disease

Von Willebrand's disease is the most common inherited haemorrhagic disorder, with a worldwide distribution and a particularly high incidence in the Scandinavian countries. The prevalence of vWD in the general population has been estimated to be about 1%, but it is possible that this is an underestimate since very mild cases may never be detected.

Von Willebrand's disease is an extremely heterogeneous disorder with more than 20 subtypes recognized, based on differences in the assembly and processing of vWF multimers. Broadly speaking, vWD types I and III represent a quantitative deficiency of a functionally normal vWF while type II variants represent the presence of a qualitatively abnormal vWF. Type I is the most common form of vWD, accounting for more than 70% of cases. The most common type II (dysfunctional) variant is type IIA, which accounts for about 15% of cases. Type III vWD is a severe, life-long haemorrhagic disorder which is clinically similar to severe haemophilia apart from the added complication of platelet dysfunction secondary to deficiency of vWF. Types IIC and III vWD are inherited as an autosomal recessive trait, whereas all other types are inherited in an incompletely dominant fashion.

Pathophysiology of vWD

Because vWF is involved in both primary and secondary haemostasis, the bleeding problems associated with vWD are highly heterogeneous. Severe type III vWD is associated with spontaneous bleeding into joints (haemarthrosis) and muscles (haematoma), and with severe and prolonged bleeding following trauma. Most cases of vWD, however, are relatively mild and significant bleeding problems may be absent. Where present, bleeding is usually manifest as mucous membrane bleeding including recurrent nose-bleeds (epistaxis), heavy or prolonged menstruation (menorrhagia) and easy bruising. Bleeding from coincident pathology such as

Von Willebrand's disease was first described in 1926 as an apparently inherited haemorrhagic condition in several members of a Finnish family from the Åland Islands in the Gulf of Bothnia. This new condition was readily distinguished from haemophilia by the presence of a prolonged bleeding time test. Von Willebrand suspected that the condition, which he named **pseudohaemophilia** but later came to bear his name, was a disorder of platelet function. The true nature of von Willebrand's disease has only recently been identified.

Table 18.1 *Classification of haemophilia*

FVIIIAct	Classification	Incidence	Manifestations
<0.01	Severe	40	Spontaneous haemarthroses and haematomas
0.01–0.05	Moderate	35	Bleeding after relatively minor trauma
>0.05	Mild	25	Bleeding after major trauma, e.g. surgery

duodenal ulcers may be unusually heavy and prolonged. Mild vWD is clinically similar to platelet disorders such as Bernard–Soulier disease.

Treatment of vWD

With the exception of the type III variants, vWD is a relatively mild haemorrhagic disorder and treatment is only required for post-traumatic bleeds and to cover surgery. The most common form of treatment involves the use of the vasopressin analogue DDAVP (1-desamino-8-D-argininylvasopressin) which triggers the release of vWF from the Weibel–Palade bodies of vascular endothelium. This therapy is suitable as a short-term measure only; the endothelial stores of vWF are exhaustible, following which further treatment is ineffective.

DDAVP treatment is most useful in types I and IIA vWD. It is ineffective in type III vWD and triggers acute and severe thrombocytopenia in type IIB vWD. These forms require infusion of cryoprecipitate which is rich in vWF.

Haemophilia

Haemophilia is the second most common inherited haemorrhagic disorder, occurring in all ethnic groups. The incidence of this X-linked recessive disorder in the UK is approximately 0.005%. Haemophilia is characterized by a decreased plasma concentration of functionally active FVIII. The plasma FVIII Act relates closely to the clinical severity of the condition, as shown in Table 18.1.

Genetics of haemophilia

The gene that encodes factor VIII is located on the tip of the q arm of the X chromosome. Haemophilia results from mutations of this gene and so is inherited as an X-linked recessive disorder. This mode of inheritance is associated with several clearly defined features:

- Hemizygous males express the disease.
- Heterozygous females are typically symptomless carriers.

Haemophilia has probably been recognized as a distinct disease since antiquity. The earliest written evidence of its recognition comes in the Babylonian Talmud which records a decision that the fourth-born son of a particular woman should be exempt circumcision if her first three sons had all bled to death following this ritual. This is a clear attempt to formally recognize the existence of a severe haemorrhagic disorder which is transmitted vertically to males by symptom-free carrier females.

- Homozygous females express the disease.
- The sons of a hemizygous male are normal.
- The daughters of a hemizygous male are obligate carriers.
- The sons and daughters of a carrier female have a 50% chance of inheriting the mutant gene.

Its large size and complexity have hampered characterization of the factor VIII gene and its mutations. The gene has been shown to span 186 kb, to comprise 26 exons which range in size from 69 to 3106 bp and are separated by 25 introns, and to occupy almost 0.1% of the X chromosome. The factor VIII gene appears to be highly susceptible to mutation: more than 100 different mutations have been identified, most of which are unique to an individual family. Precise characterization of genetic defects enables increased accuracy in the detection of female carriers and in antenatal diagnosis of haemophilia.

Carrier detection in haemophilia

One of the most common tasks of the haemostasis laboratory is to offer an assessment of the likelihood that an individual female is a carrier of haemophilia. Typically, such an investigation progresses through up to four phases:

- **Formal counselling** of the possible carrier prior to any laboratory investigation. Among the issues that must be explored are the possible implications of the results that might be obtained, the type of tests available for carrier detection and the possibility that the results might be inconclusive. The potential impact of any results on other family members should also be considered.
- **Family study.** The construction of as complete a family pedigree chart as possible may identify the subject as an obligate carrier, in which case no further assessment is required. Obligate carriers include daughters of confirmed haemophiliacs, mothers of at least two haemophiliac sons born at separate deliveries and mothers of one haemophiliac son where definite evidence of haemophilia in other members of the family exists. Possible carriers need further investigation. Using the pedigree chart, a probability of carrier status can be derived by examining the relationship of the subject to the closest affected family member and applying a factor of 0.5 for each vertical or horizontal step. For example, in the pedigree chart shown in Figure 18.1, the probability that the subject (III2) is a carrier is 0.5×0.5 i.e. 0.25.
- **Phenotypic assessment.** In theory, a female carrier of haemophilia should have approximately 50% of the normal plasma concentration of factor VIII. In practice, however, the range of values obtained is wide and overlaps with the normal range. However, measurement of the plasma concentrations of FVIII Act and vWFAg on a number of occasions permits the calculation of

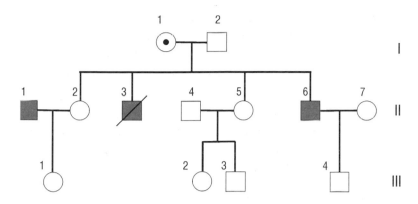

Figure 18.1 *Family study in haemophilia. I1 is an obligate carrier because she has two haemophiliac sons (one of whom (II3) is dead); II1 is an unrelated haemophiliac; II2 and II5 have a 50% chance of being carriers; III2 is the subject of the study; III4 is normal (son of a haemophiliac)*

the probability of carrier status. The probabilities obtained from the family study and the phenotypic assessment can be combined to produce a more refined assessment of the likely carrier status.

- **Genotypic assessment.** Definitive diagnosis of carrier status in most cases requires identification of the factor VIII gene mutation using DNA analysis.

Antenatal diagnosis in haemophilia

Antenatal diagnosis should only be undertaken in centres with full genetic, haematological and obstetric expertise in such matters. The steps involved in the antenatal diagnosis of haemophilia are similar to those required for carrier detection. Careful pre-investigation counselling of both parents regarding the implications and limitations of possible results is extremely important. Similarly, examination of a family pedigree chart may obviate the need for investigation.

Phenotypic assessment can be performed during the second trimester of pregnancy using direct assay of FVIII Act and FVIIIAg in foetal blood obtained directly from the umbilical cord. Genotypic assessment can be performed in the first trimester of pregnancy using foetal DNA obtained by chorion villus sampling (CVS) or, later, by amniocentesis. Some parents prefer to wait until the second trimester of pregnancy when ultrasound foetal scanning at 16–20 weeks can sex the foetus and so avoid invasive testing of a female foetus. Possible future developments for antenatal genetic diagnosis of haemophilia include screening of pre-implantation embryos as part of the *in vitro* fertilization programme and the use of foetal cells derived from the maternal circulation.

Pathophysiology of haemophilia

Primary haemostasis is normal, even in severe haemophiliacs, so bleeding from minor cuts and abrasions is seldom troublesome. More substantial tissue damage results in the formation of weak clots which are highly susceptible to mechanical or fibrinolytic

Prospective parents who are at risk of conceiving a haemophiliac son but who are unwilling to undergo antenatal diagnosis may be able to take advantage of recent developments in *in vitro* fertilization. It is now possible to sex pre-implantation conceptuses and to select only females for implantation. Using this approach, half of the children will be entirely unaffected and half will be symptom-free carriers. It is currently impossible to screen conceptuses for haemophilia.

breakdown. This explains the classical pattern of bleeding into joints and deep tissues which is delayed for some hours after trauma. Most apparently spontaneous bleeds probably result from some ill-remembered minor trauma in the preceding hours.

The most common sites of haemorrhage in haemophilia are the weight-bearing joints such as knees, elbows, ankles, shoulders, wrists and hips. In addition to bearing much of the strain of everyday movement, these joints are particularly susceptible to the knocks and bumps of everyday life. Recurrent bleeding into joint spaces is extremely painful and results in irreversible crippling joint and tissue damage. This is a major cause of illness in haemophiliacs and frequently necessitates joint replacement.

In addition to recurrent haemarthroses, severe haemophiliacs are plagued by frequent, painful bleeding episodes, which most commonly involve the large weight-bearing muscles of the thigh and calf, posterior abdominal wall and the gluteal muscles. Haematomas may take several months to resolve and frequently the affected muscle is permanently damaged with progressive contraction and loss of power.

Other common bleeding manifestations in haemophiliacs include blood in the urine (haematuria), cerebral bleeds which may be fatal, recurrent nosebleeds and gastrointestinal haemorrhage.

The pattern of bleeding in haemophilia differs according to age. If delivery is not traumatic, bleeds in the first few months of life are uncommon. However, as the child becomes mobile and increasingly adventurous, the falls and bumps that characterize this period of life frequently cause extensive traumatic bruising and haematoma formation and may result in unjust accusations of non-accidental injury. Bleeding in haemophiliacs is not faster than normal but typically continues for longer and may recur several times. For example, dental extractions may bleed intermittently for several weeks. With experience, however, the haemophiliac learns to avoid hazardous situations and to seek medical attention early, thereby limiting the damaging effects of haemorrhage. However, this 'damage reduction' is caused by alteration in behaviour, not by changes in the nature of the disease, which remains constant throughout life.

Treatment of haemophilia

Treatment of haemophilia involves the infusion of freeze-dried and heat-treated factor VIII concentrate to limit established bleeding. Prompt and early treatment is essential if secondary tissue damage is to be avoided following a bleed; so most severe haemophiliacs are taught how to administer factor VIII concentrate to themselves at home. Ancillary methods of treatment include the use of fibrinolytic inhibitors and the injection of DDAVP to stimulate the release of vWF from the vascular endothelium. Recombinant human factor VIII concentrate has recently become available and is free of the risk of viral contamination. It is very expensive, however, and is only offered to children in most centres.

Haemophilia B

Haemophilia B, also known as **Christmas disease**, results from a deficiency or defect of factor IX, occurs with a frequency of about 15–20 per 1 000 000 and is clinically indistinguishable from haemophilia. The factor IX gene spans approximately 33.5 kb of the X chromosome at the terminus of the long arm in the Xq27 region, close to the fragile X locus and the factor VIII gene. More than 50 different mutations of the factor IX gene have been characterized, including both point mutations and gross deletions.

The basic approach and underlying principles of carrier detection and treatment in haemophilia B are identical to those for haemophilia.

The possibility that haemophilia might consist of more than one defect of coagulation was first raised in 1944 when Argentinian investigators showed that the plasma of two haemophiliacs was mutually corrective. Several similar studies followed until, in 1952, Biggs *et al.* published a report of several patients with the variant form of haemophilia. Since one of the patients was called Christmas and the report appeared in the Christmas issue of the *British Medical Journal*, the name adopted for this condition almost chose itself!

Inherited thrombotic disorders

An inherited thrombotic tendency results from any alteration in the haemostatic balance that impairs the capacity of the body to combat clot formation. The two main mechanisms that oppose clot formation are the naturally occurring anticoagulants such as antithrombin III and proteins C and S and the fibrinolytic mechanism. Overall, the inherited thrombophilias are estimated to be about three times more common than the inherited bleeding disorders.

Antithrombin III deficiency

ATIII deficiency is a relatively common autosomal dominant disorder with an estimated incidence of about 0.05%. The disorder is manifest as a susceptibility to recurrent deep venous thrombosis (DVT) or pulmonary embolism which is exacerbated by pregnancy, surgery or oral contraceptive use. In the normal population, thromboembolic problems are most commonly associated with middle and old age whereas in ATIII deficient individuals, thrombotic complications typically start in the second or third decade of life. Thromboses in infancy or early childhood are uncommon in ATIII deficiency.

ATIII deficiency can be divided into two subtypes:

- **Type I deficiency** results from mutations that interfere with the rate of synthesis of ATIII and so is characterized by a relative lack of ATIII as measured by both functional and immunological assays. Typically, a thrombotic tendency results when the plasma ATIII concentration falls to less than 50–60% of normal. Up to 80% of cases of inherited ATIII deficiency are of this type.

The earliest description of antithrombin III deficiency as a cause of a thrombotic tendency was published by Egeberg in 1965. His report described a Norwegian family with an increased incidence of venous thrombosis which appeared to be associated with trauma, inflammation or pregnancy. Investigation showed that the affected individuals all had an antithrombin III level which was 50% of normal as measured by immunological and functional assays.

In 1960, Mammen, Thomas and Seegers reported the presence of an inhibitor of coagulation, which they named **autoprothrombin IIa** because they thought that it was a degradation product of thrombin. Sixteen years later, Stenflo isolated a novel vitamin K-dependent factor and named it protein C because it eluted in the third peak of a DEAE chromatographic separation. Protein C subsequently was shown to be identical to autoprothrombin IIa. The first description of an inherited protein C deficiency as the cause of a thrombotic tendency was published by Griffin et al. in 1981.

- **Type II deficiency** results from point mutations that interfere with the function of ATIII and is characterized by a lack of ATIII as measured by functional assays but a normal concentration as measured by immunological assays.

Once the presence of inherited ATIII deficiency is established, treatment typically takes one of three forms:

- Counselling about avoidable factors which are known to predispose to venous thrombosis such as obesity, venous stasis and the use of oral contraceptives which are known to lower the circulating ATIII concentration further.
- Acute thrombotic events are managed with a combination of heparin and androgenic steroids which induces a transient rise in circulating ATIII concentration. Prophylactic coumarin therapy is usually instigated as quickly as possible and may be required as a long-term measure.
- Unavoidable elective surgery can be covered by replacement therapy using specific ATIII concentrates.

Protein C

The incidence of protein C deficiency is the subject of controversy, with estimates ranging between 0.006 and 0.5%. Greater reliance can be placed on the observation that up to 8% of individuals with recurrent venous thrombosis are protein C deficient, a slightly higher incidence than that for ATIII. Protein C deficiency represents an array of genetic defects of the protein C gene which, in common with ATIII, are classified as type I (quantitative) and type II (qualitative) defects. Heterozygous protein C deficiency is typically associated with a plasma concentration between 30 and 60% of normal and is accompanied by recurrent venous thrombosis. However, an individual with homozygous protein C deficiency has recently been described who exhibited no evidence of thrombophilia, suggesting that the nature of the molecular defect and other risk factors are important determinants of disease severity.

Treatment of protein C deficiency mirrors that of ATIII deficiency. In the absence of thrombosis, counselling about the disorder and its associated problems may be all that is required. Prophylactic anticoagulant therapy is usually withheld until the first thromboembolic event, because some heterozygotes may never have a thrombosis. Surgical cover can be managed using fresh frozen plasma or specific protein C concentrate.

Protein S

Protein S is a vitamin K-dependent protein that circulates in the plasma in two forms:

- About 40% circulates as a free and haemostatically active protein.
- About 60% circulates bound to C4b-binding protein and has no recognized haemostatic activity.

The overall incidence of protein S deficiency in the general population is unknown but, in a selected thrombotic population, the incidence has been reported as between 1 and 8%. Protein S deficiency is clinically indistinguishable from protein C deficiency. About 70% of cases of protein S deficiency exhibit type I deficiency.

Factor V Leiden

Inherited resistance to activated protein C (APCR) is the most common inherited cause of thrombophilia, with an overall incidence of 2–10%. Up to 60% of Caucasians with confirmed venous thrombosis demonstrate this phenomenon. In more than 90% of cases, APCR can be attributed to a single point mutation in the factor V gene, a substitution of the arginine at position 506 by a glutamine. This mutated factor V, known as FV Leiden after the city of its discovery, is activated normally by thrombin or FX_a, but is resistant to inactivation by activated protein C, leading to a thrombotic tendency. FV Leiden is most common in populations of Caucasian origin, whereas it is not found in certain other ethnic groups such as Japanese and Chinese.

Inherited deficiency of fibrinolysis

Hypofibrinolysis may be the result of impaired plasminogen activation secondary to a variety of causes:

- Deficiency of tissue plasminogen activator synthesis or release.
- An increased concentration of plasminogen activator inhibitor.
- Deficiency of plasminogen.
- Fibrinogen abnormalities which are resistant to fibrinolysis.
- Defects within the factor XII-dependent pathway of fibrinolytic activation.

Acquired disorders of haemostasis

Acquired disorders of haemostasis are far more common than the inherited disorders described above. The acquired disorders of haemostasis are typically multifactorial and are associated with varying assortments of thrombocytopenia, platelet dysfunction, coagulation abnormalities and vascular involvement. Because of this, no attempt will be made to classify these disorders as related to one particular component of haemostasis.

Pioneering experiments designed to investigate the role of tissue damage in haemostasis were conducted during the nineteenth century and revealed apparently paradoxical findings. Rapid injection of tissue extract into animals was immediately fatal due to widespread thrombosis, while slow infusion of tissue extract prompted death due to uncontrollable haemorrhage. These results are now explicable as two facets of DIC. It was not until the 1950s that the first reports of DIC associated with human clinical conditions appeared.

Disseminated intravascular coagulation

Disseminated intravascular coagulation (DIC) is a common complication of a wide range of disorders and is characterized by the widespread activation of all of the haemostatic mechanisms. Paradoxically, although the early result of DIC is thrombosis, the most obvious feature in most cases is haemorrhage secondary to the consumption of coagulation factors and platelets. Thrombosis is manifest as the formation of occlusive microthrombi throughout the microcirculation, but especially in the kidneys, leading to widespread ischaemic damage. Bleeding manifestations typically involve the gastrointestinal tract and the sites of venepunctures, surgical wounds or indwelling catheters. Subcutaneous and deep tissue haematomas are also common. DIC may present as an acute, life-threatening thrombohaemorrhagic condition or may follow a chronic, less malevolent, course.

Pathophysiology of DIC

As shown in Table 18.2, DIC is seen in association with a wide range of conditions. The most common triggers of DIC are

Table 18.2   *Acquired conditions associated with DIC*

Obstetric complications
  Amniotic fluid embolism
  Placental abruption
  Retained dead foetus
  Eclampsia
  Septic abortion
Malignancy
  Disseminated carcinoma
  Acute leukaemia (especially M3)
Infections
  Septicaemia (especially from meningococci and other Gram-negative organisms)
  Protozoa (especially *P. falciparum malaria*)
Trauma
  Surgical (especially thoracic)
  Crush injuries (especially penetrating brain injuries)
  Burns
Liver disease
Miscellaneous
  Tissue necrosis (necrotizing enterocolitis)
  Anaphylactic shock
  Acute anoxia
  Graft rejection
  Cardiopulmonary bypass
  Acute intravascular haemolysis (e.g. ABO-incompatible blood transfusion)
  Snake bite

infection, malignancy and obstetric complications. DIC occurs in response to varying combinations of three mechanisms:

- Release of tissue factor or similar procoagulant material into the circulation stimulates activation of the coagulation cascade. This is the predominant triggering mechanism of DIC associated with obstetric complications, surgery, trauma, malignancy, transfusion reaction, liver disease, malaria, tissue rejection and some snake bites.

- Damage to vascular endothelium results in contact activation of platelets, coagulation, fibrinolysis, complement and the kinin system, and can trigger DIC in extensive burns, Gram-negative septicaemia, tissue necrosis and acute or prolonged hypoxia.

- Direct activation of platelets can occur in some forms of septicaemia or acute viral infections, in the presence of immune complexes and during cardiopulmonary bypass. Secondary platelet activation occurs in response to all forms of DIC.

Whatever the triggering event, the pathophysiology of DIC remains the same. Systemic thrombin generation triggers activation of the coagulation cascade and platelets, resulting in the deposition of microthrombi throughout the body and leading to widespread occlusion of the microcirculation. The resulting ischaemic tissue damage propagates haemostatic activation. Occlusion of the microcirculation of the brain and lungs by microthrombi may be life-threatening.

Widespread activation of platelets and coagulation rapidly and progressively lead to thrombocytopenia, a drop in the circulating levels of coagulation factors and progressive depletion of circulating antithrombin III secondary to reticuloendothelial clearance of thrombin:antithrombin complexes. Fibrin deposition and local endothelial injury trigger secondary fibrinolysis, resulting in plasmin generation and digestion of fibrinogen, factors V and VIII, and a range of other plasma proteins. Fibrin(ogen) degradation products interfere with fibrin polymerization and platelet function. To cap it all, widespread activation of the complement and kinin systems leads to an increase in vascular permeability, hypotension and shock. These secondary events in the pathogenesis of DIC explain the apparently paradoxical thrombohaemorrhagic state which typifies this condition. Once triggered, DIC can rapidly spiral out of control and result in death. The emphasis, then, must be on speed of recognition, assessment of severity and the prompt institution of effective therapy. The pathogenesis of DIC is depicted schematically in Figure 18.2.

As well as the acute and calamitous events described above, many conditions are associated with a chronic, compensated DIC. This state results from a weak, but sustained, stimulus, where the increased consumption of coagulation factors and platelets is compensated by an increase in their production. The pathophysiology of the chronic

Figure 18.2 *The pathogenesis of DIC*

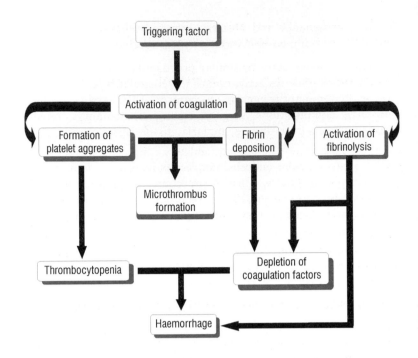

The most common cause of DIC worldwide is snake bites. The venoms of a variety of poisonous snakes act by inducing disseminated activation of coagulation. Ironically, many of these venoms have proven to be useful in the investigation of defects of coagulation. Some of these known associations are listed below:

- **X activation** by *Vipera russeli*.

- **Prothrombin activation** by *Oxyuranus scutellatus*, *Echis carinatus* and *Notechis scutatus*.

- **Fibrinogen activation** by *Bothrops atrox*, *Agkistrodon rhodostoma*, *Crotalus adamanteus* and *Agkistrodon contrortix*.

- **Fibrinogenolysin** by *Crotalus atrox*.

- **Platelet activation** by *Bothrops jararaca*.

condition is identical to that of acute DIC. Conditions associated with chronic DIC include intrauterine death, leukaemia, disseminated carcinoma, graft rejection and vasculitis.

Treatment and management of DIC

Many aspects of the treatment of DIC are highly controversial, partly because the complexity and heterogeneity of the pathophysiology of this disorder make rational treatment selection and objective assessment of effectiveness very difficult. The primary aims of treatment are to eliminate the triggering mechanism for the DIC as quickly and as completely as possible and to maintain life in the meantime by replacement therapy and, in some cases, anticoagulant therapy. Replacement therapy typically involves the administration of large quantities of fresh frozen plasma and cryoprecipitate, which are valuable sources of coagulation factors and natural anticoagulants, platelet concentrates, red cell concentrates and volume expanders such as human albumin solution.

The administration of an anticoagulant such as heparin to a bleeding patient whose blood is apparently incoagulable may seem paradoxical. The rationale for this manoeuvre is that interruption of coagulation should also slow consumption of platelets and secondary fibrinolysis and permit restoration of haemostatic function. This approach is clearly effective in cases of chronic DIC. Its efficacy is much less certain in acute DIC, however, particularly where septicaemia is involved. In certain cases of severe DIC where standard replacement therapy has proved ineffective, the use of antithrombin III concentrates may be successful.

Haemostatic disorders associated with malignancy

Disturbances of haemostatic function secondary to malignant conditions are both common and diverse but the most common is DIC. Expression of tissue factor by renal, gastric and colonic tumours commonly causes a thrombotic tendency. The monoclonal immunoglobulins that characterize multiple myeloma coat both platelets and coagulation factors, thereby preventing normal function and increasing their rate of clearance. The increased blood viscosity and restricted mobility associated with myeloma also contributes to an increased thrombotic risk. Defective platelet function is common in many haematological malignancies. Prostatic tumours have been shown to promote local fibrinolytic activity.

Haemostatic disorders associated with liver disease

The liver is the site of synthesis of most of the coagulation factors and natural anticoagulants, although factor VIII appears to be synthesized independently of the others. Acute hepatocellular failure is associated with failure of synthesis of coagulation factors and with an increased incidence of DIC and primary fibrinolysis. In the absence of DIC, the levels of circulating coagulation factors, particularly factor V, correlate well with the severity of the hepatocellular damage. The vitamin K-dependent proteins II, VII, IX, X, protein C and protein S are all reduced in concentration due to a combination of decreased synthesis and impaired γ-carboxylation. Synthesis of dysfunctional coagulation factors may also be present. Thrombocytopenia is a common finding in liver disease and may be associated with DIC or hypersplenism. Defects of platelet function are also relatively common.

Chronic liver disease is associated with thrombocytopenia, platelet dysfunction, failure of synthesis of coagulation factors, dysfibrinogenaemia and increased fibrinolytic activity. In general, the severity of the haemostatic disturbance reflects the severity of the liver disease.

Obstructive jaundice causes impairment of the vitamin K-dependent carboxylation of γ-glutamic acid residues on coagulation factors II, VII, IX, X, protein C and protein S. All other haemostatic proteins are typically normal or elevated. The presence of circulating PIVKAs is one of the earliest and most sensitive markers of hepatic failure.

Pregnancy and delivery

Normal, uncomplicated pregnancy is associated with considerable changes in haemostatic function. Most women experience a progressive rise in the concentration of fibrinogen, factor VIII and vWF and a fall in the level of protein S and fibrinolytic activity. The mild hypercoagulable state which results is probably a normal physiological preparation for the rigours of delivery and placental separation.

DIC is a common complication of a number of obstetric disorders such as *abruptio placentae*, amniotic fluid embolism, retained dead foetus, septic abortion and eclampsia.

- **Abruptio placentae** is the premature separation of the placenta from the wall of the uterus. The placenta is a rich source of tissue factor. In most cases, evacuation of the uterus results in rapid resolution of the DIC, without the need for massive replacement therapy. The most serious complications of this condition relate to shock, renal failure and thromboembolism.

- **Amniotic fluid embolism** occurs when a small amount of amniotic fluid is forced into the maternal circulation and presents as an acute and severe DIC with profound respiratory distress secondary to thrombotic occlusion of the pulmonary microcirculation, and uterine haemorrhage. Treatment options include massive replacement therapy and the administration of heparin or the fibrinolytic inhibitor ε-aminocaproic acid (EACA). The mortality rate of this complication is in excess of 80%.

- **Retained dead foetus** causes a chronic, compensated DIC with a gradual and progressive drop in the platelet count and a rise in the level of circulating fibrin(ogen) degradation products (FDP). Significant bleeding is typically absent but the danger of rapid acceleration to acute DIC is present.

- **Septic abortion**. Because of the mild hypercoagulable state which accompanies pregnancy, any severe infective complication such as septic abortion threatens to trigger acute DIC with shock and acute renal failure.

- **Eclampsia** describes a curious syndrome of pregnancy which is characterized by progressive hypertension, a raised blood urate level secondary to renal impairment, proteinuria, convulsions and chronic, compensated DIC. Occasionally, a hitherto relatively stable case may accelerate abruptly into acute DIC with Haemolysis, Elevated Liver enzymes and Low Platelets, a condition known as the **HELLP syndrome**. This clinical emergency threatens the life of both mother and baby and requires massive replacement therapy and rapid delivery.

The neonatal period

Most normal neonates show some degree of haemostatic impairment at delivery, secondary to hepatic immaturity and vitamin K deficiency. The first weeks of life are the most critical time for haemorrhage due to hereditary and acquired coagulopathies. At full term, the vitamin K-dependent factors II, VII, IX and X are at around only 40% of adult levels and fall further during the first 5 days of life. The circulating fibrinogen level is typically normal but there may be a significant proportion of the foetal variant of fibrinogen, which shows delayed aggregation of fibrin monomers.

Haemorrhagic disease of the newborn

Haemorrhagic disease of the newborn describes an acquired bleeding tendency, sometimes severe, which develops in the first days of life and is secondary to deficiency of the vitamin K-dependent coagulation factors. In the absence of supplementation, vitamin K deficiency can be expected to develop in about half of normal full-term babies because of low body stores at birth and the inadequacy of the dietary supply of this vitamin. Powdered baby milk is supplemented with vitamin K during manufacture and so provides a better dietary source than breast milk. It is standard practice to administer vitamin K to all neonates within 24 h of birth. Serious haemorrhagic disease of the newborn is rarely encountered following adequate vitamin K prophylaxis. Treatment consists of the administration of vitamin K_1 and replacement therapy using fresh frozen plasma.

A variant of haemorrhagic disease of the newborn occurs in premature babies secondary to hepatic immaturity, with failure of production of coagulation factors and consequent poor utilization of vitamin K. In these circumstances, vitamin K treatment is ineffective.

Disseminated intravascular coagulation

Neonatal disseminated intravascular coagulation may be triggered by birth asphyxia, respiratory distress syndrome, trauma, viral or bacterial infection, aspiration of meconium and amniotic fluid or hypothermia. Hepatic immaturity or liver disease may further exacerbate this condition. The pathophysiology of the condition is identical to that seen in adults.

Platelet disorders

The most common acquired abnormality of platelets in neonates is thrombocytopenia, which may be secondary to a variety of conditions including DIC, transplacental passage of maternal antiplatelet antibodies, congenital cyanotic heart disease, giant haemangioma and following exchange transfusion. Neonatal platelet dysfunction may be seen following antibiotic or other drug therapy.

Plasma concentrations of coagulation factors in neonates differ significantly from those in adults. A normal full-term infant attains adult levels by the age of 3 months. Normal neonate levels are as follows (as a percentage of adult levels):

II	30–40%
VII	10–45%
IX	10–15%
X	10–30%
XI	20–80%

In addition, ATIII is raised and fibrinolytic activity depressed.

Acquired purpuras

The acquired purpuras are a group of disorders of primary haemostasis which are manifest as mucous membrane bleeding and a tendency to bruise spontaneously or following minimal trauma. They can be divided into the vascular purpuras and the platelet-associated purpuras, depending on which component is most affected. In most cases, however, the pathogenesis of the purpura is complex and multifactorial.

Vascular purpuras

Henoch-Schönlein purpura (HSP), or allergic purpura, is a self-limited allergic vasculitis which is seen most commonly in young children and is manifest as a purpuric rash covering the arms, legs and buttocks, with renal impairment and abdominal and joint pain. Typically, a recent history of upper respiratory tract infection or of penicillin or sulphonamide therapy is present. HSP appears to be caused by IgA immune complex-mediated vascular endothelial damage.

The most common vascular purpura, senile purpura, is a benign condition of old age which is caused by a combination of loss of skin elasticity and atrophy of vascular collagen. The condition is manifest as persistent purplish patches on the backs of the hands, forearms and neck that appear spontaneously and leave permanent brown stains when they fade. About 40% of elderly people display this natural phenomenon for which no treatment is required or available.

The apparent excess of easy bruising seen in young women, for which no cause can be found, is known by the spuriously scientific title of purpura simplex. In cases of excessive bruising, for which no cause can be found, the possibility of self-mutilation secondary to psychiatric disturbance or physical abuse by carers must be considered.

Severe, prolonged vitamin C deficiency, or scurvy, is associated with defects of collagen and a bleeding tendency. Scurvy is associated with chronic malnourishment and, in the developed world, is most commonly seen in alcoholics, the elderly and the poor.

Thrombocytopenic purpuras

Thrombocytopenia is the most common acquired platelet abnormality and can result from three main causes:

- Failure of thrombopoiesis (e.g. hypoplastic anaemia, severe vitamin B_{12} or folate deficiency).
- Accelerated consumption or destruction of platelets (e.g. immune

thrombocytopenic purpura, thrombotic thrombocytopenic purpura and haemolytic uraemic syndrome).

- Splenic sequestration of platelets due to hypersplenism or splenomegaly.

Immune thrombocytopenic purpura (ITP) is characterized by antibody-mediated destruction of platelets with thrombocytopenia, extensive petechiae, bruising and mucosal haemorrhagic complications such as epistaxis and menorrhagia. The white cell count, differential count and haemoglobin concentration are typically all normal. Examination of the bone marrow reveals megakaryocytic hyperplasia with an increase in immature, hypolobulated forms. Three forms of immune thrombocytopenic purpura are recognized:

- An acute, self-limited form which is most common in children between the ages of 2 and 6 years and is often preceded by an acute viral illness such as rubella, measles or chickenpox.

- A chronic form with an insidious onset and no history of recent viral illness. This form is most common in young adults and seldom remits spontaneously.

- A self-limited neonatal form which is associated with the passive transplacental transfer of maternal anti-platelet antibodies.

In all forms of ITP, platelet destruction is mediated by the presence of platelet-bound immunoglobulin with subsequent Fc receptor-mediated phagocytosis by splenic macrophages.

Thrombotic thrombocytopenic purpura (TTP) is a rare but clinically serious disorder which most commonly affects young adults and is characterized by fever, erratic neurological disturbances such as convulsions, hallucinations and paralysis, renal failure, microangiopathic haemolysis and thrombocytopenia with haemorrhagic manifestations. The haemolysis and thrombocytopenia are secondary to the disseminated deposition of platelet-fibrin microthrombi in arterioles and capillaries. The trigger for the formation of these thrombotic lesions is unknown. It is increased platelet aggregation and consumption, rather than coagulation factor depletion, that is the major cause of morbidity and mortality in this condition. TTP has been described secondary to a variety of conditions including pregnancy, bacterial infection, autoimmune disease, neoplasia and drug ingestion.

The treatment for TTP involves intensive supportive care such as haemodialysis, artificial ventilation, plasmapheresis and transfusion of fresh frozen plasma. The administration of anticoagulants such as heparin or anti-platelet drugs is of dubious benefit. The mortality rate of TTP is about 50%.

A closely related condition, haemolytic uraemic syndrome (HUS), most commonly affects infants and young children and is associated with the localized deposition of platelet-fibrin microthrombi in the renal vasculature with thrombocytopenia, microangiopathic haemolysis and renal failure. In many cases, there is a recent

Acquired thrombocytopathies are seen most commonly in association with drug ingestion (e.g. aspirin), uraemia or grossly elevated FDPs. However, ingestion of certain foods has been shown to impair platelet function and, occasionally, may be troublesome. Many of the culinary culprits are associated with Chinese cooking, e.g. garlic, ginger and black tree fungus.

Recombinant factor VIIa has been used successfully to treat more than 50 patients with inhibitors to factor VIII or IX. Included in this group were both haemophiliacs with inhibitors induced by treatment and non-haemophiliacs with spontaneously acquired inhibitors. This form of treatment shows promise as an alternative approach to the treatment of this clinically challenging group of patients.

history of bacterial infection. HUS is triggered by immune-mediated damage to vascular endothelium.

Acquired inhibitors of coagulation factors

Antibodies directed against coagulation factors may arise following replacement therapy for deficiency states such as haemophilia or as spontaneous events. The most common inhibitors are directed against factor VIII or IX following treatment. Spontaneous inhibitors also most commonly affect factor VIII but rare instances of inhibitors directed against many other coagulation factors have been reported.

In 5–10% of haemophilia patients an IgG antibody is produced which is directed against factor VIII. Once the inhibitor is formed, further factor VIII infusion acts as an antigenic stimulus, markedly increasing the concentration of the inhibitor. The incidence of inhibitor production is highest in severe haemophiliacs. Factor VIII inhibitors can also occur spontaneously in non-haemophiliacs in association with pregnancy, autoimmune conditions such as rheumatoid arthritis and systemic lupus erythematosus (SLE), and in the elderly, sometimes in the absence of obvious predisposing factors. Males and females have an equal tendency to inhibitor production.

The presence of an acquired inhibitor triggers a progressive and complete destruction of the target coagulation factor, leading to clinical consequences similar to those of severe haemophilia. The long-term treatment of coagulation factor inhibitors is fraught with difficulty but treatment options include the use of immunosuppressive drugs, or attempting to induce immune tolerance using long-term continuous infusion of the affected coagulation factor.

Acquired thrombophilia

Thromboembolic disease is a major cause of morbidity and mortality in developed countries, rivalling malignancy as the most important cause of non-accidental death.

Arterial thrombosis

Thromboembolic events within the arterial circulation are usually secondary to vascular endothelial injury. For example, rupture of a pre-existing atheromatous plaque in a coronary artery prompts localized formation of an occlusive thrombus, leading to oxygen starvation of the left ventricle of the heart and acute myocardial infarction. Similar episodes involving the cerebral circulation result in **transient ischaemic attacks** or **thrombotic stroke**. Myocardial infarction presents as crushing tightness of the chest with sweating, nausea, breathlessness and collapse. The chest pain frequently radiates to the arms, throat and jaw. Transient ischaemic attacks are accompanied by fleeting neurological dysfunction or loss of vision. Completed thrombotic stroke is accompanied by similar symptoms which persist for more than 24 h and may be severely and permanently disabling.

Venous thrombosis

The most common thromboembolic event is a **deep vein thrombosis** of the lower limbs. The main site for this thrombus formation is within a valve pocket where there is maximum stasis and vortex-type blood flow. Vascular endothelial damage is usually absent. A venous thrombus may become dislodged, forming a circulating **embolus** which may lodge in the pulmonary microcirculation resulting in a **pulmonary embolism**. Venous thrombosis typically presents with pain, swelling, discolouration and warmth in the affected area. However, symptoms may be absent and none of these symptoms are specific for this condition. Pulmonary embolism presents as acute chest pain and breathlessness with shock, cough and haemoptysis and may be rapidly fatal.

Risk factors for arterial and venous thrombosis

A number of risk factors have been identified that are associated with an increased incidence of thromboembolic disease, as shown in Table 18.3.

The anti-phospholipid syndrome

The anti-phospholipid syndrome (APS) is caused by the spontaneous production of antibodies that are directed against anionic phospholipids. This is manifest *in vitro* as prolongation of phospholipid-dependent coagulation screening tests, which is usually

Table 18.3 *Risk factors for arterial and venous thrombosis*

Venous thrombosis	Arterial thrombosis
Increasing age	Increasing age
Obesity	Obesity
Immobility	Lack of exercise
Pregnancy (post-partum)	High saturated fat, low fibre diet
Oral contraceptive use	Smoking
Malignancy	Stress
Anti-phospholipid syndrome	Hyperlipidaemia
Postoperative period	Hypertension
Polycythaemia	Polycythaemia
Homocystinaemia	Elevated factor VII concentration
Diabetes mellitus	Elevated fibrinogen concentration
Gout	Probable genetic factors

indicative of a bleeding tendency. However, these antibodies are seldom associated with a thrombotic tendency *in vivo*. The anti-phospholipid antibodies that characterize the APS are sometimes known as **lupus anticoagulants**.

Screening for APS should be considered in patients with SLE, unexplained recurrent thromboses, a thrombosis before the age of 40 years or women with a recurrent foetal loss in the first and second trimester of pregnancy. The condition also occurs occasionally in otherwise healthy individuals and may be detected as a chance finding as part of routine pre-operative screening.

Prophylaxis and treatment of thrombosis

Anti-platelet drugs

The deposition of platelets at sites of arterial vascular endothelial damage is an important step in the pathogenesis of arterial thrombosis. The prophylactic administration of anti-platelet drugs such as **aspirin (acetylsalicylic acid)** has been shown to be effective in reducing the rate of reinfarction in myocardial infarction survivors. The major risk associated with any form of anti-thrombotic therapy is that of inducing haemorrhagic complications. Several large clinical trials have shown that the daily administration of 50–300 mg of aspirin retains the anti-thrombotic effect while minimizing the risk of haemorrhagic complications.

Oral anticoagulants

Oral anticoagulants are suitable for self-administration and so can be used outside of the hospital setting. The most widely prescribed oral anticoagulants, including **warfarin,** are coumarin analogues which act by inhibiting the normal recycling of vitamin K within hepatocytes, thereby preventing the γ-carboxylation of the terminal glutamate residues of the vitamin K-dependent coagulation factors. Because the action of warfarin relies on the inhibition of the synthesis of new coagulation factors, its anticoagulant effect is not fully expressed for about 3 days after the commencement of therapy. The required degree of anticoagulation is typically maintained by heparin therapy during this period. Therapeutic anticoagulation requires the induction of a controlled coagulopathy and is therefore fraught with dangers. Successful therapy involves treading the fine line between haemorrhagic and prothrombotic states. It is essential that the required degree of anticoagulation is established early and is subsequently closely controlled.

Heparin

Heparin is a mucopolysaccharide which is purified for clinical use from bovine lung or porcine intestine. It cannot be absorbed from

The search for new anti-thrombotic agents with improved safety and clinical effectiveness is relentless. Several new anticoagulants have been developed which show early promise and are currently undergoing clinical trials to assess their efficacy and safety. Among these is **hirudin**, a direct inhibitor of thrombin which was originally extracted from the medicinal leech but is now available in recombinant form. Hirudin has been shown to inhibit fibrin-bound thrombin more effectively than heparin:ATIII complexes and may prove to be a suitable alternative to heparin therapy.

the intestine and must therefore be administered intravenously or subcutaneously. The anticoagulant effect of heparin is instantaneous, making it the treatment of choice for acute thrombotic episodes. Heparin exerts its anticoagulant effect by binding to ATIII and potentiating its action against thrombin, Xa and other activated serine proteases.

For the treatment of established thrombosis, high-dose heparin is administered by continuous intravenous infusion. The short *in vivo* half-life of heparin (about 1 h) facilitates fine adjustment of the anticoagulant effect. Intravenous heparin therapy is associated with a severe risk of haemorrhage, which may be exacerbated by the induction of heparin-dependent thrombocytopenia.

Low doses of heparin administered subcutaneously have been shown to offer effective postoperative prophylaxis. The incidence of significant bleeding problems is much lower than for intravenous heparin therapy, although the risk of thrombocytopenia persists.

Thrombolytic drugs

Therapeutic anticoagulants are effective prophylactic anti-thrombotic agents and can prevent propagation of an established thrombus. However, they do not promote lysis of thrombi. This is the role of the thrombolytic agents such as streptokinase (SK) and tissue plasminogen activator (t-PA).

SK is synthesized by β-haemolytic streptococci and activates both free and fibrin-bound plasminogen *in vivo* to release plasmin. The resultant systemic fibrinolysis shows no specificity for the site of the thrombus and so induces a profound hypocoagulable state which is accompanied by a severe risk of bleeding. SK therapy is associated with a highly significant reduction in morbidity due to ischaemic muscle damage and reinfarction in acute myocardial infarction. The *in vivo* half-life of SK is less than 10 min. The repeated use of SK is limited by its immunogenicity and its tendency to induce febrile reactions.

Recombinant human t-PA is highly fibrin-specific and so exerts its lytic action directly on the formed thrombi and does not induce systemic fibrinolysis. Although t-PA is fibrin-specific, it is not thrombus-specific. Digestion of multiple small haemostatic plugs, which form part of the normal defence against wear and tear, may result in serious haemorrhage. Overall, the incidence of haemorrhagic complications during t-PA therapy is similar to that for SK therapy. The *in vivo* half-life of t-PA is less than 10 min.

Suggested further reading

Bick, R.L. (1996). Disseminated intravascular coagulation: Objective clinical and laboratory diagnosis, treatment, and assessment of therapeutic response. *Seminars in Thrombosis and Hemostasis* **22**(1), 69–88.

Bick, R.L. and Kaplan, H. (1998). Syndromes of thrombosis and hypercoagulability – Congenital and acquired causes of thrombosis. *Medical Clinics of North America* **82**(3), 409–460.

Boltonmaggs, P.H.B. and Hill, F.G.H. (1995). The rarer inherited coagulation disorders – a review. *Blood Reviews* **9**(2), 65–76.

Green, P. M., Naylor, J.A. and Giannelli, F. (1995). The hemophilias. *Advances in Genetics* **32**, 99–139.

Hillarp, A., Dahlback, B. and Zoller, B. (1995). Activated protein C resistance: From phenotype to genotype and clinical practice. *Blood Reviews* **9**(4), 201–212.

Lethagen, S.R. (1995). Pathogenesis, clinical picture and treatment of von Willebrand's disease. *Annals of Medicine* **27**(6), 641–651.

Self-assessment questions

1. Which of the following are inherited haemorrhagic disorders:
   (a) Bernard–Soulier syndrome;
   (b) Ehlers–Danlos syndrome;
   (c) thrombotic thrombocytopenic purpura;
   (d) pseudo von Willebrand's disease;
   (e) protein S deficiency;
   (f) Henoch-Schönlein purpura?
2. Why is the pattern of bleeding seen in von Willebrand's disease different to that in haemophilia?
3. Name three inherited disorders of platelet function.
4. Define the term obligate carrier of haemophilia.
5. What is the most common inherited thrombotic disorder?
6. Differentiate between type I and type II deficiency of antithrombin III.
7. List three obstetric triggers of disseminated intravascular coagulation.
8. What is the mechanism of action of:
   (a) warfarin;
   (b) heparin?

Key Concepts and Facts

- A haemorrhagic diathesis results from an alteration in the haemostatic balance that either impairs clot-promoting activities or potentiates clot-inhibiting activities.

- Inherited vasculopathies include hereditary haemorrhagic telangiectasia (HHT) and Ehlers–Danlos syndrome.

- Inherited thrombocytopathies include Bernard–Soulier disease, pseudo von Willebrand's disease, Glanzmann's thrombasthenia and storage pool disease.

- The clinical manifestations of thrombocytopathies include easy bruising, petechial rash, mucous membrane bleeding and excessive bleeding following minor trauma.

- The two most common inherited coagulopathies are von Willebrand's disease and haemophilia.

- Von Willebrand's disease (vWD) is caused by a deficiency or defect of vWF, while haemophilia is caused by a deficiency or defect of FVIII.

- The most common form of vWD (type I) is inherited as an autosomal dominant disorder, while haemophilia is an X-linked recessive disorder.

- Because vWF is involved in both primary and secondary haemostasis, the bleeding problems associated with vWD are highly heterogeneous.

- Primary haemostasis is normal, even in severe haemophiliacs. Bleeding results in the formation of structurally weak clots which are easily disrupted.

- The inherited thrombophilias are about three times more common than the inherited coagulopathies.

- Inherited thrombophilias include FV Leiden, deficiency of proteins C, S and ATIII and hypofibrinolysis.

- Acquired disorders of haemostasis are far more common than inherited disorders and are typically multifactorial.

- DIC is an acquired thrombohaemorrhagic condition and is characterized by widespread activation of all the haemostatic mechanisms.

- The most common triggers of DIC are infection, malignancy and obstetric complications.

- Other common acquired haemorrhagic disorders include haemorrhagic disease of the newborn, the vascular purpuras and the thrombocytopenic purpuras.

Answers to Self-Assessment Questions

Chapter 1

1. Red bone marrow is haemopoietically active and, in adults, is found mainly in the pelvis, vertebrae and sternum. Yellow marrow occupies the remaining marrow space and is inactive but can readily be recruited into its active counterpart during periods of increased demand for blood cells.
2. CFU-GEMM, myeloblast, promyelocyte, myelocyte.
3. T_H lymphocyte.
4. Chronic renal failure is associated with failure of erythropoietin synthesis and so failure of the feedback mechanism that senses tissue hypoxia and increases the rate of erythropoiesis.
5. Monocyte, lymphocyte, neutrophil, platelet, erythrocyte.

Chapter 2

1. Iron is absorbed maximally from the duodenum and upper jejunum. Vitamin B_{12} is absorbed optimally in the terminal ileum. Folates are absorbed maximally from the upper jejunum.
2. Ascorbic acid enhances inorganic iron absorption by favouring the reduced Fe^{2+} form.
3. Iron is stored mainly in the liver, tissue macrophages and bone marrow. Vitamin B_{12} and folate are stored mainly in the liver.
4. Because iron is an essential component of haemoglobin, iron deficiency is associated with anaemia with a consequent reduction in exercise tolerance.
5. The stomach plays a central role in iron and vitamin B_{12} absorption and so its surgical removal would predispose strongly to deficiency of these haematinics. The effect on folate absorption would be minimal.
6. In the absence of methylcobalamin, folate cannot be converted to a metabolically active form, resulting in a *functional* deficiency of folate and retarded DNA synthesis.

Chapter 3

1. Negative iron balance occurs when the rate of iron absorption is

insufficient to meet daily requirements. Latent iron deficiency describes a state of depleted iron stores but normal erythropoiesis. Iron deficient erythropoiesis describes the state where the red cells produced are microcytic and hypochromic but the haemoglobin level is still normal. Iron deficiency anaemia describes the state where the red cells produced are microcytic and hypochromic and the haemoglobin level is low.

2. The iron requirement is increased during growth and pregnancy, where there is chronic loss of blood or where there is loss of iron from the body.

3. Microcytosis, hypochromasia, reduced MCHC, increased free intracellular protoporphyrin.

4. In iron deficiency, haemoglobin synthesis is retarded and an extra mitotic division occurs before the erythroblast nucleus is poisoned by the increasing concentration of haemoglobin, resulting in a mature red cell that is smaller than normal.

5. Idiopathic sideroblastic anaemia is now known as myelodysplastic syndrome refractory anaemia with ring sideroblasts (RARS).

6. Haemochromatosis is a hereditary condition in which feedback control over the rate of absorption of dietary iron is lost. Haemosiderosis is secondary to chronic blood transfusion.

Chapter 4

1. Although the requirement for vitamin B_{12} is increased during pregnancy, the excess demand is insufficient to exhaust normal body stores in the 40 weeks of a normal pregnancy.

2. Normal folate body stores are sufficient to last for about 12 weeks whereas the increased demands that accompany pregnancy last for 40 weeks.

3. The folate content of an individual red cell is determined by the availability of this vitamin during its production. Thus, a sample of blood will contain red cells aged between 1 and 120 days old and provides an estimate of folate status averaged over this period of time. Serum folate estimation measures the concentration of folate in the blood at the time of venepuncture and is subject to relatively wide fluctuation.

4. Which of the following statements are true?
   (a) False.
   (b) True, although the rate of DNA synthesis is retarded to a greater extent.
   (c) True.
   (d) False.

5. The conversion of homocysteine to methionine requires methylcobalamin as a coenzyme. In vitamin B_{12} deficiency, this reaction is impaired and homocysteine accumulates.

6. Deficiency of vitamin B_{12} and folate results in an accumulation

of dUTP relative to dTTP and misincorporation of uracil into DNA instead of thymine. Suboptimal repair of this defect leads to fragmentation of the helical structure, impaired mitosis and premature cell death.

Chapter 5

1. The combination of glycine and succinyl Co-A to produce δ-aminolaevulinic acid.
2. The first and last two steps occur within the mitochondria. The intervening steps occur within the red cell cytoplasm.
3. Hb Gower 1 $(\zeta\varepsilon)_2$, Hb Portland $(\zeta\gamma)_2$ and haemoglobin Gower 2 $(\alpha\varepsilon)_2$.
4. Contact with water would result in oxidation of the central Fe^{2+} in haem to Fe^{3+} with consequent loss of function.
5. The normal alveolar pO_2 is 100 mmHg.
6. Anaemia results in decreased oxygen carrying capacity of the blood. The immediate physiological responses of the body to tissue hypoxia during exertion are to increase cardiac output and to increase oxygen intake by panting.
7. The slightly pink tinge of Caucasian skin and the red of mucous mebranes is a reflection of haemoglobin concentration.

Chapter 6

1. No. The contribution of δ globin to total globin synthesis is low, so that an absence of this molecule would be readily compensated.
2. As a reduced concentration of HbF and anaemia. As the rate of synthesis of β globin increases during the first months of life, the severity of the condition would diminish markedly.
3. The predominant form of α thalassaemia in American blacks is α^+ thalassaemia, which means that homozygous α° thalassaemia is rare.
4. The two conditions would tend to moderate each other because the result of a reduction in α globin synthesis on an individual with impaired β globin synthesis would be to bring the two synthetic rates closer to equality.
5. The bluish discolouration of the skin seen in cyanosis is caused by an increase in the concentration of deoxyhaemoglobin in the peripheral circulation. The haemoglobins M are associated with formation of methaemoglobin which exists in the deoxy form.
6. A reduction in atmospheric oxygen pressure (pO_2) would decrease the haemoglobin oxygen uptake and might trigger a sickling crisis.

Chapter 7

1. Which of the following statements are true?
   (a) False.
   (b) False.
   (c) False.
   (d) False.
   (e) False.
   (f) True.
   (g) True.
   (h) False.
2. There are three possible candidates: Phil, Glynn and Malcolm.

Chapter 8

1. A haemolytic disorder is any condition that leads to a reduction in the mean lifespan of the red cell. Haemolytic anaemias occur when the increased demand for replacement red cells secondary to haemolysis exceeds supply and anaemia ensues. A haemolytic disorder in which the anaemia is due primarily to a cause other than haemolysis is said to have a haemolytic component.
2. The major site of haemolysis in HS is the spleen. Splenectomy therefore minimizes haemolysis and leads to a reduction in spherocytosis but does not affect the intrinsic red cell defect that defines HS.
3. Common HE, HE with infantile poikilocytosis, HE with spherocytosis and HE with stomatocytosis.
4. HX is characterized by excessive leakage of K^+ from the cell, leading to progressive water depletion.
5. Haemolysis in PCH is biphasic. Exposure to cold triggers D–L antibody binding to red cells in the peripheral circulation but no haemolysis. Subsequent warming allows rapid complement-mediated intravascular haemolysis to occur, resulting in haemoglobinuria.
6. Pregnancy and birth cause foetal red cells to be transferred to the maternal circulation. If these are Rh positive, they may stimulate maternal antibody formation, which may prove troublesome in subsequent pregnancies. Administration of anti-D immediately following delivery is intended to trigger destruction of any Rh positive foetal red cells which may be present, thereby preventing maternal immunization.
7. Penicillin-type immune haemolysis is triggered by non-specific binding of the drug to the red cell surface, stimulation of IgG anti-drug antibodies and selective removal of affected cells by the spleen. Some patients on α-methyldopa, levodopa or mefenamic acid therapy produce a warm-reactive autoantibody, often with Rh specificity, which triggers binding to red cells and triggers their destruction. Innocent bystander haemolysis occurs when the drug triggers the formation of anti-drug

antibodies, which form large immune complexes. These are adsorbed onto the red cell surface, triggering complement-mediated intravascular haemolysis.

Chapter 9

1. Mature red cells have no nucleus or mitochondria and so cannot synthesize protein and are dependent upon anaerobic glycolysis for energy production and the hexose monophosphate pathway for protection against oxidative stress.
2. Oxidative phosphorylation occurs within mitochondria.
3. The conversion of ATP to ADP.
4. Three main processes within red cells are energy-dependent: the cation pump, which maintains intracellular cation balance; maintenance of cell shape and deformability; and the phosphorylation of glucose and fructose-6-phosphate.
5. 2,3-DPG binds avidly to β globin, but not to other non-α globins. Haemoglobins which lack β globin chains, such as haemoglobin F $(\alpha\gamma)_2$ therefore have a higher oxygen affinity than haemoglobin A in the presence of 2,3-DPG. The increased oxygen affinity of haemoglobin F confers its ability to extract oxygen from maternal haemoglobin A at the placental barrier.
6. Reducing power is required to combat membrane lipid oxidation, to maintain haem iron in the Fe^{2+} state and to detoxify reactive oxygen species.

Chapter 10

1. The most common defect of the EM pathway is pyruvate kinase deiciency. The most common defect of the HM pathway is G-6-PD deficiency.
2. Pyruvate kinase deficiency is moderated by an accumulation of 2,3-DPG, which acts to increase oxygen delivery to the tissues.
3. G-6-PD deficiency results from structurally abnormal enzyme variants that have impaired stability or catalytic activity. More than 350 different G-6-PD variants have been described. The variety of molecular abnormalities is reflected in clinical heterogeneity.
4. Gd^B is present in 99% of Caucasians and in about 70% of blacks. Gd^A is found in about 20% of blacks.
5. Ingestion of oxidant drugs, ingestion of fava beans and infection.
6. Favism describes extreme sensitivity to fava beans as a trigger of acute haemolysis. This condition is associated particularly with Gd^{MED}.

Chapter 11

1. Any two from each of the following:
    (a) Acute leukaemias: acute lymphoblastic and acute non-lymphoblastic leukaemias.
    (b) Chronic leukaemias: chronic lymphocytic, prolymphocytic, hairy cell and chronic myeloid leukaemias.
    (c) Myelodysplastic syndromes: refractory anaemia, refractory anaemia with ring sideroblasts, refractory anaemia with excess of blasts, refractory anaemia with excess of blasts in transformation and chronic myelomonocytic leukaemia.
    (d) Non-leukaemic lymphoproliferative disorders: multiple myeloma, Hodgkin s disease and the non-Hodgkin s lymphomas.
    (e) Non-leukaemic myeloproliferative disorders: primary proliferative polycythaemia, primary thrombocythaemia and myelofibrosis.
2. Descriptive studies involve surveys of defined populations to determine the incidence of a given disease and to investigate factors such as age, sex, race, occupation and socio-economic status, which may influence disease incidence. Analytical studies investigate evidence of apparent causal relationships.
3. Acute lymphoblastic leukaemia has a peak incidence in the children of the developed world. The occurrence of multiple myeloma is almost restricted to the elderly.
4. The increased incidence of CML, ALL, ANLL and MM in Hiroshima and Nagasaki after the explosion of nuclear weapons provides the best evidence of the leukaemogenic potential of high dose ionizing radiation.
5. HTLV-I.
6. A proto-oncogene is a normal gene which regulates cell growth and division. An oncogene is a mutated form which promotes dysregulated growth and division and may contribute to malignant transformation.

Chapter 12

1. (a) M3.
    (b) M5a.
    (c) L3.
2. (a) TALL.
    (b) Pre-BALL.
    (c) M6.
    (d) M3.
3. An allogeneic graft uses marrow from a donor. An autologous graft uses marrow from the host.
4. Graft versus host disease occurs when immunocompetent cells in transplanted marrow attack normal host antigens, e.g. skin, liver and gut. The graft versus leukaemia effect describes the

reduction in the risk of leukaemic relapse consequent upon immunocompetent cells in transplanted marrow attacking residual leukaemic tissue in the recipient.

Chapter 13

1. (a) CML.
   (b) CLL.
   (c) Hairy cell leukaemia.
2. (a) BCLL or sometimes BPLL.
   (b) PLL.
   (c) HCL.
   (d) PLL.

Chapter 14

1. Refractory anaemia (RA), refractory anaemia with ring sideroblasts (RARS), refractory anaemia with excess of blasts (RAEB), refractory anaemia with excess of blasts in transformation (RAEB-t) and chronic myelomonocytic leukaemia (CMML).
2. (a) RAEB-t.
   (b) CMML.
   (c) RAEB.
3. (a) Abnormalities of chromosome 7.
   (b) Complex or multiple cytogenetic abnormalities.
   (c) Abnormal localized immature myeloid precursors.
4. RAEB-t is the most likely and RARS the least likely MDS to transform into ANLL.

Chapter 15

1. Myeloproliferative: primary proliferative polycythaemia (PPP), primary thrombocythaemia and myelofibrosis. Lymphoproliferative – any three from: multiple myeloma, Waldenström's macroglobulinaemia, Hodgkin's disease (HD) and any of the non-Hodgkin's lymphomas (NHL).
2. Serum erythropoietin levels would be low in PPP but raised in COAD. Evidence of increased leukopoiesis and thrombopoiesis in PPP but not in COAD, e.g. WBC, Plt, serum vitamin B_{12} and serum lysozyme may be raised in PPP. Leukocyte alkaline phosphatase raised in PPP but not in COAD. Marrow smears show generalized hyperplasia in PPP but erythroid hyperplasia only in COAD.
3. Cardiopulmonary disease is associated with impaired oxygen transport which leads to tissue hypoxia and triggers erythropoietin release.

4. The inexorable accumulation of the monoclonal immunoglobulin, which is synthesized by the malignant plasma cells, leads to an increase in plasma viscosity.

5. IgM immunoglobulin is a large molecule which has a greater effect on plasma viscosity than any other immunoglobulin type.

6. Painless asymmetrical lymphadenopathy and generalized itching in the absence of a skin rash. Pyrexia, drenching night sweats, anaemia, lymphocytopenia or leukoerythroblastosis all suggest advanced disease.

7. Reed–Sternberg cell.

Chapter 16

1. Hypoplastic anaemias are characterized by failure of haemopoiesis. The cytopenia in hypersplenism is secondary to peripheral blood cell destruction.

2. (a) Fanconi's anaemia.
   (b) CDA type II.

3. Parvovirus B19.

Chapter 17

1. Vascular, platelets, coagulation and fibrinolytic.

2. The adventitia is the exterior coat of the blood vessel and is composed of collagen with a few smooth muscle cells. The medial layer is composed of elastic fibres arranged in concentric, circumferential layers in elastic arteries. In muscular arteries, the media is composed of smooth muscle cells that permit rhythmic contraction and relaxation of the artery. In arterioles and veins, the media is thin and of much less functional importance. The border between the media and the adventitia may be marked by a collection of elastic fibres which form the external elastic lamina. The intima forms the inner layer and consists of a thin monolayer of flat vascular endothelial cells mounted upon an internal elastic membrane of collagen fibres.

3. Any three from von Willebrand factor (vWF), thrombomodulin, tissue factor pathway inhibitor (TFPI), prostacyclin (PGI_2) and tissue factor.

4. (b) Thrombospondin.
   (e) Platelet factor 4 (PF4).
   (f) Von Willebrand factor.
   (g) β-Thromboglobulin (β-TG).

5. GPIb and GPIIb/IIIa.

6. II and VII.

7. FXIII.

8. Protein C, protein S and thrombomodulin.

9. Plasminogen has a very strong affinity for fibrinogen, binding via its kringle loops.

Chapter 18

1. (a) Bernard–Soulier syndrome.
   (b) Ehlers–Danlos syndrome.
   (c) Pseudo von Willebrand's disease.
2. von Willebrand's disease affects both primary and secondary haemostasis. The defective platelet function is manifest as bruising and mucous membrane bleeding. Haemophilia is a defect of coagulation and is manifest as haematoma and haemarthrosis.
3. Any three from Bernard–Soulier disease, pseudo von Willebrand's disease, Glanzmann's thrombasthenia and storage pool disease (grey platelet syndrome).
4. An obligate carrier is an individual who must be a carrier, e.g. the daughter of a known haemophiliac.
5. Factor V Leiden.
6. Type I deficiency represents a failure of synthesis of a normal protein; type II deficiency represents synthesis of a defective variant of antithrombin III.
7. Any three from *abruptio placentae*, amniotic fluid embolism, retained dead foetus, septic abortion and eclampsia.
8. Warfarin acts by inhibiting the recycling of vitamin K within hepatocytes thereby preventing the γ-carboxylation of the vitamin K-dependent coagulation factors. Heparin exerts its anticoagulant effect by binding to ATIII and potentiating its action against thrombin, X_a and other activated serine proteases.

Useful World Wide Web sites

Relevant organization sites

http://www.ibms.org The Web site for the Institute of Biomedical Science. Contains useful professional information relating to education matters, IBMS publications, CPD etc. Scheduled to expand so worth keeping an eye on.

http://www.hematology.org The Web site for the American Society for Hematology. Some first rate review articles written by acknowledged experts in the field. These are updated regularly and all can be downloaded in Adobe Acrobat®.pdf format. If you do not have the latest version of Acrobat reader, it can be downloaded free from http://www.adobe.com.

http://www.blackwell-science.com/uk/society/bsh/bshmain.htm The British Society for Haematology site gives membership information and some useful links to other sites. A relatively new site and therefore still growing.

General interest sites

http://www.ncbi.nlm.nih.gov/PubMed/ A very friendly and flexible interface for Web-based Medline® literature searches. It is accessible to all Web users, although some features require subscription and payment. Features include a MeSH Browser, Advanced Search facilities, Clinical Alerts, Clinical Queries, a Journal Browser, a Citation Matcher, Loansome Doc and Internet Grateful Med.

http://www.bids.ac.uk A Web-based literature search database, based at the University of Bath, which is a little less easy to use than PubMed. It is possible to ask for the contents pages of selected journals to be e-mailed to you as they appear. This facility is free to registered users and is a useful way to stay up to date in a particular field of interest. BIDS is also available via telnet but is currently only accessible via academic sites. Registered students may be able to access this site from home via their University ATHENS account.

http://pathy.med.nagoya-u.ac.jp/index-e.html A small but useful Atlas of Hematology, published by the Nagoya University School of Medicine in Japan.

http://www.medlib.iupui.edu/hw/hema/ The Hematology page at Indiana University School of Medicine.

http://healthlinks.washington.edu/courses/blood/ This is an excellent primer on blood morphology which is compiled by James R. McArthur, MD at the University of Washington. The article is also available as part of the 19th edition of the *Cecil Text Book of Medicine*.

http://www.geocities.com/HotSprings/5340/ This is an excellent site which is maintained by Roberto Stasi MD. It gets very busy so it is best to access this site in the morning before America wakes! The variety and quality of information accessible from this site is uniformly excellent and includes a series of case studies, teaching files, tutorials and on-line handbooks as well as a wealth of links to other relevant sites. If you only bookmark one site, make it this one!

http://www.microbes.demon.co.uk/haem.htm IBMS Southampton and Winchester Branch site which has pages for all of the main biomedical disciplines. The haematology page includes a link to the Sickle Cell Disease page at the University of Chicago (http://uhs.bsd.uchicago.edu/uhs/topics/sickle.cell.html), teaching notes on various conditions and some case studies at http://www.geocities.com/HotSprings/2255/blood.html.

http://seconde.scripps.edu/ The home page for the journal *Blood Cells, Molecules, & Diseases*. Most of the top haematology journals have Web sites which provide Instructions to Authors, contents pages, subscription information etc. This one is interesting in that the full text is published bimonthly in Adobe Acrobat® format on this site.

http://www.museum.state.il.us/isas/health/blood.html The Haematology pages at the Southern Illinois University-Edwardsville have numerous links to haematology associations worldwide and to some of the top haematology journals. Many of the journal pages include downloadable articles either free or on subscription.

http://cjp.com/blood/ This is the site for BloodLine – The Online Hematology Resource (www.bloodline.net), which claims to be the Internet's most comprehensive hematology Web site. Bloodline is published by Carden Jennings Publishing Co., Ltd, a medical publisher in Charlottesville, Virginia. The site includes abstracts and proceedings, case studies, images, reviews, e-mail discussions, journal links, meeting listings, research grant information, Web links, employment ads, publications for sale and organization information. Also available is a free subscription to BloodNews, an e-mail announcement service. This site is free but requires you to subscribe on the first visit.

http://www3.ncbi.nlm.nih.gov/Omim/ The home page of OMIM (TM), Online Mendelian Inheritance in Man. This database is an authoritative catalogue of human genes and genetic disorders and is edited by Dr Victor A. McKusick *et al*. The database contains textual information, pictures, reference information and numerous links to a database of MEDLINE articles and sequence information.

http://www.bis.med.jhmi.edu/Dan/DOE/intro.html This is a very good primer on molecular genetics, prepared by Denise Casey of the Oak Ridge National Laboratory. The material can be viewed online or downloaded in Adobe Acrobat®.pdf format.

http://www.lmb.uni-muenchen.de/groups/ibelgaufts/cytokines.html Horst Ibelgauft's famous cytokine home page at the University of Munich. The Web is an ideal medium for maintaining and presenting up to date information in this rapidly developing area. The site also includes a cytokine dictionary, cell line data and cytokine alert for the most recent announcements.

http://www.pathology.washington.edu/Cytogallery/ A primer on cytogenetics at the University of Washington.

Disease-specific sites

http://www.meds.com Medicine OnLine is a commercial on-line medical information service aimed at healthcare professionals. Most of the information at the moment is cancer-related although expansion to cover other areas is planned. There is some good information relating to leukaemias and lymphomas on this site.

http://cancer.med.upenn.edu The home page of the University of Pennsylvania Cancer Centre. This site is aimed at both healthcare professionals and patients. There is some good material on leukaemias, lymphomas and myeloma on this site.

http://cancernet.nci.nih.gov/ The National Cancer Institute Web site is aimed at healthcare professionals, patients and cancer researchers but is organized in such a way that each can find the relevant information easily. The site includes PDQ®, a comprehensive cancer information database which includes extracts from peer-reviewed articles, cancer fact sheets and other publications. Also here is CancerTrials™, a comprehensive clinical trials information resource. CancerNet can also be accessed via the University of Bonn at http://imsdd.meb.unibonn.de/cancernet/cancernet.html.

http://www.leukaemia.demon.co.uk/ The Web site of the Leukaemia Research Fund contains a wealth of patient information, details about LRF research grants and ongoing activities and a searchable database of LRF information. Numerous short introductory articles can be found at this site. The following is a selection:

Leukaemia clusters	http://www.leukaemia.demon.co.uk/leukclus.htm
Leukaemia and related diseases	http://www.leukaemia.demon.co.uk/leuk.htm
Acute leukaemia in children	http://www.leukaemia.demon.co.uk/alchild.htm
Down's syndrome and leukaemia	http://www.leukaemia.demon.co.uk/down's.htm

Coping with childhood leukaemia	http://www.leukaemia.demon.co.uk/coping.htm
Acute lymphoblastic leukaemia	http://www.leukaemia.demon.co.uk/all.htm
T Cell acute lymphoblastic leukaemia	http://www.leukaemia.demon.co.uk/tall.htm
Acute myeloid leukaemia	http://www.leukaemia.demon.co.uk/aml.htm
Chronic lymphocytic leukaemia	http://www.achiever.com/freehmpg/cll/homepage.html
	http://www.leukaemia.demon.co.uk/cll.htm
Prolymphocytic transformation in CLL	http://www.leukaemia.demon.co.uk/pll.htm
Chronic myeloid leukaemia	http://www.leukaemia.demon.co.uk/cml.htm
Eosinophil leukaemia	http://www.leukaemia.demon.co.uk/eosin.htm
Hairy cell leukaemia	http://www.leukaemia.demon.co.uk/hcl.htm
Mast cell leukaemia	http://www.leukaemia.demon.co.uk/mast.htm
Large granular lymphocytic leukaemia	http://www.leukaemia.demon.co.uk/lgl.htm
The lymphomas	http://www.leukaemia.demon.co.uk/lymphoma.htm
Burkitt's lymphoma	http://www.leukaemia.demon.co.uk/burkitts.htm
Multiple myeloma	http://www.leukaemia.demon.co.uk/myeloma.htm
Waldenstrom's macroglobulinaemia	http://www.leukaemia.demon.co.uk/wm.htm
Plasma cell leukaemia	http://www.leukaemia.demon.co.uk/pcl.htm
Solitary plasmacytoma	http://www.leukaemia.demon.co.uk/plasma.htm
Monoclonal gammopathy of unknown significance	http://www.leukaemia.demon.co.uk/mgus.htm
Aplastic anaemia	http://www.leukaemia.demon.co.uk/aa.htm
Fanconi's anaemia	http://www.leukaemia.demon.co.uk/fanconi.htm
Myelofibrosis	http://www.leukaemia.demon.co.uk/myelofib.htm
Essential thrombocythaemia	http://www.leukaemia.demon.co.uk/et.htm
Polycythaemia vera	http://www.leukaemia.demon.co.uk/prv.htm
The myelodysplastic syndromes	http://www.leukaemia.demon.co.uk/mds.htm
Paroxysmal nocturnal haemoglobinuria	http://www.leukaemia.demon.co.uk/pnh.htm
Immune thrombocytopenic purpura	http://www.leukaemia.demon.co.uk/itp.htm
Histiocytosis	http://www.leukaemia.demon.co.uk/histio.htm
Amyloidosis	http://www.leukaemia.demon.co.uk/amyloid.htm

http://walden.mvp.net/~lackritz/ A Web site written by an American academic who contracted CLL and subsequently assembled these pages as a resource for patients and professionals alike. The site is professionally presented and the variety of links is exhaustive. An excellent site.

http://www.acor.org/diseases/hematology/Leukemia/frame.html A primer on genetic aspects of leukaemia.

http://www.acor.org/diseases/hematology/Leukemia/frame.html A primer on leukaemia aetiology.

http://www.mcw.edu/gcrc/cop/powerlines-cancer-FAQ/toc.html A primer of frequently asked questions about power lines and leukaemia compiled by Professor John E. Moulder at the Medical College of Wisconsin.

http://www.path.sunysb.edu/hemepath/tutorial/ A series of tutorials and case studies on lymphomas and plasma cell dyscrasias from the State University of New York at Stoney Brook.

http://rialto.com/g6pd/ A site which provides information on the

genetic, physiological, molecular and clinical aspects of G-6-PD deficiency. Also http://rialto.com/favism/index.htm.
http://uhs.bsd.uchicago.edu/uhs/topics/sickle.cell.html The Sickle Cell Disease pages at the University of Chicago.

Index